Clinician's Guide to
Pediatric Chronic
Illness

Notice

Medicine is an ever changing science. As new research and clinical experience broaden our knowledge, changes in treatment and drug therapy are required. The authors and the publisher of this work have checked with sources believed to be reliable in their efforts to provide information that is complete and generally in accord with the standards accepted at the time of publication. However, in view of the possibility of human error or changes in medical sciences, neither the authors nor the publisher nor any other party who has been involved in the preparation or publication of this work warrants that the information contained herein is in every respect accurate or complete, and they disclaim all responsibility for any errors or omissions or for the results obtained from use of the information contained in this work. Readers are encouraged to confirm the information contained herein with other sources. For example and in particular, readers are advised to check the product information sheet included in the package of each drug they plan to administer to be certain that the information contained in this work is accurate and that changes have not been made in the recommended dose or in the contraindications for administration. This recommendation is of particular importance in connection with new or infrequently used drugs.

Clinician's Guide to
Pediatric Chronic Illness

Michael J. Light, M.D., F.A.A.P.

Professor of Pediatrics, University of Miami

Fellow of the American Academy of Pediatrics

McGraw-Hill

Medical Publishing Division

New York   Chicago   San Francisco   Lisbon   London   Madrid   Mexico City
Milan   New Delhi   San Juan   Seoul   Singapore   Sydney   Toronto

McGraw-Hill

*A Division of The **McGraw·Hill** Companies*

Clinician's Guide to Pediatric Chronic Illness
Copyright © 2001 by The **McGraw-Hill** Companies, Inc. All rights reserved. Printed in the United States of America. Except as permitted under the United States Copyright Act of 1976, no part of this publication may be reproduced or distributed in any form or by any means, or stored in a data base or retrieval system, without the prior written permission of the publisher.

1 2 3 4 5 6 7 8 9 0 DOC DOC 0 9 8 7 6 5 4 3 2 1

ISBN 0-07-134720-8

This book was set in Korinna by Keyword Publishing Services.
The editor was Martin Wonsiewicz.
The production supervisor was Catherine Saggese.
Project management was provided by Keyword Publishing Services.
The cover design was by Aimee Nordin.
R.R. Donnelley & Sons was the printer and binder.

This book is printed on acid-free paper.

Library of Congress Cataloging-in-Publication Data
Light, Michael J.
  Clinician's guide to pediatric chronic illness / author, Michael J. Light.
     p. ;   cm.
  Includes bibliographical references and index.
  ISBN 0-07-134720-8
    1. Chronic diseases in children.   2. Chronically ill children
    [DNLM: 1. Chronic Disease—Child.   2. Pediatrics.   WS 200   L723c   2001] I. Title.
  RJ380.L544   2001
  618.92—dc21   00-050018

To my parents, Mary and Dougie,
who guided me through
childhood and adolescence

To my wife, Jeannie,
the love of my life

This book is dedicated
to all who are affected by chronic illness,
and to everyone
who helps to make their lives better.

Contents

PART II. DESCRIPTION OF CONDITIONS

Preface

Pediatrics is the care of children from the newborn period to adulthood. It is the time of growth and development. Clinical pediatric care involves the diagnosis and management of wellness and illness. *Chronic illness* is usually defined as an illness or medical condition that lasts for more than three months. The spectrum of disorders is very extensive. Some affect millions of children and are very common whereas some are so rare that they may not be seen in a lifetime of clinical care. The *clinician* is the professional who provides direct patient care. In reality, everyone is involved at some level with children and adolescents who have chronic illness.

Part I describes general considerations that may affect any child with a chronic condition. It starts with an outline of the scope of the problem with some numbers that show the extent of chronic illness. Access to care and the effect of chronic illness on the child and the family are discussed. Nutrition, eating disorders, and complementary medicine are presented in the context of chronic illness. Normal and abnormal development are outlined. Physical and occupational therapy that are so important in achieving optimal outcome are only briefly mentioned. Sensory and mental health problems are often secondary effects of a large number of chronic conditions.

Although surgical and orthopedic problems could merit their own section in Part II, they are included in Part I because they also are present in multiple situations. Home care and technology dependence services are increasingly being utilized. Unfortunately, there is an increase in child abuse and neglect in the population of children that are affected by chronic conditions. There are many legal and ethical issues that are pertinent to this population.

Part II is the description of the individual conditions that affect children and adolescents. The intent is to present in detail the most important chronic conditions. The question of which conditions are important is debatable. To the families, the condition that they deal with every day is, by definition, the most important. The compromise, which is "author's discretion," is to detail the most common and well-known conditions. These conditions are fairly predictable and include asthma, diabetes, and AIDS. In addition, the majority of conditions that are included in pediatric textbooks are also presented so that there are a total of 30 or so "well-known" conditions and more than 100 other conditions.

There are two appendices. First is a listing of all of the sources of information that were used to help in providing the data for this book. The second appendix lists resources and organizations that potentially can help clinicians and caregivers (including parents) in the care of children with chronic conditions. Internet sites can act as a starting point for information about chronic conditions. These are current at the time of writing and most of them should be stable enough to be useful in the long term.

The author wishes to acknowledge the assistance of Hazelden Press, Inc., in particular Karen Chernyaev who guided him through the editorial process in the early phases of the project. Many people contribute to the publication of a book and the author is grateful to the publishers, McGraw-Hill, especially Martin Wonsiewicz, and to Alan Hunt of Keyword Publishing Services Ltd.

To improve future editions of this book, the author requests feedback from the readers. Comments or suggestions can be e-mailed to either <u>mlight@med.miami.edu</u> or <u>mlight39@yahoo.com</u>.

Clinician's Guide to

Pediatric Chronic Illness

I

Part I

General Considerations

1

Chapter One

Chronic Illness in Children

In the previous centuries health care for children was almost non-existent. In the United States and around the world, epidemics of infectious disease were common with high death rates. The industrial revolution of the 19th century was accompanied by some progress in nutritional care and an awareness of the effects of poverty and child labor. The father of pediatrics is thought to be Abraham Jacobi (1830–1919) who pioneered clinical research in children and helped to establish "milk stations" where sick children could be brought for treatment. Probably the most important measures in the first half of the 20th century resulted from improved sanitation and the pasteurization of milk. This led to a reduction in the death rate from dysentery and tuberculosis. The US Children's Bureau was established in 1912 to focus on the issues of child labor and led to the first Maternity and Infancy Act in 1921, which provided grants to state health departments to develop Divisions of Maternal and Child Health.

The Title V of the Social Security Act in 1935 resulted in federal grants to states for maternal and child health (MCH), Crippled Children's Services (CCS) and child welfare services. CCS changed its name in 1985 to the Program for Children with Special Health Needs (CSHN). Medicaid, the largest maternal-child health program, was founded in 1965 as Title XIX of the Social Security Act to reduce the health care financial barriers for the poor. In 1974 the Women, Infants and

Children (WIC) Special Supplemental Food Program was started to provide nutrition for low-income pregnant and post-partum mothers and their infants and children (to 5 years of age).

Definition of Chronic Illness

Pediatric chronic illness can be defined as a condition that causes a state of bad health of children that has lasted for more than 3 months. Using this definition, the extent of the problem is world-wide and enormous. The difficulty with the definition is that it is too vague and encompasses so many variations. The solution is to get somewhat specific and to define a number of conditions that contribute to the problem. The World Health Organization describes health as "a state of complete physical, mental, and social well being and not merely the absence of disease." In spite of this definition, health is measured in terms of mortality and morbidity so that disease does impact health.

In 1990, "Healthy People 2000" set forward the goals of increasing the health span of everyone, reducing the health disparity, and achieving access to preventive care for all Americans. The initiative contained several objectives relevant to children, including improving nutrition and infant health, reducing unintentional injuries, controlling HIV infection, preventing sexually transmitted diseases, increasing immunization, and reducing the barriers to health care.

Impact on Society and the World

Estimates of the prevalence of chronic illness of children vary from 10 to 20 percent. The numbers increase significantly (to 30–35 percent) if psychosocial or emotional disorders are included.

Children with chronic illnesses and their families have special needs that are greater than those of healthy children. Families have the central role in caring for the children. The problems families encounter in providing health care tend to be similar regardless of the specific condition that affects the child. Although the problems may be similar, the potential impact of a condition that causes chronic illness varies greatly depending on the condition, the severity of disability, the effect on development, the timing of onset and duration, the environment that the child will grow up in, and the response to therapy. It is different for a condition that is static, or improving, or worsening. In many cases, a cure or resolution is not possible and the potential for a good outcome involves a structured approach to care.

Frequency of Conditions

There are common conditions such as asthma and diabetes and there are rare conditions that a clinician may never see in a lifetime of practice. The number of children with chronic illness is increasing year by year as children are surviving because of advances in health care and technology. Medical care has become more complex and more people are involved in this care. The era of managed care has seen a shift away from costly in-patient hospital treatment to out-patient and to home care.

Incidence is the percentage of children affected with any given illness during childhood, while *prevalence* refers to the number of children with a given illness in any 1 year. It is difficult to provide an accurate figure for the incidence or prevalence of the conditions described in this book. For some, the numbers imply the chance of being born with a condition, such as cystic fibrosis (CF), which is about 1 per 2,500 Caucasian live births and less common in other populations (see "Cystic Fibrosis", Chapter 20). There are about 30,000 children and adults in North America with CF and perhaps twice that amount worldwide. Asthma is even more difficult to describe because it is a clinical diagnosis without a specific test to confirm the diagnosis. The incidence of childhood asthma is reported to be as high as 20 percent, making it one of the most common conditions. The prevalence is about 4 percent, which means that there may be 2.7 million children and adolescents with asthma in the United States.

The National Health Interview Survey (NHIS) uses a checklist and questions that ask for information concerning medical visits and activity restriction that are caused by illness or disease. At intervals, this survey collects epidemiologic data on specific topics. The 1988 Child Health supplement provided numbers of children with chronic illness and disability. Newacheck and others evaluated the impact of chronic illness in adolescents and found that 2 million (6.2 percent) of the non-institutionalized adolescent population had some limitation in daily activity caused by a chronic health condition; 3.7 percent had limitation in major activities and 0.5 percent were unable to participate in major activities (work or school) because of a chronic condition.

TABLE 1-1. CHRONIC CONDITIONS PER 1,000 CHILDREN

Total number with chronic conditions	307.6
Impairments	
Musculoskeletal disability	15.2
Deafness and hearing loss	15.3
Blindness and vision impairment	12.7
Speech defects	26.2
Diseases	
Diabetes	1.0
Sickle cell disease	1.2
Cerebral palsy	1.8
Anemia	8.8
Asthma	42.5
Respiratory allergies	96.8
Eczema and skin allergies	32.9
Epilepsy and seizures	2.4
Arthritis	4.6
Heart disease	15.2
Frequent or repeated ear infections	83.4
Frequent diarrhea/bowel trouble	17.1
Other	19.8

Prevalence rates of chronic conditions are similar for children (302 per 1,000) and adolescents (315 per 1,000). This implies that there are more than 8 million 10- to 17-year-olds who have one or more chronic conditions.

Table 1-1 lists the disabilities and illnesses that were most common in the 1988 NHIS as cases per 1,000. It needs to be remembered that these numbers are derived from filling out a questionnaire. Also note that the results are compiled so that respiratory allergies, for example, include "*hayfever or any other respiratory allergy.*" Table 1-2 lists many of the conditions described in this book with a range of incidences and prevalences that are derived from the medical literature mostly from the books that are listed in Appendix I.

TABLE 1-2. INCIDENCE OR PREVALENCE OF CHRONIC CONDITIONS IN CHILDHOOD

Down syndrome	1 in 660 live births
Achondroplasia	1 in 15,000 live births
Fragile X	1 in 1,250 males, females 1 in 2,500
Klinefelter syndrome	1 in 850 live births
Turner syndrome	1 in 2,500 live births
Phenylketonuria	1 in 10,000–15,000 live births
Galactosemia	1 in 50,000 live births
Glycogen storage disease	1 to 100,000–400,000 live births
Diabetes (Type I)	2 per 1,000 children (<18 years)
Congenital hypothyroidism	1 in 4,000 live births
Asthma	2–15 per 100 children
Cystic fibrosis	1 in 2,500 Caucasian live births
Immotile cilia syndrome	1 in 16,000 live births
Kartagener's syndrome	1 in 32,000 live births
Obs. sleep apnea syndrome	2 per 100 of 4–5-year-old children
Congenital heart disease	4–10 in 1,000 live births
Chronic renal failure	18 per 1 million children
End-stage renal disease	3–6 per 1 million children
Crohn's disease	1–7 cases per 100,000 children
Sickle cell anemia	1 in 600 African-American live births
Hemophilia	1 in 7,500 male live births
Acute lymphoblastic leukemia	4 per 100,000 Caucasian children, 2.4 per 100,000 African-American children
Attention deficit disorder	3–5 per 100 children
Mental retardation	1–2 per 100 children
Autism	4–5 per 10,000 children
Anxiety disorders	7–15% of children and adolescents

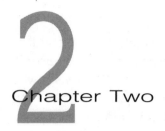

Chapter Two

Health Maintenance

The diagnosis of a chronic illness may be made at any time. Some disorders are diagnosed before birth, many in the newborn period, and others during childhood. After diagnosing a chronic illness, the next step is to address the medical issues. Who will provide care? Where will it be provided? What is the best way to access the system? When the diagnosis is made, various provider options are available but any choices made are likely to change as time goes on.

The changing environment of health care in the United States makes it difficult for the patient, who is now the consumer, and the family to understand all the choices. Managed Care Organizations (MCOs) have been established to provide optimal health care while at the same time reducing costs. MCOs cover a multitude of approaches to providing care. They include Health Maintenance Organizations (HMOs), which include Kaiser Permanente and a series of groups of physicians or providers who are united together. Examples include PPOs, which are Preferred Provider Organizations, and IPAs which are Independent Physician Associations.

The barriers of access to medical care for children are financial, system, and knowledge-based. Children with disabilities are more likely to receive physician care if they have insurance than if they do not. It would make sense that the more that health care services are needed, the more they are accessed, but in reality the poor, uninsured, minority, and single-parent children will receive less medical care. This may be because of the barriers to care as well as an unwillingness to seek care. One study showed that uninsured children received 40 percent less care than their insured counterparts. The goals of the Medicaid and Supplemental Security Insurance (SSI) programs have improved access to health care for many poor families in the last 20 years, but many more who need care do not receive it. In addition, there are many families who utilize limited resources who do not need or benefit from them.

Managed care has problems that are the result of decisions being made on the basis of cost rather than necessity. Outcome measures have been implied as justifying the sharing of cost and revenue. This does not justify withholding treatment for a specific individual who may benefit from therapy. A treatment that has the potential to reduce costs, for example an intervention that will lower hospitalization rates, should lead to its consideration, but if it is not recognized by the payor, it may be denied because the rules say so. Medicaid benefits vary considerably from state to state and while the regulations are appropriately restrictive they are impossibly complicated and the bureaucracy so involved that they do not assure that the patients and families who need the most, get the most. Within the last few years, studies have shown that a significant proportion of children were without health insurance for 1 year, and that of the children with chronic disorders, 76 percent had private insurance, 11 percent had Medicaid, and 13 percent had no insurance.

There are many levels of medical care and some of the levels may be accessed more easily than others. In- and out-patient care, drugs, home care, durable medical equipment, various therapies (e.g., respiratory, physical, occupational), mental health, dental, and eye care may all have different levels of accessibility and payment. Choosing a health plan involves learning what options are available and selecting the one that has the most potential to meet the needs. If there is a child with a chronic disorder and different options are available, it is helpful to discuss this with a clinician involved with the care. Unfortunately, the selection of the health plan is often dependent on the occupation of the parent (whose employer or insurance company provides the alternatives) rather than on the needs of the child with the chronic disorder.

The additional needs of many of the conditions described also put a burden on the health care system. Because of the complex nature of many conditions and the treatments that they require, there is a financial burden as well as a systems problem. Multiple specialists, surgical procedures, and complex therapies tend to be expensive. Capitated managed care systems are not geared to providing care for small populations of medically needy children who require technologically advanced and specialized care, which tends to be very expensive. Cost effectiveness and specialized care can be achieved but the question is where should the line be drawn as to how much care is provided and who should draw that line? In the last few years the lines have been drawn at the point where there is actually a reduction in the level of care that is provided for many patients who were able to receive it in the past. Outcomes research will reveal how much this impacts morbidity and mortality.

Primary Care Provider

In the United States, the primary care provider (PCP) has been placed in the position of coordinator of care for many patients, particularly those enrolled in managed care health plans. In many parts of the world the general practitioner functions in this role. The PCP should be an integral part of the care of a child with a complex chronic condition. The importance of this is that the PCP is in a position to be the advocate for child and family and to ensure that there is access to the care that is indicated to allow optimal growth and physical and mental development. The PCP considers all the opportunities for care for the whole child and family. This implies that they are in the best position to provide a broad approach to care. If the family is able to define an individual who is able to provide ongoing continuity of care and it is an individual with whom they have good rapport, it is an excellent basis for optimal management. If the PCP undertakes the role of coordinator of care, there will need to be a commitment to providing the resources that are necessary. This will involve time and money, because the time needed to provide care for a child with a chronic illness may be considerable and may not be reimbursed at an appropriate level.

The role of the primary care provider and the involvement in the care of health management of children has been proposed to be at different levels. Although this was inspired in the era before managed care and could theoretically be updated, it does provide a framework for provision of care.

Level 1 care is routine health maintenance for healthy children. This may exclude children with chronic conditions who will be referred to another level either because the practitioner is unwilling or unable to provide an appropriate level of care.

Level 2 care is the performance of task-oriented care which is independent of primary care but can supplement this. Examples include provision of specific care that the subspecialist requests but does not implement, such as immunizations or ordering laboratory tests. In the managed care environment this may be invoked or forced by the managed care gatekeeper so that costs can be saved.

Level 3 care is when the primary care provider is the central figure in the care of the child with a chronic disorder. The provider is experienced in management of the more complicated child but will refer for specialty care as indicated. It requires a greater knowledge base and commitment than routine healthy child management.

Level 4 care represents comprehensive primary health care incorporating the complex requirements of the chronic condition and its relationship with the child and the family. Of necessity, the practitioner will have broad knowledge of the chronic condition as well as the ability to provide excellence of primary care. The provider will utilize subspecialty expertise and access community resources that are indicated. The practitioner works with the specialists without relinquishing care to them.

Level 5 care means that the primary provider becomes the case manager for the family of the child with a chronic condition. This involves facilitating a short- and long-term plan of care and assisting in the implementation of this plan. The primary care provider is the advocate for the patient and family and evaluates the outcome. This level of care requires coordination and communication between all parties, meaning the patient and family, to the specialists and the health care professionals involved in the provision of care.

Other clinicians including physician assistants and nurse practitioners may provide primary care. Although they often work under the supervision of a physician, their roles are increasingly becoming independent and they provide much of the ongoing care that is important in the management of chronic illness. They also provide much of the education that is necessary to allow the family to understand the condition and the implications of treatment.

Specialty Care

The specialist or consultant may play a major role in the management of children with chronic illness. The specialist may be the first to consider the diagnosis or may actually confirm the PCP's suspicions. Depending on the condition, the specialist may be pivotal in defining the treatment plan and will be the one to provide follow-up for the problems that are specific to the condition. The degree of involvement will vary with the diagnosis and the organ systems involved. Many children receive the majority of their medical care from specialists and consultants. The ideal approach to management is that there is continuity provided by a primary care physician who may be a pediatrician, a family practitioner, or a generalist. On occasions the specialist will function as the primary caretaker. This has merit if the approach of the consultant is able to be broad-based and when the condition has a dominant system involvement in which the consultant is expert.

Subspecialists may have limited knowledge of so-called normal pediatric care which implies awareness of appropriate growth and development and of how to achieve this. They also need to be able to involve the various consultants that are indicated. The development of specialty services has also led to some problems. There is increased difficulty to access specialty care and care tends to be fragmented. Prior approval is often necessary before services are paid for and, in many situations that are deemed not an emergency, there may be delay before treatment is initiated. This can be frustrating to the family as well as to the caregiver.

Multidisciplinary Care

Many chronic illnesses have features that are best managed by a team of caregivers. It is useful to have a leader of the team who can be the PCP or a specialist, but it could be a nurse manager or a social worker depending on what needs to be coordinated. If the medical care is complex, a physician or nurse will usually take responsibility to ensure communication between clinicians.

Case management of complex medical problems has advantages. It improves communication and makes it easier to provide the necessary services. This becomes increasingly important as managed care impacts access to care. The case manager can be the advocate of the patient and family and this role has been incorporated into Public Law 99-457, the Early Intervention Program for Infants and Toddlers with Handicaps.

Primary care providers who are responsible for the care of children need to consider the role that is in the best interest of the child. They should consider their role, as well as how the various caregivers should inter-relate. They need to ensure that the family is aware of the many options available.

Immunizations

The overall goal of immunization in children is to prevent illness and to reduce the potential for spread of communicable diseases.

It becomes even more important to reduce the morbidity associated with chronic diseases and so plays an important role in care. The *Red Book* is published every 3 years by the American Academy of Pediatrics and updates are provided annually in the journal *Pediatrics*. The recommendations are frequently changed as new information becomes available, including better vaccines and protocols. For these reasons, specific schedules for immunization will not be detailed here. It is the responsibility of the primary care provider to ensure that the recommendations are followed and that this is modified based on the diagnosis of the chronic condition.

Immunization may be active or passive. Active immunization involves administration of all or part of a microorganism (that may have been modified) to induce an immunologic response that mimics the natural infection but does not provide a risk to the recipient. Some agents result in life-long immunity, others require re-immunization at intervals. The vaccine may be live and attenuated, or killed (inactivated). Passive immunization entails administration of preformed antibody in the form of immune globulin (gamma globulin) that is derived from pooled plasma of adults. It is used to replace immunoglobulins in antibody deficiency disorders, especially in congenital or acquired B-lymphocyte defects. It is used in certain diseases to suppress a toxin (e.g., botulism) or if a high-risk individual is exposed (e.g., leukemia patient who is exposed to varicella). There are hyperimmune globulins that are specific so that high concentrations of the desired antibody are achieved. These include hepatitis B (HBIG), rabies (RIG), varicella-zoster (VZIG), cytomegalovirus (CMV-IGIV), tetanus (TIG), and respiratory syncytial virus (RSV-IGIV). Some are given intramuscularly and some intravenously.

All immunization requires informed consent. Although they are very safe, they are not devoid of side effects. Hypersensitivity reactions are rare. Allergy to eggs has been associated with reactions to influenza and yellow fever. A history of a systemic anaphylactic reaction to egg ingestion, such as generalized urticaria, hypotension or airway obstruction, contraindicates the use of "flu or yellow fever vaccination." MMR (measles, mumps, and rubella) is not contraindicated by egg allergy, but 90 minutes' observation following administration is recommended.

Children with chronic illness may require specific recommendations for immunizations. For the most part the administration of immunizations follows the recommendations for all children. Live-bacterial and live-virus vaccines are contraindicated in patients with congenital disorders of immune function. For the child who is receiving immunosuppressive therapy, the risk of the immunization is balanced with the risk of the potential illness. For example, live-virus varicella immunization in a child exposed to varicella with acute lymphocytic leukemia in remission may be justified. Inactivated vaccines and immune globulin are not a risk to immune-compromised children. However the immune response may be diminished with reduced efficacy of the vaccine. The Red Book provides guidelines for administration of vaccinations for children who are receiving corticosteroids. In addition, children who are immune compromised following transplantation, especially bone marrow, will require specific recommendations for immunization.

HIV infection in children requires the usual routine vaccinations of DTP, hepatitis B, and Hib except that oral poliovaccine is contraindicated and inactivated poliovirus should be given. Unless there is severe HIV immunosuppression, MMR should be given but varicella vaccine should not be given.

Asplenic children, including those who have sickle cell disease or post-splenectomy, have an increased risk for fulminant bacteremia, which has a high mortality rate. *Streptococcus pneumoniae* and *Hemophilus influenzae* type b are the most important pathogens, but other bacterial infections and malaria are more common and problematic. Pneumococcal vaccine should be given to all children over 2 years of age and Hib given in the schedule recommended for all children and if previously unimmunized. Meningococcal vaccine is also indicated. Many children will, in addition, receive penicillin daily for pneumococcal prophylaxis.

Children with many chronic diseases (e.g., cystic fibrosis) are at increased risk for complications of influenza and should receive an annual "flu shot."

Health Promotion

The goal of primary care pediatrics includes helping families achieve optimal growth and development of children. This includes many activities such as growth and development as well as illness prevention. It is reasonable to recommend that the guidelines for all children should be applied in the presence of chronic illness. The medical management of the child with chronic illness is not the only component of care. There are many lifestyle and other non-medical considerations. Some of these components, such as good nutrition, need to be added and some, such as smoking and drugs, need to be avoided. Education is one of the major keys to health promotion. This needs to be included in the overall care plan and should be considered in the light of the family situation. The plan needs to be realistic and achievable, otherwise it will not be followed. It will need to be evaluated at each visit and reinforced as necessary.

A full range of preventive and therapeutic services are covered by Medicaid which include hospital care, physician and out-patient services, laboratory, and skilled nursing services. Some states include eye, dental, drugs, and home health care. Eligibility varies from state to state but the major criteria include receiving welfare or SSI. This may be through AFDC (Aid to Families with Dependent Children) which is dependent upon income relative to the poverty level.

An important program is the Early Periodic Screening Diagnosis and Treatment Program (EPSDT). This enables children who are eligible for Medicaid to receive health screening and, if health problems are identified, the costs of diagnosis and treatment are covered.

Managed care programs associated with Medicaid may be more beneficial for children with chronic conditions than straight Medicaid. This is because there may be a wider range of services with better coordination of care; however, access to specialists may not be as easy.

Children who are dependent on mechanical ventilation or other technologies may be eligible for home-care coverage under the Medicaid Model Home and Community Based Waiver. The purpose for the coverage is to provide home health nursing and services to reduce the need for continued hospitalization. This program should lead to considerable cost savings.

Supplemental Security Income (SSI), Title XVI of the Social Security Act, was extended in 1976 to include children under 16 with disabilities. This is designed to help recipients to become as self-sufficient as possible. Although there is no direct payment of costs for medical care, the recipients are eligible for care under Medicaid which then helps pay for the medical care of the child with a chronic condition.

The requirements for eligibility are complex. The financial level is set at a level below the poverty line (in 1994 it was 74 percent) and dependent on the cash level of the applicant's resources.

Disease Prevention

There is potential to reduce or prevent chronic disease in children which may be achieved by awareness and education. Unfortunately, the majority of chronic conditions are not able to be predicted or prevented. The management of chronic illness includes measures to avoid further complications that increase morbidity. Examples include anticipatory guidance, which involves discussing age-appropriate interventions that should be part of routine pediatric care. Careful consideration of the specific immunization needs is essential.

Preventive medicine tends not to be a high priority and it needs to be. Acute care medicine dominates medical teaching and prevention that may take years to achieve may be difficult to sell to those who pay the bills. Also the consequences of risky behaviors and the later development of illness may not be taken seriously enough.

3

Chapter Three

Impact on the Child and Family

Impact on the Child

There is a direct impact of a chronic illness that affects the child by altering the developmental potential. This varies with the illness and the limitations that result as well as the severity and duration. There are indirect effects that result from these changes and that affect the social and psychological behavior of the child. If the illness does not have potential for cure, the goals of therapy are to minimize the effects so that the child can function as near to normal as possible.

Illnesses that produce physical changes that are visible to others tend to produce more difficulties than illnesses that cannot be recognized. Therapy for an individual child must take into consideration the treatment of the condition as well as the indirect effects which may not be so obvious.

Disability can be measured in terms of time away from school or confined to bed. On average, a child loses 5.3 days per year because of illness (acute and chronic).

There is increased morbidity in children who do not have access to medical care. This includes the homeless, children living in poverty, children with chronic illness and foreign-born children.

Impact on the Family

It is usual for a child's chronic condition to impact the rest of the family. After the diagnosis of chronic illness there is a period of adjustment. There is an intense emotional period that results from learning that there is a chronic illness. The extent varies with the condition and its expression. The adaptation over time may lessen or worsen the situation. Parents who have children with special needs have more stress than those who do not encounter such problems.

There are several emotional stages that family members may experience. Not everyone goes through all the stages and it is sometimes difficult to progress to the next stage. The typical emotional reactions are shock, anger, resentment, guilt, denial, and sadness. If family members progress to the positive stages, then acceptance and a resolution to make the best of the situation results. "Emotional baggage" of the earlier reactions may persist and get in the way of the healing.

The additional burden of a child with a chronic illness can have either a positive or a negative impact. The positive impact can be the ability to look after a child who needs help and to provide that help. The negative relates to the inability to provide for the emotional, physical, or financial needs of the child.

Divorce continues to be very common in the United States, although the rate peaked in 1979. Almost one-half of divorces affect children and about 1 million children each year are involved. Divorce has a major effect on children. Although chronic illness of the child does not seem to be a major factor on the decision to divorce, it certainly will impact the child.

The numbers of dual-earning parent families also has increased recently. The role of working mothers will become more difficult if the demands of care of a chronically ill child require their presence at home.

Single-parent status results from divorce, separation, or death. There may be birth or adoption of a child by a single person. The number of children who are being raised in single-parent households is increasing yearly. Children acquire stepparents if the parent remarries. The involvement with the stepparent varies with the custody issues so that if the parent who is rearing the child remarries the stepparent will acquire the role of parenting.

The financial impact of a child with chronic illness can be considerable and increases the stress on the family. Expenses for direct health care, home care, special diets, counseling, and equipment may only be partly covered by insurance. The extras, which include transportation, utilities and loss of time from work, will not be reimbursed. There may be health care "caps" on insurance that limit the amount of reimbursable services.

Foster Care

Children tend to be placed in foster care because their parents are unwilling or unable to provide for their emotional and developmental needs. This results most commonly because there is a single parent, poverty, and inability to provide the basic needs. Many children are placed in foster care because they have been exposed to illegal substances or they have been abused or neglected. Children who are in foster care may have chronic illness and some are technology-dependent which means that the foster parents need to be capable of providing extra care.

Foster care is usually with good parents, but children in foster care tend to be shorter and have a higher incidence of chronic medical problems. In addition, there is a higher incidence of emotional problems and school difficulties. The emotional problems vary with age. Very young children may have eating and sleeping problems. Early school-age children may have hyperactivity and discipline problems. Adolescents may exhibit risky behaviors including substance abuse, sexual experimentation, and violent activities. Depression is common, especially in older children. It must be remembered that physical and sexual abuse and child neglect are not uncommon in foster homes.

Adoption

There are about 150,000 adoptions each year in the United States. More than half the children adopted from foster care are adopted by the foster parents that have been looking after them. Domestic newborn adoptions have potential maternal and infant problems. The mother may have a history of mental illness or of sexually transmitted or other infectious diseases. The infant may have prematurity, a congenital anomaly, a genetic disorder, or have been exposed to drugs or toxins. In many cases, the medical and other previous history before coming to the foster family is not available. Many foster children have chronic medical conditions that have been inadequately diagnosed or treated.

International adoptions imply that the child was born in a foreign country. Although it is intuitive that there should be testing for hepatitis B, HIV, syphilis, TB, and so on, it is not recommended to insist on this before the child comes to the United States. Use of contaminated needles places the child at risk and the results may be unreliable or even fabricated. A videotape of the child may provide information about the development of the child. Many children have undiagnosed chronic illness and developmental delay is common.

Educational Goals

Education provides the child with the means to live and to work in the adult world. School dominates the life of a child and more time is spent there than anywhere else except home. Schooling is important for children with chronic conditions as many children do not get a chance to socialize with other children except at school. Integration of children with chronic conditions may be associated with resistance from the school or other parents. Schools may not have the facilities to safely provide for the needs of the medical condition. Many schools do not have school nurses. Children with disabilities are entitled to receive therapy that will help in their overall education. This includes speech, physical, and occupational therapy. Unfortunately, the children with mild disabilities may not be eligible for special services.

■ SCHOOLING

In most cases education at school is preferable to education at home. Participation in school activities can build self-esteem. This is important for children with chronic conditions who may not have the opportunity to interact as much with other children. Parents may need to communicate with the teachers and school nurse to ensure that they are aware of the medical conditions and special needs of the child.

■ CHILDREN WITH DISABILITIES

Public Law 94-142, the Education of All Handicapped Children Act of 1975, had a number of specific objectives. First was that all children (5–18 years of age) had the right to receive a free and appropriate education. The education should be in the least restrictive environment based on individual needs. This also implies special education should it be necessary. The law was amended in 1986 (Public Law 99-457) to cover the whole of childhood from birth to 21 years of age. The intent of the laws is to identify children who are at risk and to provide services that will optimize the developmental potential of the child. The problems that result include funding for services, who is responsible, and will the services actually be provided to the child who needs them. Unfortunately, the laws were unclear as they related to the various conditions that lead to handicap and disability. This meant that the child with severe cognitive dysfunction would be eligible for special education, whereas children with milder handicaps or other chronic conditions may not be eligible for services. In 1990 the Individuals with Disabilities Education Act specified conditions causing disability, although children less than 5 years of age were classified as severe developmental delay without specifying the condition. The 1997 amendment now classifies disabilities broadly as shown in Table 3-1.

Medically fragile and technology-dependent children may not be able to receive the services that are needed within the school system. Many schools do not have health nurses and their skills

TABLE 3-1. CLASSIFICATION OF DISABILITIES UNDER 1997 AMENDMENT

(A) *In general:* The term "child with a disability" means a child
   (i) with mental retardation, hearing impairments (including deafness), speech or language impairments, visual impairments (including blindness), serious emotional disturbance, orthopedic impairments, autism, traumatic brain injury, other health impairments, or specific learning disabilities; and
   (ii) who, by reason thereof, needs special education and related services.
(B) *Child aged 3 through 9:*
   The term "child with a disability" for a child aged 3 through 9 may, at the discretion of the State and the local educational agency, include a child
   (i) experiencing developmental delays, as defined by the State and as measured by appropriate diagnostic instruments and procedures, in one or more of the following areas: physical development, cognitive development, communication development, social or emotional development, or adaptive development; and who, by reason thereof, needs special education and related services.

may not include management of a child with complex medical conditions. Nowadays, tracheostomy care, nebulized medications, tube feedings, and administration of medications may be performed by school personnel (teachers, for example) who are not trained to perform such tasks. They may not be trained in first aid or cardiopulmonary resuscitation (CPR).

It is certainly true that children with chronic conditions may have difficulties related to education. Many schools do not have the additional resources either on the healthcare side (nursing or equipment needs) or to provide an appropriate education even though it is mandated by law.

■ INDIVIDUAL EDUCATION PROGRAM

The Education for All Handicapped Children Act provided for an Individualized Education Program (IEP) for each child referred for special education. These services may be provided in a regular classroom, a special classroom or facility, at home, or in the hospital setting. "Mainstreaming" implies that a child is receiving special-education services within the regular school system. This allows the greatest educational potential for the child who spends most of the time in the regular classroom but may receive extra services such as speech or occupational or physical therapy in another setting.

The IEP requires that each child be evaluated by a multi-disciplinary team to define the specific educational goals. There needs to be a measurable goal and time line for achieving these objectives.

■ SCHOOL ISSUES

If medications need to be given during the time at school there has to be a legal prescription and written permission from the parents. There needs to be provision for safe storage and means of access so that they can be given at the appropriate time. Some medicines, especially asthma medications, will be prescribed to be given when necessary and there needs to be arrangements so that they can be given. There may be problems of access, particularly if the school campus is large or if the child avoids going to the school nurse because of "not wanting to be different."

Absence from school because of chronic illness may make it difficult for the child to keep up with the class. Stress and anxiety may result in school phobia with subsequent absenteeism. If prolonged absence is necessary, home instruction should be arranged. Mobility in the school may be a problem. If the child is unable to walk between classrooms or buildings, a wheelchair may be useful.

■ HOSPITALIZATION AND SCHOOL

Many chronic conditions require hospitalization and it is necessary to consider schooling in this context if the time away from school is significant. Often the hospital will have some resources for education but it is sensible to involve the school officials so that the specific needs of the child are met. Education within the hospital environment has the potential to reduce the stress and disruption of the hospital stay.

■ **TERMINAL ILLNESS AND SCHOOL**

Children and adolescents who have a terminal illness may benefit from continuing in the school because of the benefits of socialization, but expectations should be realistic. It is useful to have a plan to allow the teachers and other pupils the opportunity to understand the medical situation and to be aware of the course of the illness.

If there is awareness of the potential for a crisis to occur at school, it is necessary to define the responsibility of the school personnel in the event that an emergency situation arises. If it is appropriate, a DNR (Do Not Resuscitate) order is written so that the child is not subjected to a resuscitation that is not indicated, should a cardiac arrest occur. There should be a physician order as well as permission from the parents in writing. It is sensible for the child to wear an ID bracelet indicating the DNR order. The school does not legally have to honor the DNR order and, at the beginning of the school year, parents should present the case to the school board for approval.

Death and Dying

Infant mortality is the death rate during the first year of life. The rate varies from country to country. At the beginning of the 20th century in the United States the rate was about 200 infants per 1,000 live births and in 1994 it was 7.9 per 1,000 live births. Despite these numbers the United States lags behind many developed countries. Japan has the lowest infant mortality rate and the United States does not figure in the 20 lowest mortality rate countries. After 1 year of age there is a dramatic change in the causes of death with injuries being the most common cause. The death rates have increased since the early 1900s among African-Americans and males. Mortality rates have declined in most areas in childhood except for injuries. Drowning and burns are the second and third leading causes of death in boys aged 1–14 years and these diagnoses are reversed in girls. Firearms are a major cause of death in boys but not in girls.

Children who have been ill for a long time often understand more about death and dying than would be expected by their age. This is particularly so if the child has been attending a clinic or has been hospitalized and there has been exposure to other children who have died, perhaps of the same condition. How much information about dying and death is communicated to the child by clinicians is usually discussed with the parents. Adjustment after a child dies may be a very difficult and long process for the family. It is usually considered that after an interval of time, resumption of activity and work are beneficial.

Hospice

The first true hospice was opened in Sydenham in Southeast London in 1967 and named St. Christopher's. It was described by Dame Cicely Saunders, who founded the modern hospice movement, as a "safe haven for the dying." The role of hospice has been to manage pain and the symptoms of disease and to provide grief support for the terminally ill and their families. Hospice means care for the dying. Its role is to help patients and families make the most of the time that remains and to make the process of dying more comfortable and bearable. It is implied that hospice is not going to cure disease and that dying appears inevitable. Medical care that has been directed toward fighting a disease or an illness is no longer going to be necessary.

There has been a major change in the last few decades about how and where we die. There is more discussion about issues of dying and terminal care has more options. Having said this, the picture for children could be better. It used to be that the majority of children with a terminal illness died in the hospital. Hospices do wonderful work with terminally ill patients and their families and may be a consideration for a child. It is often difficult to make a decision in the midst of a crisis and it helps to have the opportunity to make a decision in advance. One of the problems with choosing hospice is coming to the realization that death may be imminent and accepting the finality of the situation.

The admission policies for hospice may be complicated and should be looked into in advance. There are specific criteria that need to be met and there are exclusions which vary from institution to institution. For example, if the level of nursing care is beyond the capabilities of the hospice, admission will be refused. Although hospice is a place that cares for patients who are dying, their philosophy is to make the time of living as positive and comfortable as possible. Hospice provides comfort or palliative care which is directed at the symptoms of the illness. The technology that is used in conventional medicine is not going to be available in the hospice setting and CPR is not appropriate.

The majority of patients who seek hospice have cancer. It is not intended to be an environment for neurologically devastated children who are stable and may have a long life span. Although only 1 percent of admissions are less than 18 years of age, many hospices will accept children. The usual admission criteria are: (1) a medical diagnosis of a terminal illness that is likely to end in death within 6 months; (2) the patient is seeking comfort-oriented care rather than attempting to cure a disease or illness; (3) the patient and the family as well as the physician consent to care; and (4) consent is given for DNR (do not resuscitate) that implies that CPR will not be given.

Hospice functions with an interdisciplinary team. There is a medical director and nursing and social work staff who coordinate the services. Hospice provides much of the care in the home with home visits at least weekly. The nurse will communicate with the physician. If the child is at home, much of the responsibility of the nurse will be to provide education to the caregivers. Between visits, the family will have access to an on-call nurse who will be able to assist.

The social worker responds to issues related to the family and the environment. Much of the work will involve insurance issues, financial issues, legal questions, and helping with the arrangements after death. It is likely that the social worker will provide counseling for the patient and family. This will mostly focus on the present situation, resolving conflicts and fears related to dying.

The hospice team may include an aide who functions in many ways. Aides provide care for those unable to look after themselves. This may include bathing, mouth or hair care, skin care and generally helping in the activities of daily living. Aides will tend to visit the home a few times a week for 1–2 hours per visit depending on the needs of the family.

Most hospices will have a chaplain who is able to provide spiritual care for the terminally ill. This tends to be nondenominational and nonsectarian. Alternatively there will be someone on call in the community who can provide assistance that is appropriate for the family.

At some point there may be a consideration that the care can no longer be provided in the home and in-patient hospice services may be appropriate. In-patient hospice care may be in a freestanding structure or may be part of a hospital or nursing home that has been designated for such care. Such units usually are able to admit patients for short periods.

There are various types of hospice. They may be community-based, independent nonprofit corporations that are governed by a community board of directors. Home health agency-based hospices are part of home-care agencies which may be a separate unit within the organization or integrated into the home-care program. Hospital-based hospices are part of the parent organization but still may provide services in the home.

Certification of hospices implies that they are eligible to participate in Medicare and if the state has a Medicaid hospice benefit (half do) then they are eligible also for Medicaid. Joint Commission on Accreditation of Healthcare Organizations (JCAHO) no longer accredits hospices and so there is no national program for evaluation of hospices. Medicare benefits are paid on a per diem basis depending on the level of service. It is implied that all of the services that are needed will be paid from this flat rate.

Chapter Four

Nutrition

The relationships between nutrition and biological growth are complex and poorly understood. Certainly calorie and protein intake relate directly to outcome but there are many indirect factors that come into the overall picture. Socioeconomic status also impacts growth and development. Nutrition costs money and the impact of chronic illness may worsen an already difficult financial situation.

Nutritional problems are common in children with chronic illnesses. Poor nutrition can contribute to alterations in growth and development. Malnutrition may result in decreased immune function, which increases susceptibility to infection. Malnutrition may result from decreased calorie intake, maldigestion or malabsorption, increased metabolic demands, or nutrient losses. In addition, appetite may be poor and treatments may alter the metabolic rate.

It may be difficult to achieve the necessary caloric intake in a variety of chronic illnesses such as congenital heart disease, chronic renal disease, as well as chronic infections. Anorexia is common for a variety of conditions and nausea, vomiting, or abdominal pain may lead to decreased intake.

Diet

The requirements for calories and fluid vary with age. The goals for an individual patient can be defined. It is important to evaluate protein, fat, and carbohydrate intake. A poor diet is one with excessive calories combined with nutritional deficiencies. A poor diet could be described as a high intake of fat, simple sugars, sodium and chemicals with a low intake of fiber, essential fatty acids, vitamins and minerals. With the availability of prepackaged foods and fast-food restaurants, the prosperous nations of the civilized world may have a much poorer level of nutrition than the deprived third-world countries. Heart disease is much more common in the industrialized nations of North America and Europe than it is in Asia and South America.

It is possible that the widely held belief that a very-low-fat diet with low-cholesterol foods will reduce heart disease is incorrect. It is important to remember that the effects of poor nutrition in children may not become evident until they are adults. Many problems of suboptimal nutrition may not be clinically evident. Reimbursement for nutritional supplements may be difficult from private insurance and impossible from state or federally funded programs.

A well-balanced diet is not as simple to achieve as it seems. Three "square" meals a day does not guarantee good nutrition. Many foods, including fruits and vegetables, do not have the nutritional value that they had in the past and modern processing has altered their content. The US Department of Agriculture developed the Food Guide Pyramid, as shown in Figure 4-1, to help choose healthful food in the right proportions. The lower part of the pyramid includes the grains which constitute the largest part of the diet. These include breads, pastas, rice, and cereals and comprise 6–11 servings per day. The next level is the fruits and vegetables which should have 3–5 and 2–4 servings, respectively. There should be 2–3 servings of milk, yogurt, and cheese and 2–3 servings of meat, poultry, fish, eggs, dried beans,

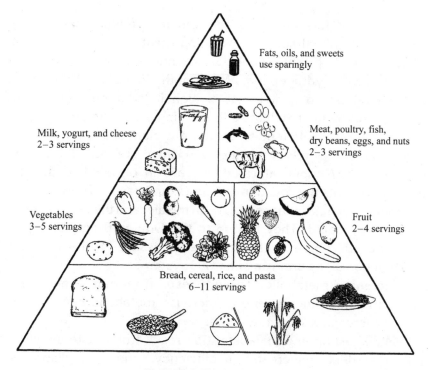

Figure 4-1. The food pyramid.

and nuts. The top of the pyramid is fats, oils, and sweets that should be eaten sparingly.

The major food source of a nutritional diet is carbohydrate. Fruit, vegetables, and whole-grain carbohydrates constitute about 40 percent of the diet. There should be a reduction in the amount of refined carbohydrates which include white bread, sugar, pastries, cookies, and candies. The amount of cereals, rice and pasta, and starchy vegetables should not be excessive.

Protein comprises about 30 percent of the calorie intake including fish, lean meat, tofu, beans, seeds, nuts, milk, and eggs. It is probably reasonable to balance protein derived from animal and plant although, obviously, the vegetarian diet limits the former.

The intake of fats and oils is more debatable. A reasonable approach is to have 30 percent of the diet as fats. The caloric density of fats (9 cal/g) is about twice as high as protein and carbohydrate (4 cal/g).

Saturated fats are solid at room temperature and mostly derive from animal sources including meat and dairy products. They are called saturated because their chemical bonds are saturated with hydrogen ions. Much of the increase risk for heart disease relates to a diet that is high in saturated fats which predisposes to atherosclerosis (hardening of the arteries).

Unsaturated fats tend to come from plant sources (and fish) and tend to be oily meaning that they are liquid at room temperature. Monounsaturated fats are in olive oil, and poly-unsaturated fats are found in fish, nuts, and seeds. There are two essential fatty acids that need to be in the diet and these are linoleic and linolenic acid. They belong to the Omega-6 and Omega-3 groups of oil, respectively, and are necessary for the structure and function of the brain and nervous system.

Increased metabolic demands result from many conditions. Infections and cancers tend to increase metabolic demands as well as increase work of breathing.

Maldigestion and malabsorption result from gastrointestinal (GI) disorders, pancreatic insufficiency, and liver disorders. Management can include altering the intake or replacing pancreatic enzymes. Malabsorption can result from chronic small bowel disease.

Children after the first year of life tend to eat 3 meals and 2 snacks per day. Whole cow's milk is usual after 1 year, although some will continue to breastfeed. Milk intake should not exceed 1 quart per day because more than this will lead to loss of interest in other foods. Cholesterol and fat should not be limited until after 2 years of age.

Children who eat well during infancy may become poor eaters as toddlers. Even though they are presented meals that they should like, favorite foods may be refused. Behavior problems related to eating are common in the pre-school age.

■ ORAL INTAKE

In infancy it is possible to increase the caloric density of formula. Standard formulas are 20 Cal/oz and can be increased in older infants to 30 Cal/oz. Increased calories can be achieved by using less dilute formulas or by adding carbohydrates (e.g., polycose) or fats (e.g., medium-chain triglycerides or vegetable oil). Human milk is the best nutritional intake for babies with immunologic and psychosocial benefits.

The intake should not exceed 4 g/kg/day of protein and the fat content should not exceed 60 percent of calories. It is usual to recommend introduction of supplemental foods at 6 months of age.

■ BREASTFEEDING

Breastfeeding is only contraindicated in a few situations. Medications that should be considered contraindications include chemotherapeutic agents, radioactive isotopes, lithium, ergotamine, and drugs of abuse. Relative contraindications include anticonvulsants, antihistamines, sulfa drugs, and salicylates, all of which have the potential to affect the infant. Other reasons to recommend avoiding breastfeeding include infections such as HIV and TB and metabolic disorders such as galactosemia and tyrosinemia.

■ NUTRITIONAL ASSESSMENT

A dietary history is essential for defining the nutritional plan. In infancy the dietary history should include the formula or breastfeeding intake with the type and amount of intake as well as the duration of feeding. For older children, a 1–3-day intake provides information of the amount of fluid and calories that are consumed.

Measures of nutrition include height, weight, and head circumference. Measures of arm circumference and triceps skin fold provide information of body composition. Weight should be naked weight (without diapers) and height should be crown–heel length. Head circumference should be above eyebrows and ears and around the back of the head. During the first year of life, birthweight doubles at 4 months, triples at 1 year, and then quadruples at 2 years. Length increases by 50 percent in the first year but does not double until 4 years. Although there is a lot of variability, the average child from 2 years to puberty increases weight an average of 2–3 kg and 6–8 cm per year.

The growth curves referred to should be age and sex appropriate. Some growth curves are specific and can be used for defined populations. The most commonly used curves are the National Center for Health Statistics (NCHS), which are predominantly for bottle-fed infants. Breast-fed infants grow slower than bottle-fed infants, which may need to be considered. African-American children were included in the sample and they are accurate for this group. Asian children have different growth rates and merit a separate chart. Medical conditions lead to different growth rates and there are charts available for Down syndrome and other conditions that show more realistic growth patterns for the population.

Vitamins and Minerals

The daily requirements for vitamins and minerals are usually met when there is a balanced diet. Recommended Daily Allowances (RDAs) have been developed for vitamins based on the intake of infants and children who are healthy with some extrapolation from the effects of deficiency of vitamins. The effects of vitamin deficiency, or excess, have been evaluated from laboratory and biochemical effects of vitamins at the tissue level as well as epidemiologic observations of nutritional status in humans. There has been some extrapolation of animal data, the validity of which is questionable. Much of the data for children has been derived from intravenous vitamins given with parenteral nutrition. Even when there is wide variation in intake from any source, the measured levels of plasma vitamin levels do not vary greatly.

The need for specific vitamins varies with storage and depletion so that A, D, E and the B-vitamins 4 (folic acid), 6 (biotin), and 12 deplete slowly over 6–36 months, and vitamin C and the remaining B-vitamins deplete over a few weeks if they are eliminated from the diet. Current recommendations include supplementing the diets of preterm infants and adding vitamin D to the diet of solely breast-fed infants.

Vitamin A, called retinol, is necessary for growth, skin and epithelial tissue, and vision. Vitamin A exists in several forms and may be derived from beta-carotene, the most important vegetable carotenoid. Vitamin A deficiency results in growth failure, apathy, mental retardation, and skin and cornea changes. The eye changes are described as xerophthalmia, and vitamin A deficiency is the most common cause of blindness in children throughout the world.

Excess of vitamin A causes intracranial hypertension which results in vomiting, headache, and stupor. This can be from short-term intoxication as well as prolonged ingestion of excessive amounts of vitamin A. Other effects include skeletal changes and skin rashes. It is noted that excess dietary carotenoids do not get converted into vitamin A and a diet high in carrots and sweet potatoes, for example, results in benign carotenemia which is characterized by yellow pigmentation of the skin. This is distinguished from jaundice because the sclera will not be yellow.

Vitamin A analogs are effective treatments for acne (see Chapter 28) and widely used by teenagers. The treatment of acne with retinoic acid in females who may become pregnant is cause for concern. The treatment may lead to multiple congenital deformities of the fetus and so pregnant or potentially pregnant females are advised to avoid such therapy. Vitamin D deficiency results in rickets if it occurs before the epiphyses of bones have closed, and osteomalacia after they have closed.

■ VITAMIN SUPPLEMENTATION

The recommendations state that children who have a balanced, adequate diet do not need supplemental vitamins. Children at risk, including those who have inadequate nutrition either from neglect or an inadequate diet, should receive vitamins. Chronic illness, including cystic fibrosis, inflammatory bowel disease, or liver disease, should receive supplemental vitamins. It is not indicated to use megadose levels of vitamins.

■ MINERALS

Eating a diet rich in calcium together with exercise helps to build strong bones. The amount of calcium needed in the diet at various ages:

First 6 months	400 mg
7–12 months	600 mg
1–10 years	800 mg
After 10 years	1,200–1,500 mg

Enteral Feeding

If the caloric needs cannot be met by oral nutrition the result will be failure to thrive. Strategies to increase the intake should be tried before resorting to enteral feeds. Enteral feeds can be achieved by feeding a tube through the mouth to the stomach or small intestine or by percutaneous placement of an ostomy tube.

The most common procedure is the percutaneous endoscopic gastrostomy, which may be performed in one or two stages. The two-stage procedure involves placing the tube endoscopically and allowing a tract to form. When there has been adequate healing the tube is replaced with a "button." In the one-step procedure, the button is placed at the original operation.

Consideration for the need of a fundal plication should be made at the time of the placement of the gastrostomy tube. The difficulty is that assessment of gastroesophageal reflux is not always reliable. The complications of fundal plication in the pediatric patient are significant and so it should only be done if it is clearly indicated. Although it is reasonable to evaluate reflux after the gastrostomy tube is in place, it is usually preferable to do both procedures at the same time to avoid the need for a second anesthesia.

When the caloric intake is not sufficient to achieve a desirable rate of growth, alternative strategies are necessary. Enteral feedings can be provided by nasogastric tube but this is not a long-term solution. Percutaneous endoscopic gastrostomy tube (PEG) is a means of providing supplemental calories or total caloric intake if necessary. Feeding can be given continuously or by bolus.

Parenteral Nutrition

Parenteral nutrition may be necessary if adequate calories cannot be administered enterally. This occurs with severe GI dysfunction and with short gut syndrome. Parenteral nutrition requires venous access and is expensive. It also increases the risk for infection and metabolic problems. This is discussed in detail in Chapter 12.

There are two categories of failure to thrive: organic and non-organic. Organic causes include many of the disorders described elsewhere. Non-organic causes include cases where no specific cause is found.

Definition of failure to thrive is weight below the third percentile for age or a sudden deceleration in growth rate. There tends to be delay in developmental milestones and there may be significant psychosocial problems.

Hypoallergenic Diets

Hypoallergenic diets are considered if there is possible intolerance to certain foods. The foods that most commonly result in problems include shellfish and peanuts but the ones that require a specific diet may be more difficult to achieve because they are constituents of many items in the diet. A food should be removed from the diet for 2 weeks to demonstrate an elimination benefit. This is difficult for gluten (grains and cereals containing wheat, etc.), eggs, or milk products which are present in many foods. In this situation a diet is derived that excludes the potential allergens. The allergist, often in conjunction with the nutritionist, can suggest an appropriate diet.

Severe food allergies are rare but can provoke life-threatening anaphylaxis. Even small quantities may produce a devastating effect so that a trial of a suspected food (especially peanuts or lobster) should only be considered in a controlled environment (e.g., hospital rather than home).

Blood Sugar

The pancreas secretes insulin which takes glucose from the blood-stream and delivers it to the liver and muscles where it is stored as glycogen. The insulin is secreted in response to sugar that is absorbed following eating. If the glucose level in the blood is low, glucagon is secreted which releases glucose from glycogen in the liver to restore blood glucose to the normal range.

Choking

Children less than 4 years of age are more likely to choke on food than older children. The commonest cause of death from airway obstruction is the hot dog, although grapes, raw vegetables, popcorn, nuts, and hard candy are also potential problems. Children with neurologic problems are at increased risk.

5

Chapter Five

Eating/Elimination Disorders

Anorexia nervosa (AN) and bulimia nervosa (BN) are similar disorders that are often challenging to the clinician. When the two conditions are present in the same individual it is called bulimorexia. It is often difficult to understand the motivation for self-induced starvation or vomiting. The caregiver, as well as the parents, may feel frustrated because there appears to be a simple and logical solution to the problem but it is rarely easy to manage. One of the major differences between AN and BN is that individuals with BN tend to be outgoing and they are aware that the behavior is abnormal so that they are self-conscious about it. There appears to be increased depression and addiction in both conditions.

Anorexia Nervosa

Anorexia nervosa (AN) is often characterized as an intense fear of becoming obese that does not diminish even when weight is lost. Body image is distorted so that the patient may complain of being overweight despite obvious emaciation. It is important to exclude medical conditions such as diabetes or thyrotoxicosis associated with weight loss. The DSM-III required a weight loss of 25 percent of original body weight or for a growing child, weight that is less than 25 percent of expected. The DSM-III-R modified the weight

TABLE 5-1. CRITERIA FOR DIAGNOSIS OF ANOREXIA NERVOSA AND BULIMIA NERVOSA

Anorexia nervosa
Refusal to maintain body weight at or above minimally normal weight for age and height
Weight loss so that body weight is less than 85% expected
Intense fear of being overweight or getting fat despite being underweight
Amenorrhea for 3 menstrual cycles in postmenarchal girls

Bulimia nervosa
Recurrent episodes of binge eating followed by purging. Purging may be self-induced vomiting or misuse of laxatives, diuretics, or enemas
Behaviors occur at least twice a week for 3 months
Lack of control of eating during binge episodes
Distorted perception of body shape or size

loss to 15 percent to allow for earlier diagnosis. Absence of 3 menstrual cycles in children expected to be menstruating was also added.

The current (DSM-IV) diagnostic criteria are shown in Table 5-1. There are now two types of AN called *binge-eating/ purging*—who lose weight as a result of laxatives, diuretics or self-induced vomiting, and *restricting*. The restricting subtype is associated with weight loss resulting from severe calorie restriction and/or exercise. The prevalence appears to be about 0.5–1 percent of adolescents between 12 and 18 years of age. Only 5–10 percent of those diagnosed are male. The disorder is considered to be multifactorial with psychological being only a part. There are contributions from cultural issues that are more common in Western societies that embrace the slim and trim body. There are developmental and family factors so that picky eaters and young children with digestive disorders are more likely to have symptoms of AN. There is also an association with major depression.

The approach to management of AN involves refeeding and psychotherapy. Initial treatment involves weight gain and, in the early phases, psychotherapy is postponed until weight gain is established. Before managed care, patients were often admitted to psychiatric hospitals but now they are admitted to medical or pediatric wards. The psychotherapy phase is then conducted as an outpatient. The insurance companies are apt to deny admission for the initial weight gain maintaining that it can be achieved as an out-patient. A team approach to management in a supervised environment is more likely to be successful than out-patient care.

Electrolyte abnormalities are common in severe cases. Refeeding may be difficult and small gains should be sought with goals for weight gain that are realistic. It is reasonable to start with 250 cal above the previous intake and gradual increase as tolerated. A low but significant (0–5 percent) mortality has been reported.

Bulimia Nervosa

Bulimia nervosa (BN) is binge-eating with aggressive measures to prevent weight gain, including self-induced vomiting or use of laxatives or other medications. There may be periods of fasting between the binges. The most recent diagnostic criteria are shown in Table 5-1 and two subtypes were created in the DSM-IV which included *purging* and *non-purging* which referred to the current episode. The prevalence reported in the DSM-IV is in the range of 1–3 percent.

The etiology is unclear and appears to be most related to personality and family characteristics. It seems to be a coping strategy for many patients. Most patients can be successfully treated as out-patients and many seek help for the condition. The approach to treatment is to establish a regular eating pattern and cognitive behavioral therapy is employed to help patients modify their habits.

Obesity

The definition of obesity is difficult to establish and most consider that greater than the 90th percentile for weight is appropriate. Eighty percent of obese children are obese as adults whereas less than 20 percent of normal weight children are obese as adults.

There are many health risks related to obesity including orthopedic problems, amenorrhea, growth delay, glucose intolerance, and elevated blood pressure and cholesterol.

Only about 5 percent of cases of obesity are related to endocrine and other medical conditions. Genetic, psychological, and environmental conditions account for most of the development and continuation of obesity. Many children have obese parents and their food consumption is greater and activity level less than non-obese children.

Management involves behavioral modification which is more likely to succeed if there is parental involvement, reduced calorie intake over a long period of time, and an exercise program.

Failure to Thrive

The diagnosis of failure to thrive (FTT) is made when weight is less than the 3rd and 5th percentile or there has been significant deceleration in the rate of growth and crossing of 2 major percentiles on the growth curve. Causes are nonorganic, which includes calorie deprivation that is often associated with neglect, and organic. Nonorganic FTT may be from financial constraints, lack of understanding of child feeding needs, poor feeding habits, or a combination of factors. Care of infants and children should include measures of growth at each clinical encounter.

Growth is rapid during the first year of life and failure to gain weight requires early identification. Type I growth deficiency is associated with normal head growth and greater depression of weight than height. It usually results from an inadequate calorie intake but may also result from excessive loss or utilization of calories. Type II growth deficiency is accompanied by proportional reduction in height and weight with preservation of head growth. Causes include genetic disorders, endocrine disorders, as well as constitutional growth delay. Type III growth deficiency results in depression of height, weight, and head circumference. It is associated with central nervous system abnormalities, chromosomal defects, and insults that occur during fetal life or the perinatal period.

In most cases, the history and physical examination suggest the diagnosis. It is usual to avoid a costly work-up and a complete blood count, urinalysis, and electrolytes will serve as a good screen. If there is potential for physical abuse, a chest X-ray may be indicated. The principal causes of organic FTT include chronic renal disease, congenital heart disease, and thyroid disease.

The best way to differentiate nonorganic FTT is to provide an appropriate environment and allow the child to feed a decent calorie intake. In all but the most severe cases, there will be weight gain. If the child returns to the same environment, close follow-up is indicated because relapse is likely. A multidisciplinary approach is beneficial in the management of FTT.

Enuresis

Enuresis is the repeated voiding of urine in inappropriate places that may be voluntary or involuntary. Toilet training is a ritual and results in behavior that urine is voided in the toilet rather than in the clothes during the day and the bed at night. By definition, enuresis does not exist until the child is 5 years old. Primary enuresis occurs if the child has never been "dry" and secondary enuresis implies that there has been a period of "dryness" (at least 1 year) followed by "wetting." Again by definition, enuresis is functional in etiology and therefore is not caused by a medical condition. The major cause of enuresis or delay in toilet training is conflict over the use of the toilet between the child and the parent.

Non-functional enuresis is also called organic enuresis and is urinary incontinence on the basis of a medical explanation. Table 5-2 lists some of the organic causes of enuresis and these should be ruled out in a child who presents with enuresis. Mental retardation is a major cause of primary enuresis and psychopathology and stress are important causes of secondary enuresis. Enuresis may be the presenting

TABLE 5-2. ORGANIC CAUSES OF ENURESIS

Urinary-tract infection
Neurogenic bladder
Spinal cord anomalies
Hypospadias (ectopic urethra)
Constipation
Diabetes
Sickle cell disease or trait
Psychosocial/emotional disorders

symptom of a urinary-tract infection and it is more common if diuretics are being taken.

The prevalence of enuresis decreases during childhood so that 15–20 percent of 5-year-olds, 5 percent of 10-year-olds, and 2 percent of 12–14-year-olds have nocturnal enuresis. Boys are twice as common as girls to have nocturnal enuresis but girls more commonly have daytime enuresis. A genetic component seems likely because 70 percent of enuretic children have a first-degree relative with the disorder.

Enuretic episodes typically occur at night during the first 4 hours of sleep. The evaluation should include a careful history, including family history, and physical examination. The majority of children with functional enuresis are not emotionally disturbed, and the majority of children with emotional problems are not enuretic. There is a higher incidence of enuresis among emotionally disturbed children which might be expected if one of the factors causing enuresis is stress. The most common problems are anxiety, family stress, and immaturity.

Treatment for functional enuresis involves waiting for spontaneous improvement, which occurs with time. Behavioral therapy includes restricting fluids before bedtime, bladder training exercises, and midsleep awakening for toilet use. Rewarding "dry nights" may be helpful in some children. Night alarms consist of electrodes that activate a buzzer or bell when they become wet. They have been successful in many cases (50–90 percent) but there is a high relapse rate (25–40 percent) when they are stopped.

Pharmacologic treatment is useful in the management of enuresis and imipramine (Tofranil) has been widely used. Initial improvement (50–90 percent) may be followed by relapse (20–60 percent) when stopped. Tricyclic antidepressants require monitoring of drug levels and electrocardiogram, and they may have significant anticholinergic effects resulting in urinary retention, constipation, orthostatic hypotension, and sedation. There could be a risk of accidental or intentional overdose by the patient or sibling. Treatment with anticholinergic agents such as oxybutin, propantheline, or terodiline may be beneficial for those patients with small bladder capacity or an irritable or neurogenic bladder. The synthetic analogue of the antidiuretic hormone vasopressin (desmopressin) has been shown to be useful in the treatment of enuretic symptoms and may help some cases.

Constipation

Constipation is one symptom of many disorders. In the majority of children with constipation the cause is functional or behavioral. There is no one definition of constipation but a combination of reduced frequency, discomfort or difficulty in passing stool, or a feeling of incomplete evacuation. Breast-fed babies may not pass stool for 5–10 days and it is normal for babies to strain to try to pass stool. Children may have large stools every 3–4 days and in the absence of abdominal distension or discomfort and no soiling it is probably normal.

Encopresis

Toilet training leads to bowel control before bladder control. By age 4 years, 95 percent of children have attained bowel control. The intentional or involuntary passage of feces in inappropriate places (e.g., clothing or floor) after the age of 4 years is encopresis. The definition requires at least 1 event a month for 3 months. Primary encopresis implies that there has not been a 6-month period of bowel continence and secondary encopresis results when continence precedes the symptom.

Encopresis is by definition not due to a general medical condition except through a mechanism involving constipation. Fecal incontinence can be categorized as soiling with or without fecal retention. Table 5-3 lists some of the causes that may be present. For most of these conditions encopretic symptoms are unlikely to be the only or presenting symptom.

The major cause of encopresis is overflow incontinence. Stool is retained in the distal colon and rectum and the internal sphincter becomes dilated and functionally incompetent. The external sphincter cannot hold the impacted stool and there is leakage.

TABLE 5-3. CAUSES OF CONSTIPATION THAT MAY LEAD TO ENCOPRESIS

Functional (non-organic)

Organic

  GI
    Hirschsprung disease (congenital aganglionosis)
    Anal defects (e.g., fissure, stenosis)
    Colonic stricture

  Neurologic
    Cerebral palsy
    Meningomyelocele, spina bifida
    Hypotonia

  Endocrine
    Hypothyroidism
    Pregnancy

  Psychological
    Depression
    Anorexia nervosa
    Stool withholding

  Dietary/pharmacologic
    Inadequate fiber intake
    Antacids
    Iron
    Opiates
    Bismuth

The child may be unaware that soiling has occurred. Any condition that causes persistent constipation may be associated with fecal soiling. Children with encopresis tend to have large stools that may block the toilet. Soiling tends to occur in the afternoon and is less likely to occur at night. Non-organic encopresis may occur with oppositional (defiant) behavior pattern, toilet phobia, and anismus. Anismus is dysfunctional anal sphincter control in which the anus contracts rather than relaxes on defecation.

A careful history should be taken and the examination includes the rectal exam and evaluation of the external sphincter. Evaluation of neurologic function is important and plain abdominal X-ray may confirm the presence of constipation. The treatment starts with education of the parents and child. Explanation of the circumstances is important because there is a considerable stigma placed on the problem. Treatment is directed toward clearing the bowel and then reestablishing good bowel function. The maintenance program may take several months particularly if the bowel dilatation has been severe. The maintenance regimen involves dietary changes including a high-fiber diet with increased fruit and vegetables, grains, and cereals. Mineral oil with vitamins, because of fat-soluble vitamin malabsorption, or another stool softener may be useful. Young children benefit from a regimen of sitting on the toilet after the morning and evening meal to get into a routine of keeping the bowels clear.

6

Chapter Six

Complementary Medicine

This title was chosen rather than alternative medicine although the NIH has a section of complementary and alternative medicine (CAM). Alternative medicine can be defined as that which is not usually practiced by traditional physicians or taught in Western medical schools. Complementary medicine can be defined as therapies that supplement conventional treatments so that they are utilized in addition to, rather than instead of, conventional treatment. CAM has become sufficiently widely used that it is important that clinicians are aware of the benefits and risks. It is clear that we do not understand whether many treatments are useful, do not have any benefit, or are harmful. Integrative medicine implies that CAM and allopathic (Western) medicine are combined to provide optimal health.

CAM is used or tried by one-third to one-half of the population including many children. The use of conventional (Western) medicine for chronic illness has not been as useful as it has been for acute medicine and surgery. Alternative medicines are often used by cancer patients; in fact, it is estimated that $10 billion is spent on unproven cancer therapies every year. Heart disease, diabetes, asthma, and cancer have been helped by conventional medicine but there are many areas where complementary medicine can be useful, although much of the information regarding efficacy and safety has been from adult studies and there are relatively few studies of children.

It is clear that alternative medicine therapies are being used by many families with a view to improving the medical condition and/or the quality of life. There are various reasons for this; some are sensible and many are not. It is likely that there are alternative therapies that will improve how the patient feels but whether they alter the course of the illness is often difficult to establish.

The reasons people turn to alternative medicines include:

- Frustration with conventional medicine.
- Awareness of the usefulness of nutritional, emotional, and lifestyle strategies.
- Desire to avoid side effects of conventional medications.

Complementary or alternative therapies are chosen for ailments ranging from stress to life-threatening illnesses. It is an axiom that unless one can scientifically prove that a therapy is beneficial it should not be used as a treatment. By this criterion acupuncture should not be used to treat asthma, and indeed many practitioners do not believe that it should. Despite the fact that there are few studies that confirm that acupuncture benefits asthma, both the World Health Organization and the National Institutes of Health consider acupuncture to be a complementary therapy for asthma.

Children with chronic illness may well receive alternative treatments, particularly when there is a perception that conventional medical treatment is not going to alter the course of the illness. Specific recommendations are difficult to make because of the diversity of childhood illness. It is considered that the clinician should keep an open mind because some therapies are beneficial in ways that we do not understand. It is important that the communication between family and caregiver be good. If it is perceived that the practitioner is firmly against alternative medicine and the family wishes to try something, it is likely that they will not inform the practitioner because of the anticipated response. This is obviously hazardous if there is a potential conflict between the various therapies that the child is receiving. It makes sense that there is good communication that will allow the therapies to complement one another. As previously noted, we do not understand how or whether many therapies work, and we also do not have data in many cases of the relationship between standard and complementary treatments. This means that the clinician has to weigh the benefits against the potential harm.

Although many physicians are unaccepting of alternative medicine because of the lack of scientific data to support its use, there are many who embrace alternative medicine and recommend therapy for their patients.

Conventional medicine tries to be evidence-based which implies that there are valid scientific studies that document the efficacy of the treatments. Complementary medicine works on the principle that if it seems to help it has the potential to be useful. This is exemplified by acupuncture, a practice which has been around for thousands of years and seems to work. The qualifications of alternative medicine doctors are difficult to understand and the credentials vary from an advanced oriental medicine doctoral program to a certificate given following a Caribbean cruise.

The approach to CAM is holistic, which views health as the whole person and includes body, mind, and spirit. Many of the approaches to CAM utilize the natural ability of the body to heal itself. The most commonly used CAM treatments are vitamins and health foods, herbal therapy, chiropractic, relaxation techniques, massage, and acupuncture.

One of the advantages of CAM has been suggested to be prevention. In reality, conventional medicine has played an important role in prevention although it has not always been embraced by the agencies who pay the bills for medical care. Considerations for prevention for conventional medicine include immunizations, screening tests, and physicals. Exercise and change in health habits, with smoking cessation and cholesterol reduction as examples, are commonly recommended.

One of the major problems with CAM is the lack of controls and safety of alternative medicines. It would be wrong to say that, by definition, alternative or natural medicines are safe. Many natural substances and herbal remedies interact with prescription medicines and the actual effect in an individual patient may be difficult to predict. As more natural treatments are used it is likely that some of these interactions will be identified. Examples that are important include herbal medications taken at the same time as anesthetic agents, which can be a dangerous combination.

Medicines manufactured in certain countries may be contaminated and the dosage is not always accurate. Also the claims of the effects of CAM treatments are not always truthful.

It is sensible to discuss with the treating (conventional) physician CAM treatments that are considered before they are tried. If they are tried without prior consultation and symptoms develop it is important to "own up" to what is being taken because keeping quiet may be detrimental. It is important to be able to identify herbal treatments and secret ingredients should be considered to be hazardous. Injections of alternative treatments are unusual and may be unsafe.

It is important to separate the placebo effect from a treatment effect. The placebo or sugar pill effect is improvement that results from the power of suggestion. This effect is very powerful and in an individual patient may result in effects that are mistakenly attributed to the actions of the drug. This is more likely in children than adults.

Acupuncture and Chinese Medicine

Chinese medicine dates back several thousand years. It comprises acupuncture, diet, exercise, and herbal therapy. Traditional Chinese medicine shares similar philosophies with other older medicines, including Japanese, Indian (Ayurvedic), and Greek, primarily the concept of life force as a living energy that embodies the organism and its spirit. The Chinese refer to this as *qi*, or *chi*, the Japanese call it *ki*, the Hindus refer to it as *prana*, and the Greeks call it *pneuma*. When the life force is blocked or weakened, the energy is reduced in the tissues and organs. This leads to disease and healing results from correcting the blockage.

It is difficult to compare Western medicine to traditional Chinese medicine because the concepts are so different. Yin and yang refers to the balance of positive and negative forces. Yin is passive, cool and moist, and is female. Yang is active, hot and dry, and is male. Much of life relates to opposites and disease is related to imbalances. *Qi* flows through the body in 26 meridians (12 paired and two single) or channels although no anatomic structure has been identified. Figure 6-1 shows the five Chinese seasons and the elements that are associated, and the relationships between them. Figure 6-2 shows the meridians. The premise of acupuncture is that stimulation of the meridians at specific points called acupoints causes a physiologic change. The effect is thought to be related to release of endorphins which are naturally occurring opiates. Traditional acupuncture involves insertion of needles at specific

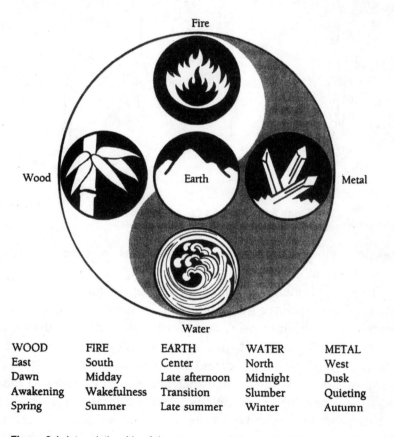

WOOD	FIRE	EARTH	WATER	METAL
East	South	Center	North	West
Dawn	Midday	Late afternoon	Midnight	Dusk
Awakening	Wakefulness	Transition	Slumber	Quieting
Spring	Summer	Late summer	Winter	Autumn

Figure 6-1. Interrelationship of the seasons and elements of Chinese medicine.

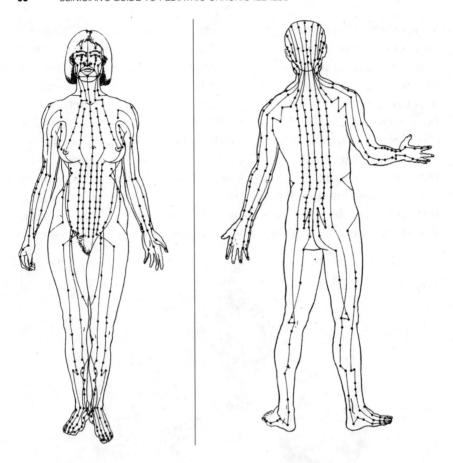

Figure 6-2. Diagram of the meridians of the body.

sites depending on the problem with 10–30 needles that are in place for about 20 minutes.

The most beneficial indication for acupuncture is pain and so the practice does have the potential to be useful in many chronic illnesses that result in pain. Success is often increased with the skill of the acupuncturist. In Eastern medicine, acupuncture is used to treat all manner of disease states and illnesses. There are plenty of studies to document that acupuncture works in many conditions. The list of conditions includes adult-onset diabetes, sinusitis, asthma, high blood pressure and so on, although the effects are variable. In some cases acupuncture treats symptoms and in others it alters the course of the disease. It is probably reasonable to consider a trial of acupuncture and if there is no improvement after six treatments it is unlikely that it is very beneficial. It is a safe treatment and most therapists use disposable needles, reducing the risk of infection.

There are differences in the training and ability of acupuncturists. Many states do not have formal licensing procedures. Medical doctors are allowed to practice acupuncture without formal licensing whereas licensed (fully trained) acupuncturists undergo thousands of hours in training.

Chiropractic Medicine

Chiropractic medicine involves restoration of the spinal biomechanical balance which affects the musculoskeletal, neurological, and vascular health systems of the body. Treatment is applied by manipulation of the spine to remove mechanical stress. The main reason for chiropractic treatment is relief of pain and reduction of tightness especially of the neck and spine.

The origination of chiropractic medicine is credited to Daniel David Palmer who opened an office of osteopathy and magnetic flow in the 1880s. In 1895 Palmer performed vertebral manipulation on a janitor who had been deaf for many years and restored hearing that had been lost 17 years earlier. Palmer reasoned that improper alignment of the spine presses on nerves that leave the spinal column at various levels to supply virtually every organ in the body. This disrupts the normal flow of nerve impulses which results in organ dysfunction. Correction of the misalignment releases the pressure on the nerve and restores health.

There are various categories of chiropractors. The "straights" contend that virtually every illness is due to subluxation and therefore can be corrected by correction of these slippages. The "mixers" understand that other factors are involved in disease and add nutrition, massage, and other holistic measures for treatment. A third category, as yet unnamed, restricts their therapy to non-surgical musculoskeletal disorders.

There are 50,000 licensed chiropractors in North America, and it is the fourth largest health profession (after physicians, dentists, and nurses). There continues to be difference of opinion between chiropractors and medical doctors. The latter consider that it is unlikely that subluxation of the spine contributes to many non-skeletal conditions.

Herbal Treatments

Many medications are derived from herbs and most of the world's population relies on herbal treatments for medical care. Herbal medicine is thousands of years old with the more recent significant work by Nicholas Culpeper, published in 1652. Today, herbal medicine is a blend of traditional medicine and modern science. Herbal medicines tend to be a mixture of many constituents rather than an isolated substance, which means that the therapeutic effect results from the whole preparation. Herbs may be prescribed as teas, liquids, or as powders in a capsule, as well as creams, oils, and ointments. Herbalists may advise which specific treatment is most beneficial for a specific condition. Many herbal preparations are available for purchase in general food stores and pharmacies and by mail order.

Some herbal treatments that are widely used include garlic (to lower cholesterol and blood pressure), ginger (for motion sickness), chamomile (for a calming effect), and valerian (a mild sedative). Echinacea has been shown in studies to be beneficial for colds and flu and to stimulate the immune system. *Ginkgo biloba* is thought to be a potent antioxidant that improves blood flow especially to the brain, heart, and legs. It has been promoted as an improver of short-term memory.

There is a PDR (Physicians Desk Reference) for Herbal Medicines. The FDA (Food and Drug Administration) does not regulate herbal medications and this PDR catalogues the German

Regulatory Authority's herbal watchdog agency, commonly called "Commission E." There is assessment of 300 botanicals with an additional 300 that are not reviewed by Commission E. There is an extensive bibliography.

Homeopathy

Homeopathy was the creation of a German physician Samuel Hahnemann, who lived from 1755 to 1843. He was disillusioned by the horrors of medieval medicine, which included blood-letting and the use of toxic substances (e.g., antimony and mercury), which often did more harm than good. Various principles formed the basic concept of the therapy. The most important was that the smaller the dose of medicine the greater is the potency. This is an anathema to scientists who point out that anything that is diluted 10-fold 30 times will not contain a single molecule of the original substance. Despite this, homeopathic remedies are widely prescribed and there is a large body of literature that documents an effect that is greater than placebo.

Hippocrates showed that large amounts of certain natural substances result in symptoms resembling disease that in small quantities result in relieving the same symptoms. This is the Law of Similars. Hahnemann demonstrated this by taking cinchona (active ingredient quinine) and within a few days developed the symptoms of malaria. The second principle was the Law of Infinitesimals that showed that the more dilute the greater the healing power. The homeopathic practitioner considers that the preparations are pharmacologically inert but biologically active and so they are safe and effective.

The bible of homeopathy is the Homeopathic Pharmacopeia, which was first published in 1897 and is regularly updated. There are many preparations that are listed that are derived from plant and animal sources (e.g., snake and bee venom) and minerals. Remedies may be prescribed as single or multiple and they are available as liquids, tablets, ointments, or granules. They are available without a prescription. While they are reported to help almost any symptom or illness they should not replace con- ventional treatment particularly in a life-threatening situation.

Hypnosis

Hypnosis is one of the mind-body therapies. In many ways it should be considered part of mainstream medicine but because we do not understand how it works, it tends to be considered as an alternative therapy. There is also the stigma of stage hypnosis, which suggests that people can be made to perform strange acts that appear entertaining with the result that it is difficult to take hypnosis seriously.

Clinical hypnosis has an important role to play in medical care and is probably underutilized. Clinical hypnosis has many potential uses including psychological, behavioral, and medical, and dental. When a trance is induced the hypnotized subject appears to be profoundly relaxed and the EEG supports this because the tracing is different than when one is asleep. During the trance state the patient is intensely focused and responds to post-hypnotic suggestion. These suggestions can be directed to reduce pain and stress, and to help with phobias, habits, skin disorders, asthma, and other conditions.

Hypnosis is a powerful tool that should only be used for clinical reasons by trained health providers. In pediatric chronic illness it is useful in helping children cope with their condition. For example, children with cancer or leukemia can learn self-hypnosis which allows them some control over their symptoms.

Meditation and Prayer

There is considerable comfort in meditation and prayer and there is a sense of relaxation and uplifting that studies claim have healing powers.

Clinicians who advocate for children need to ensure that conventional medical care is not withheld on the basis of the religious beliefs of the parents or guardians if the child is endangered by this practice.

Yoga

Yoga originated in the ancient Vedas, scriptures sacred to all Hindus. There are several types of yoga and the one most recognized is hatha yoga, which involves various postures known as asanas and breath control (pranayama). "Ha" means sun and "tha" means moon. Hatha balances movement and stillness, activity, and rest. It is excellent for relaxing and releasing body tension.

Yoga is involved with mainstream medicine in various disorders including arthritis, cancer, AIDS and others. Although it is not widely used in children it may have some benefit.

7
Chapter Seven

Developmental Issues

New parents observe their baby very closely and they anticipate that the child will develop normally. Each time that a clinician has an interaction with a child the issue of development should be considered. Developmental disorders are very common chronic problems in children and may be barely detectable or very severe.

Parents tend to notice subtle changes and will often report them. Many of these, such as crying, sleeping, erratic feeding patterns, or other behaviors, will be normal and reassurance is sought that everything is progressing as it should. Even in the first few months of life, babies are developing personality and each baby is different. Some will be quiet and some will be irritable. The significance of the findings varies but the presentation of developmental disorders is often discovered because of delay in acquiring skills. It is important to recognize the delay early because training and education may reduce the impact of the disorder.

The pediatrician who sees the child regularly is in the best position to identify problems as the child is seen in a longitudinal progression. Development is the sequential maturation of central nervous system (CNS) function within the environment of the child. Many factors are the result of genetics, which include intelligence and temperament, and to these are added the interaction with parents and caretakers and the stimulation of the home and surroundings.

Developmental Milestones

There are various stages in biologic development that can be arbitrarily defined. The neonatal period is birth through 28 days, infancy is to 1 year, preschool age is 1–4 years. School age is 5 years and beyond leading to adolescence during the teenage years. It is helpful to have some simple indicators of development at different ages. Chronic illness may result in alteration of the normal physical and mental development stages.

The majority of children may be expected to achieve certain developmental milestones at the respective age. There is considerable variation among children, which is in part genetic and in part environmental.

At 2–3 months

- Can turn over

At 4–6 months

- Can sit with support

At 7–12 months

- Can crawl
- Starts to babble

At 13–15 months

- Walks unaided
- Climbs furniture and stairs
- Drinks from a cup
- Picks up and places an object

At 16–18 months

- Walks up stairs holding someone's hand
- Walks backward
- Turns book pages
- Sorts out shapes

At 19–21 months

- Can kick and throw a ball
- Puts lids on containers
- Builds a tower of 3–4 blocks
- May show right- or left-hand preference

At 22–24 months

- Walks up and down stairs alone

At 2–3 years

- Runs well
- Pedals a tricycle
- Dresses

At 3 years

- Knows shapes and colors
- Counts to 10
- Says the alphabet
- Rides a tricycle
- Copies a circle

At 4 years

- Walks up and down stairs without holding on
- Throws a ball
- Dresses and undresses
- Hops on one foot
- Can copy capital letters

At 5 years

- Skips
- Uses a fork and spoon and maybe a knife easily
- Can print letters
- Can draw a person with several body parts

Adolescent Growth and Development

The progression of maturation of the genitalia and secondary sexual characteristics were originally described by J. M. Tanner. There is a considerable range of normal variation of onset of puberty and progression through the stages. The earliest sign of puberty in girls is the appearance of the breast bud that occurs at about 10.5 years of age. This is thelarche and indicates Tanner stage 2. The progression through breast development to Tanner 4 or 5 usually lasts 4 years, whereas pubic hair develops from stage 2 to 4 or 5 over 2.5 years. Menarche, which is the onset of menstruation, occurs at 12.5 years of age and is preceded by the maximal growth spurt.

Boys tend to mature about 6 months later than girls with the onset of testicular and scrotal enlargement occurring at 11.5 years. The growth spurt in males coincides with Tanner 4 development of genitalia. Nocturnal emissions (wet dreams) occur at Tanner 3 and the voice deepens between Tanners 3 and 4. Axillary hair develops at Tanner 4 pubic hair development and about 1 year later facial hair develops. Chest hair growth tends to follow puberty.

Emotional development also occurs during adolescence with the early adolescence (12–14 years) associated with increasing self-consciousness and the importance of peer relationships. Middle adolescence (15–17 years) is the stage of greatest turmoil with experimentation and a feeling of immortality. There is risk-taking behavior and parental conflicts. Increasing sexual awareness may lead to sexual activity. Late adolescence (18–21 years) is the time of separation from parents and leads toward emotional and financial independence in the real world.

Developmental Assessment

The most commonly used assessment tool is the Denver II, which covers the ages from 1 month to 5 years. There is also a Denver

Short Form, which allows comparison of development for age as a percentile. These assessments evaluate gross motor, fine motor, language, and social/behavioral skills. The primary care provider will usually perform the assessment at each health maintenance visit sharing the developmental milestones with the parent. Future goals can be discussed in anticipation of continuing development.

Despite the usefulness of development screening tests it is estimated that only 30 percent of pediatricians actually perform sequential tests for routine evaluation of children. Many rely on their observational skill, which unfortunately is an unreliable way of picking up subtle signs. If parents voice concern about their child's progress, it is important to take the information seriously.

Evaluation of intellectual function is difficult in the early years. There may be some indication of problems by assessment of the developmental quotient (DQ), which is the developmental age expressed as a percentage of the chronological age. The developmental age is based on the achievement of milestones during the first few months of life. Clearly, DQs below 75 percent indicate delay but are not an accurate predictor of later intellectual function.

Developmental Disorders

The major developmental disabilities, which include cerebral palsy, mental retardation, sensory impairment and learning disabilities, are present in 10–17 percent of American children. This includes disorders that are less common, such as severe cerebral palsy (1–2 per 1,000) and severe mental retardation (3 per 1,000). Mild or moderate mental retardation occurs in 2–3 percent and visual and hearing impairment in 1.2 and 1.5 percent respectively. High prevalence disorders which are usually mild include ADHD (5 percent) and learning disabilities (7–10 percent).

Developmental disorders may be global, affecting all areas of development, or specific, in which case some developmental areas are affected and some are normal. There can be a developmental diagnosis, such as mental retardation or language disorder, or a medical diagnosis, such as a chromosomal disorder or metabolic disease. The disorder may be static resulting from CNS abnormality with a delay in achieving milestones with the severity of the delay fairly constant over time. Less common is the progressive delay, with loss of milestones over time associated with regression in development.

The classic static global developmental delay is mental retardation, which is discussed in more detail in Chapter 26. The cause of mild and moderate mental retardation is unknown in about half the cases. It is necessary to perform a comprehensive evaluation because a medical condition is the possible cause. The more profound mental retardation is more commonly associated with an identifiable cause: chromosomal abnormalities account for 30 percent, injury to the central nervous system 15–20 percent, structural brain malformations 10–15 percent, and endocrine and metabolic disorders 3–5 percent. Abnormal CNS development may result in severe developmental delay independent of the environment. It may be influenced by other factors or these factors may result in delay with normal underlying CNS function. Abuse or neglect, or chronic illness, may result in delay with or without underlying CNS dysfunction.

Progressive global delay results from inborn errors of metabolism, neurodegenerative disorders, AIDS encephalopathy, and congenital hypothyroidism. The most recognizable syndrome associated with developmental delay is Down syndrome. Most of the syndromes with developmental delay also have dysmorphic features that help to identify the cause.

Language disorders may be part of global developmental delay but if they are isolated they may not be associated with motor delay or dysmorphic features. There may then be no earlier signs of difficulty until language milestones are not achieved. Hearing disorders should be immediately assessed if there is delay in language.

Autism is the most common pervasive developmental disorder and is characterized by delay in communication skills. It is not an easy diagnosis to make and should be considered in children who have delayed language, poor eye contact, unusual interactions with other children, and strange speech patterns. Girls with Rett syndrome may have autistic-like symptoms. One to two percent of children with fragile X syndrome may have autism. Landau–Kleffner syndrome is acquired epileptiform aphasia and after 3–7 years of normal development there is loss of language and seizures.

It is helpful to consider motor delay as gross and fine motor. Gross motor problems tend to result in difficulty with ambulation and involve mostly the lower extremities. Fine motor is more involved with manipulation and involves mostly the upper extremities. Motor delay may be central, peripheral or both. Central involves abnormal function of the CNS whereas peripheral tends to result from neuromuscular disorders. The prototype of central static motor delay is cerebral palsy, which results in abnormalities of movement and posture. Peripheral neuro-muscular disorders include anterior horn cell of the spinal cord disorders, peripheral neuropathies, muscular dystrophies, and congenital myopathies. Most of the peripheral disorders are associated with normal cognitive function.

Chapter Eight

Pediatric Rehabilitation

The definition of rehabilitation services is to help ill, physically impaired, or handicapped individuals to reach their potential recovery after illness or injury. It is implied that the therapies include physical, occupational, and speech therapies. Therapy may be initiated in the hospital but many of the services are provided in the clinic or at home.

The initial treatment is frequently an evaluation followed by the development of a treatment plan. The physician who specializes in rehabilitation medicine is called a *physiatrist*, and the two main areas of therapy are physical and occupational. There are nurses who specialize in rehabilitation and child life specialists who help with the psychosocial aspects of care. Physical therapists work mostly with motility issues including motor development and strength of the back, legs, and feet. Occupational therapists work with the upper extremities, especially arms and hands, and help with activities of daily living. Speech and language therapists manage understanding language and development of speech. The orthotist makes braces and the prosthetist makes artificial limbs.

The conditions that benefit most from rehabilitation in pediatrics include cerebral palsy, rheumatoid arthritis, spina bifida, traumatic and asphyxial brain (and spinal cord) injury, burns, and muscular dystrophy.

Motor Development...

Movement promotes cognitive and perceptual development and the three work together to form the basis for functional development. This means that motor development does not progress in isolation. The early stages of motor development are designed to achieve the upright posture (standing), mobility (walking), and manipulation (hand movements). As these stages progress, children develop the skills needed for independence in the activities of daily living. For infants and young children, these activities include feeding, self-care, and play. The milestones that are achieved start with functional head control and then upright trunk control. In the second half of the first year mobility increases with crawling and creeping, and pulling to standing, leading to independent walking, which usually occurs between 9 and 15 months of age.

Fine motor activity development involves control of the hand to reach and grasp, and object manipulation and release. The achievement of the stages to improve coordination will be in part dependent upon the tools (toys) and objects that are available. The progression is from holding to rotating objects. When a child shakes a toy such as a rattle, the feedback in the form of noise makes the toy more interesting. The next progression is holding objects in both hands and then transferring objects from hand to hand. At about 7–8 months of age, the infant learns to bend, to squeeze, and to tear or pull objects apart.

The preschool-age child progresses through skipping, running, and hopping, which demonstrate gross motor development. Sports and playground games are an important part of motor development of school-age children. Fine motor activity improvement is shown by learning to feed and to dress oneself.

Infants tend to have motor development disorders that may lead to contractures. The management of the disorder is destined to improve strength and to increase range of motion. The preschool child has more complex motor development with coordination. Language is progressing and communication skills improving. School-age children are prone to traumatic brain injury resulting in psychomotor delay in addition to motor disorders. Adolescents are at risk for spinal cord injury.

Assessment

Classification of functional performance in the presence of disabling conditions may be from the World Health Organization's International Classification of Impairment, Disabilities, and Handicaps and integrated by the National Center for Medical Rehabilitation Research. The result is a five-dimensional classification of pathophysiology, impairment, functional limitation, societal limitation, and disability.

The motor milestones discussed in the previous chapter provide the means to document development. The Alberta Infant Motor Scale is an observational scale that is used between 1 and 5 years of age to assess gross motor milestones. The Denver II score remains the most widely used screening tool used by pediatricians. The Peabody Developmental Motor Scales assess gross and fine motor function up to 42 months of age.

There are a number of tests that have been derived for children with disabilities although no specific tests have been identified to be particularly outstanding. They include the Gross Motor Function Measure (GMFM) and the Pediatric Evaluation of Disability Inventory (PEDI). The Functional Independence Measure for Children (WeeFIM) assesses self-care, sphincter control, movement, and communication. One of the most important questions parents of children with motor disorders ask is, "Will my child walk?" There are many factors that result in the ability to walk and research has analyzed the components. With an improvement in understanding of the normal gait, the mechanisms of the pathological gait have become clearer.

The physical therapist will assess the range of motion and the universal goniometer is the most widely used measuring instrument. This is more useful in older children and adults than infants and young children. Manual muscle testing is used to assess strength.

Physical Fitness

Physical fitness combines health-related fitness and motor fitness. Although there is evidence that physical fitness benefits adults by preventing heart disease, it is not clear whether childhood activity results in adult benefits. Healthy Children 2000 was put forward in 1990 and includes specific objectives to increase the physical activity and fitness levels of youth. The proposals defined goals to increase the amount of exercise and the proportion of children participating, as well as to reduce the problem of obesity.

Exercises include those for range of motion which are used to increase joint mobility and to reduce contracture. These can be diagrammed so that the caregivers can provide ongoing therapy. Exercises can be passive range of motion, in which the patient allows the caregiver to perform the movement. Active range of motion means that the patient performs the motions without assistance. Resistive range of motion implies that weights or physical resistance are added.

Conditioning is the process whereby exercise repeated over time results in changes in the body and in the ability to perform exercise. Training is exercise that is designed to improve performance in a specific activity by repeated exercise. Improvement in fitness results in improved muscle strength and endurance. Muscular strength can be affected by training especially at or after puberty. Most training programs require several weeks before benefits are seen. Health-related benefits of exercise are important for all children whether or not they have a disability. There are limitations for participation in sports activities that are indicated for chronic conditions in children (Table 8-1).

Physical Therapy

It used to be that the physician would evaluate and refer the child for physical therapy that would be indicated for the specific condi-

TABLE 8-1. LIMITATION OF SPORTING ACTIVITIES FOR MEDICAL CONDITIONS

Contact or Collision	Limited Contact	Non-contact
Basketball	Baseball	Archery
Boxing*	Bicycling	Badminton
Diving	Cheerleading	Body building
Field hockey	Canoeing/kayaking (white water)	Bowling
Football	Fencing	Canoeing/kayaking
Ice hockey	Field	(flat water)
Lacrosse	High jump	Crew/rowing
Martial arts	Pole vault	Curling
Rodeo	Floor hockey	Dancing
Rugby	Gymnastics	Field
Ski jumping	Handball	Discus
Soccer	Horseback riding	Javelin
Team handball	Racquetball	Shot put
Water polo	Skating	Golf
Wrestling	Ice	Orienteering
	Incline	Powerlifting
	Roller	Race walking
	Skiing	Riflery
	Cross-country	Rope jumping
	Downhill	Running
	Water	Sailing
	Softball	Scuba diving
	Squash	Strength training
	Ultimate Frisbee	Swimming
	Volleyball	Table tennis
	Windsurfing/surfing	Tennis
		Track
		Weightlifting

* Boxing not recommended for children.
 Notes: (1) Contact or collision should be avoided with absence or persistent abnormality of eye, kidney, or testis. (2) Caution necessary for spinal cord injury, bleeding disorders, carditis, enlarged liver or spleen, poorly controlled convulsive disorder. (3) Other medical conditions should be evaluated on an individual basis.

tion. Nowadays the physical therapist often participates in the multidisciplinary team that performs the evaluation. The therapist makes diagnostic decisions related to impairment and functional limitation. After deciding that treatment is indicated the next decision is to define the therapy and the duration. The justification for treatment is easier if there is an endpoint that can be reached. Unfortunately, many chronic conditions do not respond very well and so secondary effects, for example, the prevention of contractures, may be important.

Pediatric physical therapy is designed to achieve optimal motor function for mobility and to aid in the activities of daily living. Early identification of infants and children who will benefit from therapy is important. The objective is to reduce the effect of chronic illness upon developmental milestones. Screening of motor development milestones may not pick up mild abnormalities and careful history and physical examination is necessary for full evaluation. Parents notice movement of their children and may be able to find abnormalities if they are told what to watch for.

Although physical therapists do not require a specific referral in most states it is usual for the physician to write orders for therapy. It is important for the therapist to be aware of other medical problems in designing a therapy. This includes seizures, cardiac or respiratory problems, and other conditions that may impact the therapy.

Physical therapy has in the past used clinical experience to justify its usage. In the era of managed care, there needs to be scientific justification for recommendation of a particular therapy for a specific condition. The initial consultation results in the development of a treatment plan which is individualized to manage the specific problem areas. For example, the plan might include what exercises are indicated and which appliances or devices may assist. Outcome measures should be defined and assessments made to evaluate success and cost effectiveness.

Conditions that can be evaluated include loss of motion, weakness, and deformities. Treatment strategies can be devised based on the disability. Musculoskeletal impairment, which results in contractures, may respond to exercise and splinting. Weakness can be managed by strengthening exercises including weights or by exercising in a pool using water as resistance. Treatment is focused on interventions that reduce impairments and optimize functional potential. Learning and re-learning motor tasks is a major part of rehabilitation of neurologic and orthopedic impairment. The acquisition of skills of motor performance is a complex process.

Assistive Technology

Equipment and devices are used extensively in physical therapy to aid in improving function. There are a wide range of assistive devices which vary from simple splints to computer-controlled functional limbs. There are four major types of devices: postural support, wheeled mobility, environmental control units, and alternative communication devices. The first three are discussed here and the fourth is presented in Chapter 9.

The team evaluating the individual patient will make recommendations for specific devices. Justification for the expense needs to be made to the provider. Providers of rehabilitation equipment are a section of the National Association for Medical Equipment Suppliers. There is a national registry of suppliers who meet standards of practice.

Performance and skills are assessed and the equipment that has the potential to help the problem is identified. Realistic goals should be established to demonstrate improvement. Funding is applied dependent upon the various options which include federal, state, and local agencies as well as private insurance.

■ POSTURAL SUPPORT SYSTEMS

Adaptive seating systems are designed to provide postural support to achieve stable sitting particularly if there is poor muscle control or musculoskeletal misalignment. There is flexion of the hips, knees, and ankles to 90° although if there are contractures or deformity, particularly of the spine, the right angle may not be appropriate. There are different levels of support. First is the planar system, which is a flat seat and back, and the next level is the contoured system. The latter provides improved lateral support. The third level is the custom-molded system, which conforms to the body of the patient. The purpose is to provide support and to relieve pressure. The seat is improved with some lateral contouring and the back is slightly curved for lateral stability. If pelvic stabilization is necessary, a seat belt, either over the thighs or in front of the hips, will help. Additional support may be needed laterally for the legs and the head.

■ WHEELED MOBILITY

For some patients the primary purpose will be to achieve independent mobility. For others it is a means of transportation in which someone else provides direction and control. The wheelchair may be manually propelled or electric. The standard manual wheelchair has two large wheels with two forward swiveling wheels for direction. Newer lightweight models are designed for recreational use and athletic competition. Powered wheelchairs tend to be restricted to older children who have no potential for walking.

■ ENVIRONMENTAL CONTROL UNIT

An environmental control unit (ECU) is a device that helps to operate electrical or mechanical devices for patients with motor impairment. The equivalents are the remote-control devices used to control garage doors and electronic equipment. The purpose of an ECU is to improve the capabilities of the disabled individual. There are direct devices as well as radio-controlled (wireless) devices that can be activated by touch, voice, computer, or even eye movement. They need to be age-appropriate and feedback is sometimes necessary to show that activation has occurred.

Occupational Therapy

In pediatric occupational therapy (OT) there is considerable overlap with physical therapy. Many children with disabilities related to cerebral palsy or spina bifida are easily recognized to need OT. There are, in addition, many children with more subtle defects that interfere with fine motor, sensory, or cognitive development that might benefit from OT. The emphasis of the therapist is to help in the overall functional performance that is age appropriate.

The two theoretical approaches to OT are sensory integration (SI) and neurodevelopmental therapy (NDT). SI dysfunction relates to abnormal sensory function related to touch, proprioception, and kinesthetics as well as to vision, hearing, and taste. The concept relates to developmental dyspraxia, which results in poor skills in dressing and eye–hand functions. NDT relates to functional movement that results from reflex and postural responses. Neonates are evaluated using the Brazelton Neonatal Behavioral Assessment Scale. Infants are evaluated using the Bayley Scales of Infant Development and the Peabody Motor Scales.

Positioning strategies are used in the neonatal intensive care unit to help posture and muscle tone. The therapist can help the family to become comfortable in infant feeding and handling. In the first few years of life, the problems relate to fine motor coordination skills especially of the hands. The therapist will assist by devising specific exercises that involve games and play to learn the skills to achieve the developmental milestones.

Preschool children benefit from interventions that ready them for school activities. Using paper and pencil and dressing and eating are skills that should be able to be learned during this time. The school-age children and adolescents who need OT will often be identified by the school. Interventions in the area of coping in activities of daily living and developing independence may be indicated.

Chapter Nine

Sensory Disorders

Vision

In the newborn period, the pediatrician should routinely examine the eyes and high-risk infants should be evaluated by an ophthalmologist. Visual acuity screening should be done on all children by 3 years of age. At 5 years of age, there should be vision evaluation and alignment.

In the first few months of life, the parents usually will be able to tell how much interest their baby has in the environment. Reaching for objects and responding to the surroundings gives a clue as to the visual capability of the infant.

Examination of the eyes, to include shining a light and observing the response of the pupils, indicates that the retina, optic nerve, and visual pathways are intact. A red reflex indicates that the cornea, lens, and vitreous are clear. A white or yellow reflex indicates that there may be a cataract, retinal detachment, or tumor in the eye. Eye movements can be evaluated in small children by moving a toy around the visual fields. The eyes should be evaluated for squint and nystagmus. Nystagmus is small movements of the eye back and forth, which may indicate a CNS disorder or difficulty fixating. Visual acuity can be estimated in small children using Allen cards that are pictures of items that should be recognized by a 2–3-year-old (a house or tree) that are held at a distance from the eyes.

Vision tends to be 20/30 at 3–4 years improving to 20/20 or better at 6–7 years. Young children tend not to complain if there are visual problems. If one eye is involved it may be difficult to notice any sign that there is a problem. Myopia is near or short sightedness and hyperopia is far sightedness.

There are various tests that are available for routine visual assessment. By 3 months of age, most children can follow objects with both eyes. Evaluation of this shows whether one eye fails to follow throughout and deviates from the point of fixation, indicating strabismus. Amblyopia results from suppression of the vision from the weak eye. It is important to test for this because if the suppression of the "lazy" eye continues beyond 5 or 6 years of age then blindness can result.

The corneal light reflex is performed with the light shone directly into the eye from a distance of about 16 inches (40 cm).

Using the Snellen Letter charts, the child stands 20 feet from the chart and if he or she can read line 7, the vision is 20/20, or normal. If only the second line can be seen clearly, the vision is described as 20/100. The National Society to Prevent Blindness recommends that 3-year-old children with 20/50 or worse vision in either eye and older children who have 20/40 or worse vision in either eye be referred for further evaluation.

Color vision should also be tested because about 8 percent of white males and 4 percent of black males have color vision deficit. The gene is on the X-chromosome and only 0.5–1 percent of females have any problems with color vision. Color vision can be tested with the Ishihara test for older children and the Hardy–Rand–Rittler test for young children.

■ STRABISMUS

Strabismus is the term used to describe misalignment of the eyes. The Hirschberg test involves shining a light at the cornea and if the reflex is deviated inward in one eye then that eye is actually turned out. This is exotropia and the opposite is esotropia, when the light reflex projects on the outside of the cornea. Congenital esotropia results in the eyes being turned toward the nose which is usually evident at 2–3 months of age. Surgical treatment is usually performed before 1 year of age.

In children less than 7 years of age with strabismus, one of the images (from the deviated eye) tends to be suppressed, which leads to amblyopia. Amblyopia is a significant decrease in visual acuity when there is no sharply focused image on the retina. It mostly results when there is a significant difference between the two eyes. The causes include opacities of the cornea, lens or vitreous, strabismus or high refractive defects. The first 2 months after birth are most critical for visual development so that defects occurring in the young infant need to be diagnosed to reduce long-term morbidity. In adults with strabismus, the complaint is usually diplopia (double vision).

Pseudostrabismus is confused with congenital esotropia. In fact, the eyes are in correct alignment but appear to turn in because of prominent epicanthal lid folds. It is important to be aware that strabismus may result from CNS disorders. Cranial nerve palsies involving the 3rd and 6th nerve merit further investigation.

■ MANAGEMENT OF VISUAL IMPAIRMENT

Learning that a child has severe visual impairment can be a major shock for the family. The impact of the diagnosis depends on the degree of visual loss and the prognosis for sight. There are many organizations that assist with education of children and helping the family. Many causes of blindness result from disorders that are congenital or acquired during infancy. Others are acquired later and these children have experienced sight and therefore are likely to be frightened and confused in their new environment.

Children who are visually impaired have the potential to become independent. If development in other areas is able to be achieved then the child needs help to learn the skills required. Navigation using a white cane and tapping allows for movement and human and canine guides can help children get around.

Learning the skills to integrate into society can be difficult. Children have the ability to adapt if they are given the right tools. They can learn to socialize and to do well in school if they are given non-visual aids. Braille is a system of raised dots that symbolize letters and numbers and allows the child to read. This does not help in communication with family and friends and alternate strategies need to be developed. Cassette and tape recordings can be useful and the computer is increasingly able to change written text into the spoken word.

■ LEUKOCORIA

Leukocoria is "white pupil" or "cat's eye," when the normal bright red reflex of light reflected back from the retina is replaced by a white or yellow color. Leukocoria is seen with galactosemia and diabetes mellitus and occasionally with retinal detachment. The most important cause of leukocoria is retinoblastoma. This lethal tumor is due to a genetic disorder and the prognosis varies with the stage at which the tumor is diagnosed. Any child who shows leukocoria should be immediately referred to an ophthalmologist.

■ CATARACT

A cataract is any opacity of the crystalline lens. Congenital cataract is present at birth but may not be recognized for several months. About one-half of congenital cataracts are of unknown cause and about one-third are inherited. Intrauterine infections (TORCHS, varicella, and HIV) are associated with cataracts and they are prominent in the congenital rubella syndrome. Long-term systemic steroid therapy may result in cataract development. Conditions that require more than a few months of oral corticosteroids (e.g., asthma or nephrotic syndrome) should lead to ophthalmologic evaluation with a slit-lamp. Early identification is important because the cataracts may still be reversible.

Hearing

A hearing test is a formal evaluation of auditory function. An audiogram is a graphic representation of auditory sensitivity for pure tones. The pure tones are single-frequency sounds and the audiogram extends from 125 to 8,000 Hz, spanning the usual sounds of everyday life. Both air (headphones) and bone (vibrating oscillator) conduction can be tested. An air–bone gap implies a difference between the two. Bone conduction should be the same as, or better than, air. An air–bone gap greater than 10 dB of 2 or more frequencies (with normal bone conduction) implies a conductive hearing loss of that ear. If there is no air–bone gap and both air and bone conduction are abnormal then a sensorineural hearing loss is present.

Brainstem auditory evoked potential or response (BAER) and otoacoustic emissions (OAEs) are used to evaluate hearing in infants. The OAE is easy to test with a minitransducer in the ear canal. It is cheaper than the BAER but not as reliable. The BAER is performed by placing electrodes on the head and recording electrophysiologic activity following auditory stimulation.

Tests of hearing basically define whether hearing is impaired or not. The audiogram allows classification of hearing loss (HL) as:

0–15 dB HL:	normal
15–30	mild hearing loss
30–50	moderate hearing loss
50–70	severe hearing loss
> 70	profound hearing loss

■ HEARING LOSS

The reported incidence of hearing loss in neonates and infants is between 1.5 and 6 per 1,000 live births. Screening of high-risk infants is performed and about half are not found during screening. Conductive hearing loss implies a defect in the ear, the ear canal, the tympanic membrane, or the ossicle. Sensorineural hearing loss results from problems of the cochlea or in the neural pathway from the cochlea to the brainstem.

The types of hearing loss are classified according to the location of the defect. It is imperative to diagnose a hearing disorder of infancy within the first 6–12 months to allow treatment that can reduce the impact of the impairment. The decision to assess hearing is based on identification of high-risk children and behaviors that indicate possible hearing loss.

■ MANAGEMENT OF HEARING IMPAIRMENT

If hearing impairment is diagnosed, there are various interventions that may be indicated to improve hearing and communication. Hearing aids are available for infants. Some are worn on the body with a connection to the ear, some are integrated into eye-glasses, and some are worn in or behind the ear. As children grow older, they tend to become self-conscious about the more obvious devices. Young children often do not tolerate them at first, and many caretakers are reluctant to keep the devices in place. It is important to be aware of the batteries and their location and accessibility because children are prone to remove them from the device and to swallow them.

Communication is possible through lip reading, although much of the spoken word is difficult to interpret. Sign language is useful for enhancing the ability to communicate between the child and the caretaker. Speech therapy is essential especially if there is profound hearing loss. Learning to talk is a challenge because of the need to provide feedback and to train the child in the art of diction.

Computers have opened up a new world for communication. Computer programs that can convert voice to text are increasingly used with accurate translation. Unfortunately, the more sophisticated devices can be very expensive. Special telephones and flashing lights that signal doorbells are not as costly and yet can be most useful.

The combination of deafness and blindness in a child will result in extreme difficulty in learning and communication. Although there may be potential for adequate motor development, even this is difficult. It is beneficial for such children to learn to speak and may be possible if there is some residual sight or hearing. Unfortunately, many children have additional neurological deficits that impair the ability to develop skills and independent living is not possible.

■ MUTISM

Children who are non-verbal benefit from augmentative and alternative communication (AAC) devices that allow them to express their needs. WordPlus and TouchTalker use motion from the hand or movement from the eyes or head to control the computer screen. This results in pre-recorded phrases being "spoken" by the computer. The messages can be written on the screen or synthesized into speech. The ability to communicate allows additional skills to develop.

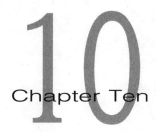

Chapter Ten

Mental Health Problems

Psychological conditions that result in chronic disorders in children are discussed in Chapter 26. This chapter will focus on global issues of chronic illness and the resultant mental health problems. Chronic fatigue syndrome and fibromyalgia are included because their causes are unknown, not because they are mental health disorders.

Behavior Patterns

Both normal and abnormal behavior of children and adolescents comprise a major amount of routine pediatric care. Behavior is influenced by genetic, neurologic, and biologic factors and even more so by social and environmental factors.

Biologic factors affecting behavior include:

- Genetic (hereditary traits for temperament, for personality, and for cognitive ability)
- Genetic disorders
- Congenital CNS infection
- CNS injury (asphyxia or bleeding)
- Psychomotor retardation
- Chronic illness

Social and environmental influences include:

- Parents and siblings
- Home environment and discipline at home
- School
- TV, computers

Behavior problems:

Young children

- Sleep disorders
- Temper tantrums

Older children

- Sexual conduct
- Substance or alcohol abuse
- Cigarette smoking
- Weapons (guns or knives)

Stress

Stress in childhood takes many forms but the symptoms displayed may be similar to those of children who are abused or depressed. Children are vulnerable to changes in the family situation and the environment. Disruptions, such as divorce, moving, or changing schools may be associated with turmoil within the family that results in stress in the child. The stress of childhood is varied and considerable. There may be stress that is specific to the child, such as a chronic illness.

Coping is the term used to describe the response to stress and individuals react differently. Children develop coping strategies to help them manage stress in many ways similar to adults. The problems relate to the fact that they may not be able to change their situation as easily and so may not be able to avoid stressful situations. Children do cope by reading or playing video games as well as by becoming more introspective and withdrawn. Some children resort to risky behaviors in response to stress and may lie or cheat to avoid stressful situations.

The response to the media has changed how children respond to the environment. Role models are not necessarily the parents but may be the latest personalities or characters on television shows or video games. Comic books are not felt to exert as much influence on children's behavior as movies and television. Television has the most impact on behavior with programs and commercials designed to modify thoughts. The average child in the United States spends more than 20 hours per week watching television. It is likely that TV has both beneficial (educational) and adverse effects on the child's development.

Mortality and Suicide

The leading medical cause of death in the adolescent is malignancy. This cause only ranks fourth overall with injuries, homicide, and suicide all being more common. Half of adolescent deaths are due to injuries and many of these are alcohol-related. Younger adolescents are more likely to die from drowning and from weapons of violence including guns and knives.

Suicide is the third leading cause of adolescent death. In many cases there is a history of depression and often a conflict either with the family or of a romantic nature. Adolescents who attempt suicide should be hospitalized. The risk behaviors in adolescents that lead to morbidity, rather than mortality, include substance abuse and sexual activity.

Sexual Disorders

Sexual activity is common in high school students with over 60 percent of males and about 50 percent of females participating in sexual activity. This leads to unwanted pregnancies, sexually transmitted diseases, and HIV infection.

All sexually active teenagers should be considered for regular syphilis screening. There should be yearly Papanicolaou smears to evaluate for human papillomavirus, cervicitis, and malignancy. Cervical cultures for gonorrhea and chlamydia test should be performed regularly. If there is vaginal discharge, this should be checked for yeast or bacterial vaginitis and trichomonas. If there are multiple sexual partners, testing should be done more frequently than once a year. If pregnancy is suspected, the beta-human chorionic gonadotrophin (BHCG) should be measured. If the over-the-counter urine pregnancy test is positive, BHCG should be checked if confirmation is required.

Teenage males require urinalysis and the leukocytesterase test is positive in sexually acquired urethritis. If there are symptoms with penile discharge or dysuria, gonorrhea culture and chlamydia test are indicated.

If vaginal or penile lesions are suggestive of herpes infection, a Tzanck test and culture should be performed.

An adolescent who requires treatment for sexually transmitted disease (STD) is entitled to confidential care in the United States. The sexual partner(s) also require treatment and there should be follow-up after treatment to ensure that there has been resolution. This is important because of the potential for failure to comply with the treatment prescribed.

Teenage Pregnancy

About 1 million teenage girls become pregnant in the United States each year. One-third of them are less than 15 years of age. Half continue to term and half choose elective termination.

The pregnancy outcome needs to be discussed with the teenager and a social worker is usually helpful in outlining the options. Adolescent pregnancy is, by definition, high risk and associated with a higher-than-usual rate of complications, including low-birth weight and premature delivery. If the pregnancy is planned to continue to term, prenatal care needs to be initiated. Contraception is recommended after completion of the pregnancy.

Pain Control

Pain management is often an important component of care. It is difficult to assess pain because it is subjective and there are no objective measures of pain. Children are more difficult to manage because their response to pain is so varied and they have problems verbalizing exactly what they are feeling.

There are various means of assessment of pain in children which vary especially with the age of the child. Children can often indicate the severity and location of pain if the questions are appropriate. It is important to reduce the stress and emotional component so that the specific problem of pain can be separated. Pain often induces fear in the child. It must be remembered that some children will deny pain if they are likely to receive an injection for treatment and may deny it to a stranger but admit it to the parent.

By 3 or 4 years of age, children may be able to accurately point to the site of pain or to indicate the position on a drawing and at this age can use a pain scale to indicate severity. The commonest pain scales for young children involve facial expressions (Figure 10-1). It is important that the clinician not make a judgment about the amount of pain that a child might have based on behavior alone. Older children may be able to rate pain on a score of 1 to 10 and then changes in the pain will usually relate to changes in the number that they assign to the pain.

It is important to be aware of symptoms of pain in the child who is non-verbal. This includes the child who is very young or neurologically impaired. In this situation, abnormal movements or behaviors, such as agitation or restlessness, may indicate pain. Crying or verbalization may suggest pain. Physiologic changes may be useful signs, including increased heart rate, blood pressure, or respirations. There may be sweating or pupillary changes. All of these indicators may be present when there is pain and absent when the pain is gone or controlled.

Fear of addiction is realistic if there is going to be chronic use of opiate medications. For acute or short-term usage, addiction is unlikely in children.

Which Face Shows How Much Hurt You Have Now?

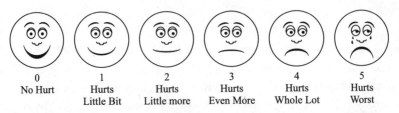

0	1	2	3	4	5
No Hurt	Hurts Little Bit	Hurts Little more	Hurts Even More	Hurts Whole Lot	Hurts Worst

Explain to the person that each face is for a person who feels happy because he has no pain (hurt) or sad because he has some or a lot of pain. **Face 0** is very happy because he does not hurt at all. **Face 1** hurts just a little bit. **Face 2** hurts a little more. **Face 3** hurts even more. **Face 4** hurts a whole lot. **Face 5** hurts as much as you can imagine, although you do not have to be crying to feel this bad. Ask the person to choose the face that best describes how he is feeling.

Rating scale is recommended for persons age 3 years and older.

Figure 10-1. The Wong–Baker FACES Pain Rating Scale. (From: Wong, D. L., Hockenberry-Eaton, M., Wilson, D., Winkelstein, M. L., Ahmann, E., and DiVito-Thomas, P. A., *Whaley and Wong's Nursing Care of Infants and Children*, 6th ed., St. Louis, 1999, p. 2040. Copyrighted by Mosby, Inc. Reprinted by permission.)

Substance Abuse

Surveys of older adolescents indicate that almost all (95 percent) try alcohol and about half have tried marijuana. Only a small minority of teenagers progress to substance abuse with the potential for addiction. Individuals who abuse one drug or substance are likely to abuse others as well. Adolescents with chronic illness, especially mental health, and disabilities have the potential to abuse alcohol and drugs.

Alcohol has two major problems for adolescents. Ingestion during pregnancy is associated with effects on the fetus and may result in physical malformations and mental retardation (fetal alcohol syndrome). The other problem results from risky behaviors that are exacerbated by alcohol. Fast driving and motor vehicle accidents are often precipitated by alcohol. Alcohol results in more deaths of adolescents than all illicit drugs combined.

Illicit drugs (excluding marijuana) are used by up to 5 percent of adolescents. Cocaine and stimulants (especially amphetamines) are the most common.

It is important to recognize substance abuse disorders at an early stage. There is often a delay because the symptoms may be nonspecific and there may be medical or mental health problems which camouflage the substance abuse.

Urine or blood may be screened for drug metabolites. Urine tests can reveal cocaine, methadone, amphetamines, diazepam, opiates, and barbiturates. Alcohol can only be tested in the blood or by breath test. It is controversial whether it is acceptable to perform drug testing without consent.

Management of alcohol and substance abuse problems is fraught with difficulty. Adolescents tend to deny that they have a problem. Therapy is expensive and motivation to succeed is often lacking.

Chronic Fatigue Syndrome

This condition of prolonged periods of debilitating fatigue that interferes with daily living is seen in adults and children. Chronic fatigue is seen commonly after infectious mononucleosis and so the causative agent, the Epstein-Barr virus (EBV), was thought to contribute to the picture of chronic fatigue syndrome (CFS). After much debate, the role of EBV in CFS is unclear. Fatigue may be central when it affects people after intense concentration over a period of time or associated with depression or apathy. Fatigue is described as peripheral when it results from intense muscular activity at work or play.

■ CLINICAL FEATURES

There is no diagnostic test for CFS and the diagnosis is made from the presence of 4 symptoms (Table 10-1). These criteria are applied after the major criteria have been satisfied. First, there is

TABLE 10-1. CHRONIC FATIGUE SYNDROME SYMPTOMS AND CRITERIA

1. *Clinically evaluated, unexplained persistent or relapsing chronic fatigue.*
2. *The concurrent occurrence of 4 or more of the following symptoms which must have persisted or recurred during 6 or more consecutive months of illness and must not have predated the fatigue.*
   - Substantial impairment in short-term memory or concentration
   - Sore throat
   - Tender lymph nodes
   - Muscle pain
   - Multi-joint pain without swelling or redness
   - Headaches of a new type, pattern, or severity
   - Unrefreshing sleep
   - Post-exertional malaise lasting more than 24 hours.

Conditions that exclude a diagnosis of CFS:
   - Any active medical condition that may explain the presence of chronic fatigue
   - If the persistence of a condition could explain the presence of chronic fatigue, and if it cannot be clearly established that the original condition has completely resolved with treatment, then such patients should not be classified as having CFS
   - Any past or current diagnosis of a major depressive disorder with psychotic or melancholic features; bipolar affective disorders; schizophrenia of any subtype; delusional disorders of any subtype; dementias of any subtype; anorexia nervosa; or bulimia nervosa
   - Alcohol or other substance abuse, occurring within 2 years of the onset of chronic fatigue and any time afterwards
   - Severe obesity as defined by a body mass index equal to or greater than 45.

a new onset of a debilitating illness that lowers the activity ability to below 50 percent of previous for a period of at least 6 months; and second, any other clinical condition that could cause the symptoms has been excluded. The conditions most commonly associated with fatigue include malignancy, neuromuscular disorders, endocrine disorders, chronic infectious conditions, autoimmune disease, psychiatric disease, and drug usage.

Fibromyalgia (FM) tends to be confused with CFS and patients with FM can have CFS. In principle, the major difference is that FM causes pain and tenderness in muscles, ligaments, and tendons (but not joints).

The difference between adults and children with CFS is that children tend to have a relapsing illness rather than the persistent illness seen in adults. Children tend to have more somatic than psychiatric symptoms. Depression in children is quite difficult to diagnose on occasions and must be excluded.

The history is most useful for making the diagnosis. The physical examination and laboratory tests tend to be normal.

■ MANAGEMENT

There is no specific treatment for the disorder although tricyclic antidepressants could be tried. The most effective strategy has been cognitive-behavioral therapy with an active rehabilitation program.

Fibromyalgia

Fibromyalgia is a syndrome of aches and pains and fatigue. The cause is unknown, there are no diagnostic laboratory tests, and the existence of fibromyalgia as a specific entity is questioned by many. The best description of fibromyalgia is that it is muscular rheumatism with tenderness, pain, and muscle spasms. The pain tends to be present all the time, with soreness and tenderness at specific points on the muscles. The fibromyalgia tender points are close to the muscular attachments and have been defined by the American College of Rheumatology (Figure 10-2). An appropriate evaluation includes checking each tender point and failure to check usually implies that the clinician is unaware of these points. The diagnostic criteria for fibromyalgia include symptoms of aching all over and tenderness at at least 11 of the 18 points. The majority (>75 percent) of patients also have difficulty sleeping, characteristically very light sleeping, are easily awakened, and have the feeling of not having had a good night's rest. Tension headaches (50 percent) and temperomandibular joint (TMJ) disorder (25 percent) are common and both produce debilitating pain. Half the patients suffer from irritable bowel syndrome which results in crampy diarrhea.

The cause of fibromyalgia is thought to be a metabolic or immune system dysfunction and genetics may contribute. Stress appears to impact the course but the reality is that no one under-

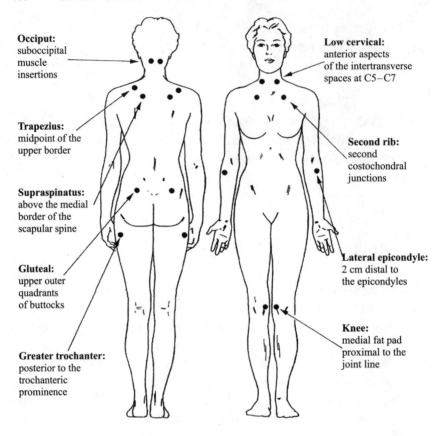

Figure 10-2. The 18 points of fibromyalgia.

stands this condition. It certainly seems to be present in childhood, and, in the classification of the disorder, primary fibromyalgia is described to start at 4–5 years of age often presenting with random aches and pains. It is possible that the growing pains reported by some children may be fibromyalgia. Secondary fibromyalgia is associated with a medical condition, for example hypothyroidism, and post-traumatic originates following an illness or accident.

The condition has been most recognized following Dr. Don Goldenberg's paper in JAMA (257: 2782, 1987) reporting the findings of 118 patients with the condition. There is a report that 6 percent of 338 children between the ages of 9 and 15 met the criteria for the diagnosis and it is increasingly being diagnosed in children. It may follow a flu-like illness and may present as a sleep disorder. The symptoms may affect cognitive tasks in school and the teacher may notice symptoms similar to ADHD, although hyperactivity is not usual.

The prognosis for fibromyalgia is better in children than adults and tends to improve over time. The goals of therapy are to improve nutrition and sleep and to control pain.

11

Chapter Eleven

Surgical and Orthopedic Problems

Children with chronic medical problems may have an increased need for surgery. Surgery may be needed to improve the underlying chronic condition or may be for causes independent of the chronic condition. For example, appendicitis may affect a child with asthma or diabetes.

The most common surgical procedures for children are repair of inguinal hernia, orchiopexy, and placement of ear tubes. Most of these procedures are performed under general anesthesia on an out-patient basis. Children with chronic disorders may have anesthetic risks beyond those of normal children so it may be prudent in some cases to perform the procedures as in-patients.

Organ Transplantation

End-stage failure of some organ systems may be amenable to replacement. Kidney, heart, lung, and liver are the predominant organs that have been transplanted in children. Additional transplants include pancreas, small intestine, and increasingly multiple organ transplants are being performed. Patients accepted onto a hospital's transplant waiting list are registered with the UNOS (United Network for Organ Sharing) Organ Center where a centralized computer network links all organ procurement organizations and transplant centers. Various factors are involved for donor selection including blood type, tissue type, and size of the organ, and each organ has specific criteria.

In 1997, the UNOS reported 3,565 children and 76,526 adults were waiting for organ transplants. According to the International Pediatric Transplant Association, children in the United States receive 11 percent of total heart transplants, 7 percent of lung transplants, 13 percent of liver transplants, and about 5 percent of kidney transplants. A higher percentage of children than adults die waiting for transplant.

The importance of immunosuppression regimens in the improved survival of transplants cannot be overstressed. Regimens usually involve prednisone, cyclosporine or tacrolimus, and mycophenolate mofetil or azathioprine. The major complications include infection, rejection, and malignancy, in addition to surgical problems.

■ KIDNEY TRANSPLANTATION

There is an almost 40-year history of renal transplantation. Kidney transplants are the second most common organ transplant (corneal transplant is number 1) in the United States with over 9,000 cases (adult and pediatric) per year. Indications for pediatric renal transplantation include symptoms of uremia not responsive to standard therapy, failure to thrive, delayed psychomotor development, fluid overload, and metabolic bone disease due to renal osteodystrophy. There are many kidney disorders that result in end-stage renal disease but the major indication is chronic glomerulonephritis.

Between 80–90 percent of transplanted kidneys are functioning 2 years after the operation. The main problem is graft rejection. Living-related 1-year graft survival is 90 percent, with 85 percent 2-year and 75 percent 5-year survival. The corresponding figures for cadaver transplants are 76, 71, and 62 (1992). The half-life of a cadaveric kidney is about 8 years. This compares poorly with the average of 12 and 26 years for living-donor kidneys matched for one and two haplotypes (tissue-typing factors) respectively.

The longer a patient with kidney disease remains on dialysis while waiting for a kidney transplant, the more likely the patient is to die prematurely even after receiving a new kidney.

■ HEART TRANSPLANTATION

About 75 percent of children requiring heart transplant under 1 year have serious congenital heart defects that cannot be repaired by corrective surgery. The remaining 25 percent have cardio-myopathy. Of children aged 1 to 5 years, half have inoperable congenital heart disease and half have myocarditis or cardio-myopathy. Of patients over 5 years, more than 60 percent require transplant for cardiomyopathy and less than 40 percent for congenital heart disease.

■ LUNG TRANSPLANTATION

Pediatric lung transplants are typically performed on cystic fibrosis (CF) patients who make up about 70 percent of pediatric lung transplant patients. Primary pulmonary hypertension, interstitial lung disease, and bronchopulmonary dysplasia make up the rest of the pediatric lung transplant population.

Double-lung transplant is bilateral, sequential, single-lung transplant which means that one lung is removed and then replaced and then the second lung is removed and replaced. Both lungs have to be replaced if there is chronic lung infection. CF does not develop in the transplanted lung. One-year survival approaches 90 percent and 5-year survival is about 65 percent. Living-lobar transplantation involves replacing the diseased lungs with lobes from a living donor.

■ LIVER TRANSPLANTATION

Various surgical techniques have been developed to address the problem of the lack of cadaver livers. Reduced-size or cutdown-and-split liver transplants, in which only a portion of a liver is utilized for the transplant, have been successful. Biliary atresia accounts for at least 50 percent of pediatric patients undergoing liver transplantation. The second most common reason for transplantation is liver disease due to inborn errors of metabolism, with α_1-antitrypsin deficiency being the most common, and others including tyrosinemia and Wilson's disease.

■ BONE MARROW TRANSPLANTATION

Bone marrow transplantation is increasingly being performed for several hematologic, oncologic, metabolic, and genetic disorders. The healthy bone marrow may be taken from the patient (autograft) or it may be taken from a donor (homograft). Donated bone marrow must match the patient's tissue type. The donor may be a living relative (usually a brother or a sister—allogeneic), or from an unrelated donor found through the national marrow donor program which lists more than 700,000 potential donors. Donors are matched through HLA tissue typing.

Indications for bone marrow transplant include blood cell disorders, especially aplastic anemia, leukemia, or lymphoma, as part of aggressive cancer treatments (chemotherapy, radiation therapy), and many immunodeficiency syndromes. It may be useful in managing hereditary hemoglobinopathies and metabolic storage diseases.

Orthopedic Problems

Orthopedic problems in children are common and are present in many chronic illnesses. A common problem in pediatrics is gait disturbance. Difficulty walking may be caused by various disorders. Some of the conditions are more common at specific ages. Legg–Calves–Perthes disease occurs from 4–9 years of age; slipped capital femoral epiphysis from 10–17 years of age. Congenital dislocation of the hip is more common in females (6 : 1).

■ LEGG–CALVES–PERTHES

This is a rare condition (1 : 18,000 live births) and occurs mostly in Caucasian children aged 4–9 years with a sex predominance of boys (5 : 1). It is avascular necrosis of the femoral head of unknown cause. It is thought to be related to repeated trauma to the femoral head, which already has poor vascularization. It is more common in children with delayed growth and is bilateral in 10–18 percent of cases. Examination shows limitation of hip movement and X-rays of the hips show the abnormal femoral head. It is important to consider the diagnosis in a child who has a limp. Treatment involves physical therapy and reduction of weight bearing.

■ OSGOOD–SCHLATTER DISEASE

This is osteochondritis at the point of insertion of the patellar tendon of the upper tibia. It commonly affects boys and results in pain below the knee. The pain is worse with movement and improves with rest. There is usually swelling and tenderness. The X-ray shows fragmentation of the tibial tubercle because of partial avascular necrosis. The disease is self-limiting so that it improves when bone growth stops. Treatment is symptomatic with avoidance of maneuvers that bring on the pain. This includes cycling and basketball where quadriceps contraction stresses the tendon. Activity can be resumed when the pain improves.

■ POPLITEAL CYST (BAKER CYST)

This is an out-pouching of the synovial capsule of the knee joint under the medial head of the gastrocnemius muscle. It is usually asymptomatic and the main issue is that there is a 30 percent recurrence rate after surgery.

■ SCOLIOSIS

This is a curvature of the spine of greater than 10 percent in the coronal (side-to-side) plane. There are many different causes. Idiopathic scoliosis is the most common cause and occurs during the adolescent growth spurt. It is more common in females and is painless. If the curve is less than 25 percent, observation is indicated. If the curvature is 25–40 percent, bracing should be considered and surgery is usually indicated for curves greater than 40–50 percent.

Congenital scoliosis usually results from abnormal vertebrae and the progression usually does not improve with bracing. Many are associated with renal, cardiac, or other anomalies which should be looked for. Paralytic scoliosis results from neuro-muscular disorders. If there is scoliosis with progression, it is usual to follow with X-rays every 6 months. The main reason to perform surgery is to stop the progression of the curvature. Usually, posterior spinal fusion will be sufficient in idiopathic scoliosis. Neuromuscular disorders associated with scoliosis may require anterior as well as posterior fusion. Metal rods, with hooks or wires, may supplement the fusion.

■ KYPHOSIS AND LORDOSIS

Kyphosis is curvature in the antero-posterior direction, usually in the thoracic region. There is a problem with ossification of the anterior portion of the vertebral body (Scheuermann kyphosis). Back pain is common and worse when standing. Bracing is usually successful in controlling the curvature. Minor degrees of kyphosis may occur in adolescent girls that can be corrected by improving their posture. Lordosis occurs in the lumbar region and tends not to be a major problem.

■ DEVELOPMENTAL DYSPLASIA OF THE HIP JOINT

This is a continuum of disorders and includes the term congenital dislocation of the hip which is not an accurate term because the dislocation tends to occur after birth. Developmental dysplasia of the hip joint results in an abnormal relationship between the proximal femur and the acetabulum (of the pelvis). The incidence is 1 per 1,000 live births. It is important to recognize the condition because if the hip is dislocated and not treated there may be permanent deformity. Ortolani described the maneuver of flexion of the hip to 90° and then abduction, with the middle finger over the hipjoint and the thumb applying pressure to the medial aspect of the thigh. If the head of the femur slips out of the acetabulum it can be felt.

Dislocation or dysplasia can be treated by splinting the legs in a position of flexion and abduction. Treatment is indicated for months and when initiated early is very successful. If dislocation is not recognized until the child starts to walk, a limp and lurching to the affected side will suggest the diagnosis.

■ CLUBFOOT

Congenital clubfoot occurs in 1 per 1,000 live births. It may be idiopathic, neurogenic, or associated with a syndrome (such as arthrogryposis multiplex congenita). It is called talipes equino-varus which means plantar flexion at the ankle joint with inversion of the foot at the heel and the forefoot. Treatment with splinting should begin a few days after birth. Initially, this can be by splinting with strapping and later with casts that stretch the foot towards the normal position. The cast should be changed frequently, sequentially correcting the forefoot, heel, and then ankle deformities. About 50 percent will require an operative procedure to lengthen structures within the foot.

■ SLIPPED CAPITAL FEMORAL EPIPHYSIS

There is separation of the proximal femoral epiphysis through the growth plate so that the head of the femur becomes displaced medially and posteriorly. Most cases (80 percent) result from a progressive chronic slip of the femoral epiphysis and 20 percent have the injury acutely following a traumatic event. It occurs in early adolescence and is most common in obese males. The presentation is a painful limp that may last for months. The pain commonly is referred to the thigh or even the medial side of the knee. There is usually a limitation of internal rotation and abduction of the hip. The diagnosis is confirmed by X-ray.

Treatment is similar to that of a fracture of the neck of the femur. If there has been an acute injury, traction may help and, in chronic cases, pinning the slip as it lies is preferred. Reduction of the chronic slip may lead to avascular necrosis of the femoral head. About 30 percent of patients have bilateral involvement so that slipping of the opposite side may occur and this could be 1–2 years after the initial injury.

12
Chapter Twelve

Home Care and Technology Dependence

Home care for children with chronic illness involves a number of considerations. The concept of providing care at home for children with chronic illness has resulted from a desire to save costs as well as to look after children in an environment that is more conducive to optimal development. There can be nursing visits to provide care, especially after discharge from the hospital. There can be hospice care for the terminally sick. The need for technology-dependent home care has increased as a result of improved survival of trauma and severe illness, improvements in cancer outcome, and more aggressive care for neuromuscular disorders. Although the costs of providing medical care in the home are considerable, there are major cost savings when it is compared to the cost of providing care in the hospital. The other main advantage of home care has been that the results have been successful.

The family needs to want to manage the child in the home setting. They must be motivated to provide care and often they will have to make sacrifices to make it work. There is a need for trust between the provider and the family. This may be difficult if there is a rapid turnover of staff. The family may take time to learn to trust the nurse and once they do they may be reluctant to trust others. Many families learn a great deal about the child's condition and may feel that the nurse that comes for an 8-hour shift may not be as committed as they would like. It is helpful to have case management so that there is an individual who is responsible for the coordination of care. The family needs someone they can contact should there be a disagreement about the treatment of the child.

The benefits of home care in addition to cost reduction include:

- A shorter hospital stay
- Improved quality of life
- Involving patient and family in care
- Allowing technology-dependent patients to be managed in a comfortable and familiar setting

Home Intravenous Therapy

Home intravenous (IV) therapy programs started in the 1970s and are spreading annually as the cost savings compared to hospitalization increase. Advances in technology have resulted in the ability to manage patients at home safely with IV therapy. Many patients prefer to receive infusion therapy at home rather than the hospital. Infusion therapies include antibiotics, pain therapy, chemotherapy, and parenteral nutrition (PN). Blood transfusions and blood products tend to be given in the hospital because of the higher risk of complications. The physician is the medical case manager with responsibility for ordering the plan of care and usually writes the orders.

Peripheral PN regimens can only be used for low-osmolarity solutions (300–900 mOsm/L). Higher osmolarity solutions must be in larger veins with faster blood flow to avoid sclerosis and inflammation of the vein wall. Central lines may be placed percutaneously and the peripherally inserted central catheters (PICC lines) are increasingly being used for intermediate (days to weeks) usage. Central lines also may be surgically inserted, often with a subcutaneous tunnel to reduce the chance of skin bacteria infecting the vein. The Hickman and Broviac catheter can be inserted surgically or through a needle. Catheters such as the mediport or portacath may be implanted under the skin. These catheters are best used when there is intermittent need for IV infusion, such as a course of antibiotics or chemotherapy. The Groshong catheter has a patented 3-position valve near the closed tip which opens inward during blood withdrawal and outward during infusion. The valve closes automatically when not in use because venous pressure is not enough to spontaneously open the valve inward. The result is that if the catheter becomes disconnected, blood loss or air embolus is prevented.

Catheter-related complications are not uncommon. It is important to check the position of the tip of the catheter before solutions are infused. Air embolus is an infrequent complication as filters and connections have reduced this occurrence. Thrombophlebitis is common with peripheral catheters and thrombus formation may occur with stasis associated with central catheters. Infection related to central catheters is a major complication. If there is fever, catheter-related sepsis must be considered. Blood cultures can be drawn from the line and peripherally at the same time. If there is evidence of fungal line sepsis, the catheter needs to be removed. Sometimes antibiotic treatment can be given to eradicate bacterial colonization of the catheter, but it is often necessary to remove the catheter.

Monitoring of laboratory parameters needs to be planned. Blood levels of antibiotics or other medications should be checked at appropriate intervals and hematology and biochemical studies can be drawn during a home visit or the patient can go for blood drawing at a clinic or hospital.

IV tubing should be changed every 24–48 hours. Central catheters should be flushed monthly to reduce the potential for blocking off by thrombus formation.

The gravity system is the simplest for home infusion therapy. The solution is hung on a pole and the rate of flow is adjusted by using an in-line clamp and by watching the number of drips in a drip chamber to estimate the rate. This is not an accurate method and there are no alarms. Some systems use an ambulatory infusion pump which is portable and battery-powered. Complications of IV therapy can be minimized with careful protocols. Infiltration of peripheral lines is common in children with pain and swelling at the site. Phlebitis is more common if the fluid is hypertonic or irritating.

If antibiotics are to be continued for more than 3 weeks, some form of central line is necessary. If there is a history of allergy, the initial dose of an antibiotic should be given in an environment where anaphylaxis can be treated.

Patients with diseases involving kidneys, liver, heart, lungs, or blood should be monitored more closely for side effects. Chemotherapy is usually administered in an infusion center initially and some chemotherapy medications should always be administered in the presence of personnel who can handle emergency situations. Unused drugs should not be disposed of down the drain or toilet but should be treated as hazardous waste.

Pain medications can be administered by IV, IM, subcutaneously, intrathecally, and by epidural catheter. Infusion pumps for narcotics can be set up so that the patient can activate the pump at intervals depending on the need for pain control. The pumps are called patient-controlled activation (PCA).

Pediatric Respiratory Home Care

The respiratory care practitioner (RCP) provides an important role in home care for many pediatric patients. It is usual for the RCP to have at least 1 year of acute care experience before working with home care. Experience in pediatrics is necessary as this comprises an important part of home care. It is important that RCPs providing home care be licensed (states have different regulations).

The main population receiving home care is the patient who is being discharged from the hospital and still requires ongoing care. Many patients are serviced by home care companies and many of the companies are durable medical equipment (DME) vendors. The RCP who is employed by the DME company will select, deliver, and set up the equipment in the home. The family will be educated in the requirements for monitoring and maintaining the equipment. The treating physician is responsible for prescribing the therapy. The RCP spends much of the time during the home visit teaching the family the safe and effective use of the equipment. A treatment plan is individualized and documentation is important. Appropriate follow-up is indicated.

Medicare does not reimburse for the RCP service whereas they will do so for a nursing visit. As a result, many companies utilize nurses to do the evaluation and education for patients on Medicare.

RCPs employed by a hospital are often part of the discharge planning team that orders specific home care treatments for children. Team members also include nurses and social workers who are responsible for evaluating the suitability of the caregivers and the home environment before the plan is initiated. The home environment needs to be evaluated for safety against fire or other hazards, particularly if home mechanical ventilation is to be used. One of the issues includes the electrical system, as there may be various appliances connected to the same electrical circuit. Awareness of the amperage of the appliances reduces the chance that the circuit will be overloaded. It is necessary to check the fuse boxes. Some older homes have inadequate circuit breakers and inappropriate fuses. Space for the equipment and circuits is necessary and they need to be placed so that there is safe distance from heaters or any source of flame. Functioning smoke detectors are essential and fire extinguishers should be available and accessible.

Categories of home respiratory equipment include:

Category I: No prescription needed.

Category II: Prescription needed but the equipment is not considered life supporting. This includes oxygen delivery devices, nebulizers, suction machines, and oximeters.

Category III: Prescription needed and the equipment is considered life supportive. This includes apnea monitors, pressure support for respiratory failure, and invasive or non-invasive mechanical ventilation.

■ HOME OXYGEN

Liquid Oxygen

Liquid oxygen systems store oxygen at $-273°F$ in a tank that is called a dewar. As the oxygen passes through warming coils it becomes gaseous. The flow can vary from $\frac{1}{4}$ to 15 L/min. The standard liquid oxygen tank lasts for a week at 2 L/min and is refilled as needed. The main advantage of the liquid system is that a small lightweight tank can be filled from the stationary system that allows the system to be ambulatory. The small tanks last for 8 hours with a flow rate of 2 L/min and they are fairly heavy; the smaller units last correspondingly less time.

The other advantages of the liquid system include quietness and no need for electricity. The system is more costly than other oxygen systems but the convenience makes it the best choice for the child who wants to be able to travel away from home. If the flow rate is more than 4 L/min, refills need to be made frequently. There is continued evaporative loss so that there is some wastage. Reimbursement for liquid systems may be less than optimal for the DME company.

Oxygen Concentrator

This is an electrical device that removes nitrogen from room air and delivers oxygen to the patient at rates of $\frac{1}{4}$ to 6 L/min. The concentrator is quite large and noisy and does require electricity to function. The advantage over the liquid system is that there is no need to refill. Running the unit increases the monthly utility bill by approximately $25. It is most useful for patients who use oxygen only at night or for those who remain in bed.

Compressed Oxygen Systems

The compressed oxygen tanks used in the hospital may be used in the home. The largest is the H tank which lasts for two days at 2 L/min. The H tank is useful as a back-up for the concentrator. It is not good as a primary source because of the need to replace the tank every few days. Smaller tanks are E and D tanks. The D tanks are small enough to carry in a shoulder bag. The E and D tanks are useful for people who only spend a limited time away from home. Cylinders and tanks containing compressed gas are the most economical method of delivering oxygen. The container must be supported either by a chain or in a base or cart. The tanks must be placed or stored away from any heat source.

Some devices are equipped to conserve oxygen to extend usage. These include the reservoir cannula, the pulsed-dose system, and the transtracheal oxygen system. The reservoir cannula stores the continuously flowing oxygen during expiration so that a bolus is available for the next inspiration. Pulsed-dose systems deliver an increased amount of oxygen during the beginning of inspiration and can reduce the amount of oxygen utilized overall. Transtracheal oxygen systems have not been used much in pediatrics. They involve insertion of a catheter into the trachea percutaneously (from the neck), which delivers oxygen directly into the trachea.

Oxygen is delivered to the airway by facemask or by cannula. The nasal cannula can be connected to the source by tubing that can be as long as 50 feet to allow some mobility. Oxygen masks are less used in the home than in the hospital. They can deliver higher concentrations of oxygen than cannulae. The simple mask requires a high flow rate (5–10 L/min) and the non-rebreather and Venturi need even higher flow rates. The prescription for oxygen usually will define the flow rate and the duration (number of hours). On occasions, oxygen will be required only during sleep and activity. It is useful to evaluate whether the oxygen can be discontinued for brief periods (e.g., during a shower or when eating). Continuous pulse oximetry is usually not recommended in the home because of the frequency of false alarms. It is helpful if there is intermittent checking of oxygen saturation to maintain an appropriate level.

■ AEROSOL THERAPY

Many children with asthma, reactive airway disease, and bronchopulmonary dysplasia will utilize bronchodilator or anti-inflammatory medications. Patients with cystic fibrosis commonly use aerosol antibiotics and mucolytics. Medications may be delivered by metered dose inhaler (MDI, also known as a puffer) or by nebulizer. MDIs need to be used correctly and the technique should be reviewed at each clinic visit. A spacer should be used with the MDI in children and a mouthpiece or facemask, depending on the patient's age and ability. Using a spacer with the facemask allows medication to be delivered even to infants.

MDI therapy allows delivery of medicine in children and has the advantage of portability and convenience. Compressor-driven nebulizers are used to deliver larger volumes of medication. The two components of the system are the compressor and the nebulizer. The compressor produces a flow rate of 8–15 L/min at about 20 psi. It can be electricity or battery-driven.

■ AIRWAY CLEARANCE TECHNIQUES

Chest physiotherapy (CPT) is indicated for clearance of airway secretions. Airway clearance techniques can be utilized in the home. The concept of postural drainage, percussion, and vibration is that the secretions are mobilized by the chest wall movement in a position that uses gravity to aid drainage. Percussion is performed using a cupped hand or a device such as a plastic or rubber handheld substitute. Vibration is usually applied with a mechanical device with increased pressure during expiration. Infants and small children can be held on a pillow or the lap of the treater. Older children can be tilted using a board or bed or can learn to self-administer. Caregivers need to be taught the techniques.

If the secretions are moved from the periphery of the lung toward the central airway, they can then be coughed out. Huffing is coughing with an open glottis. It is thought to be more efficient in removal of mucus and is also called forced expiratory technique. It is usual to perform percussion or vibration for 1 minute per segment except that extended therapy is recommended for cystic fibrosis patients and 2 minutes per segment is used. Additional methods for ACT include the flutter valve, positive expiratory pressure (PEP) valve, and autogenic drainage.

It is usual to utilize bronchodilator medications prior to starting chest PT. The contraindications to CPT include hemoptysis and pneumothorax. Chest pain and rib tenderness may be significant and lead to modification of the therapy. Coughing may be difficult if there is pain in the chest or abdomen.

Suction machines are used at home for aspiration of secretions. A tonsillar or Yankauer catheter is used for oropharyngeal suctioning and suction catheter for endotracheal secretions. It is sensible to have both electric and battery-operated machines.

■ NON-INVASIVE HOME MECHANICAL VENTILATION

Nasal positive pressure ventilation is applied by nasal or face mask. It is commonly used for night-time ventilation in neuromuscular diseases or obstructive sleep apnea. Positive pressure is applied at intervals or continuously. The former is intermittent positive pressure ventilation and the latter is continuous positive airway pressure. The system often used is BiPAP, or bilevel positive airway pressure. Some children tolerate this well but others do not.

Negative pressure ventilation is applied by an iron-lung or by a cuirasse (chest shell). Negative pressure, which results in movement of air into the lungs, is applied to the chest. The iron-lung, which saved so many lives in the polio era, has limited use. The cuirasse may be useful in neuromuscular weakness disorders but may worsen obstructive apnea.

■ HOME VENTILATION

Indications for mechanical ventilation at home include respiratory disorders such as BPD, control of breathing disorders such as central apnea, and neuromuscular disorders such as muscular dystrophy. Most children who require long-term ventilation will undergo tracheotomy. Non-invasive ventilation is mostly used for nocturnal ventilation. The majority of ventilators used at home are volume-cycled machines, which deliver a set tidal volume. Many machines are microprocessor controlled and can be used with a wheelchair.

It is important that back-up systems are available. This includes a means of applying bag ventilation and usually a back-up ventilator in case the first one fails. Various power sources are available for the primary system. These include standard AC power, back-up rechargeable battery, and additional battery power which may include an automotive-type battery.

■ HOME INFANT APNEA MONITORING

Home monitors measure beat-to-beat heart rate and will alarm, usually within 3 seconds, if the rate is below a defined level. The heart rate alarm is usually set at 80 beats per minute (bpm) on discharge from the nursery and 60 bpm after about 3 months of age. There is usually a delay for apnea, which implies absence of respiration, for 20 seconds. The monitors are impedance pneumographs which monitor chest wall movement. They provide information about central apnea (no chest wall movement and no air movement) but do not distinguish obstructive apnea. Caretakers are taught to respond to monitor alarms by initially checking the baby. If there is apnea, the baby is stimulated to alter state, which usually restores respiratory effort. Rarely, it is necessary to initiate CPR. Current monitors document the alarms and provide an event log that allows the clinician to evaluate the significance of the episodes.

■ TRACHEOSTOMY

Tracheostomy is performed for airway abnormalities such as subglottic stenosis or tracheomalacia. Infants who require long-term assisted ventilation usually will have a tracheostomy. Tracheostomy tubes can be cuffed or non-cuffed. Non-cuffed tubes are preferred in infants and small children. A fenestrated tube has openings in the curve of the tube that allow air to be expired through the glottis (voicebox).

Suctioning is performed when the patient is unable to cough out secretions. The tracheostomy tube is changed at intervals, usually every 2–4 weeks. Young children tend to be lying down with a towel behind the shoulder blades to make visualization of the neck easier. Older children may manage better sitting up for the change. Caregivers need to feel comfortable with tracheostomy changes. If there is an emergency situation it may be from a blocked tube and caregivers need to be able to change the tube immediately. On occasions, if there is difficulty reinserting the tube, one size smaller should be used because it is easier to insert.

13

Chapter Thirteen

Child Abuse and Neglect

The 1962 landmark article by Kempe and others, "The Battered Child Syndrome," heralded the modern era of child abuse. One of the major risk factors for child abuse and neglect is chronic illness. There are several reasons for this (Table 13-1). Child abuse occurs in all social and ethnic groups. The outcome may be a minor injury to the body, such as a bruise, or major injury that may result in death. There may be psychological or emotional effects that can be devastating to the child. Abuse takes on many forms including physical (injury and neglect), psychological (verbal), and sexual. More than 2,000 children die each year in the United States as a result of abuse or neglect. The number of children maltreated each year is staggering and estimated to be more than 1.5 million, with over 200,000 children being sexually abused.

The risk factors for child abuse are well defined. Chronic illness in the child may be additive to the other factors or be the primary risk. The abuse may be from the parents who may consider that the child is a burden to them. It may be caregivers, such as foster parents, day-care workers, residential home staff, and others, who find the child easy prey for abuse. If the child is in a home with parents who have been abused (as a child or as a spouse), the child is more at risk.

Clinicians need to be aware that chronically ill children may be at risk and need to watch for symptoms and signs of abuse. If the child presents with an injury that has the potential to be non-

TABLE 13-1. CHRONIC ILLNESS RISK FACTORS FOR ABUSE

Physical abuse and/or neglect
  Graduate of NICU, especially low birth weight and prematurity
  Irritable child
  Hyperactivity (ADHD)
  Developmental delay/mental retardation
  Impaired mobility
  Impaired communication (language) skills
  Craniofacial deformities
  Financial burden
  Social isolation of caretaker

Sexual abuse
  Developmental immaturity

accidental, a careful history and physical examination is necessary. The history should include the events leading to the injury and the timing of evolution of the symptoms. Were there precipitating events leading to the injury, such as problems with feeding, excessive crying, or a parental dispute? The response of the family to the injury may be important, for example, if there was a delay in seeking care.

The major factors include the family, the child, and the environment. The parental characteristics have been well described and include a history of abuse by their parents. Unfortunately, even though there may be many risk factors that can be identified, it is still difficult to predict the child that is at risk for serious harm. Intervention may not be possible in many cases until definite harm has been demonstrated. Social isolation is an increasing risk factor in our present culture. There are fewer close relationships within families. Young parents may not have the skills necessary to look after a child.

Although it is possible to identify risk factors, child abuse covers all ages and social levels and the statement that the "mother could not have done it—she is so nice" may in itself be a red flag. The child is vulnerable in various circumstances. Graduates of neonatal intensive care are at higher risk. The life-and-death environment, the inability to bond to the parents, the separation which may be for weeks or months, and the needs of the infant after discharge all contribute. The child may be fussy or have special medical needs and be difficult to manage leading to frustration of the caretakers.

The environment that is associated with high risk for abuse could be described as low socioeconomic, poor, crowded, inadequate time to provide for the child, and exposure to drugs and alcohol. It must be remembered that the rich and wealthy may abuse their child and also the child may spend time with other caretakers who potentially may abuse the child.

In all 50 states, if a physician suspects that a child has been abused, it is mandatory to inform the child protection agency. In some states, failure to report could lead to loss of medical license, a malpractice suit, or jail. When a case is reported to child protective services, the agency has the responsibility to investigate the case. If there is sufficient evidence for abuse, then the court will be petitioned regarding custody of the child and the decision will depend upon the potential for harm to the child. The physician may be responsible for testifying in court.

If a child presents to an emergency room or clinic with an injury that is non-accidental, the perpetrator does not typically confess to the crime but may present a fabricated history to try and explain the findings. On further questioning, the story may change, which is a major red flag. Because child abuse may occur at all social levels, all races, and at any age, it is important to think about the potential. It is not meant to imply that everyone is guilty before being proven innocent but rather that if the findings are possibly due to non-accidental trauma, the child's safety must be considered.

The definition of neglect is fairly broad. The definition is the failure of caretakers to provide the basic needs of their children. Emotional neglect may be failure to provide a loving environment.

It is important to distinguish symptoms of the medical condition. Table 13-2 lists some of the illnesses that are mistaken for abuse on occasions. The commonest conditions are associated with easy bruising so that relatively minor trauma results in tissue bleeding.

TABLE 13-2. ILLNESSES SOMETIMES MISTAKEN FOR ABUSE

Easy bruisability
  Coagulation disorder, e.g. hemophilia
  Presentation of leukemia
  Platelet dysfunction
  Ehlers-Danlos (cutis laxa—loose skin syndrome)
  Hemorrhagic disease of the newborn (vitamin K deficiency)

Dermatology (skin conditions)
  Epidermolysis bullosa (looks like a burn)
  Mongolian blue spot
  Capillary hemangiomas
  Eczema
  Contact dermatitis

Infections
  Purpura fulminans (meningococcemia)

Ethnic treatments
  Coining (Cao Gio)
  Cupping
  Moxibustion

Clues that the injury may not be accidental include:

- the history does not match the findings
- it may be developmentally unlikely
- the story changes on questioning
- the story from the two parents is different
- there is a long time lapse between the injury and seeking help
- the parent's reaction or behavior may be inappropriate

Physical Abuse

■ BRUISES AND BITES

The commonest outward sign of child abuse is bruising. Moving children tend to accidentally bruise themselves on the front of the body—the chin, the knees, and the shins are most common. Bruises of the buttocks, the groin, face and ears, lip and frenulum, and the "black eye" are suspicious for abuse. Hand marks and pinches, as well as bites, are non-accidental. Bruises caused by abuse will often have bizarre marks, such as a belt buckle or rope coil. They tend to be multiple and the bruises may be of different ages.

It must be remembered that many conditions, both acute and chronic, are associated with easy bruising. The implication of child abuse is that the injury involves excessive and inappropriate trauma to the child. Many ethnic treatments produce lesions that may have the appearance of child abuse. Examples include *coining*, a Vietnamese and Cambodian practice of rubbing hot coins over the chest or back (Cao Gio), and *cupping*, a Latin American practice of placing a hot cup over the back, abdomen, or chest, which results in a circular burn.

Human bites may be seen as punishment in infants and small children and may indicate sexual abuse in older children and adolescents. Bite marks have three components: the bite mark is an ovoid area with tooth imprints, the suck mark caused by pulling the skin into the mouth, and the thrust mark caused by the tongue pushing against the skin that is trapped behind the teeth. Bruises can be the surface sign of deeper injury. The bruise tends to be red to blue initially, turning to purple or black in 1–3 days, and green to brown over days 3–6. The change in coloration relates to the blood pigments under the skin and from 6–15 days it changes to tan then yellow and then fades. Although the days are specified, the younger the child the quicker the cycle and there is a wide variation so that declaration that a bruise that is green has to be 3–6 days may not be true.

When bruises occur in areas of the body that are unlikely to be injured accidentally, abuse should be considered. Multiple bruises, bruises of different ages, and bruises of the buttocks and genitals are usually not accidental. Bruises should be photographed and the pattern noted. If there is a pattern that matches a recognizable object, for example a handprint or a loop from a rope or belt, it is non-accidental.

■ FRACTURES

Fractures may be caused by accidental and non-accidental trauma. Many chronic conditions are associated with brittle bones which make fractures possible following minor trauma. This is true of premature babies and any condition that reduces mobility so that the bones become osteopenic. The presence of fractures at different phases of healing is very suspicious for abuse if there is no logical explanation for the findings. Multiple fractures at different sites are also suspicious for abuse.

Fractures of the medial one-third of the clavicle and of the acromial apophysis of the scapula are suspicious of abuse as they are rarely caused accidentally.

Fractures that involve the growth plates at the end of the bones are called metaphyseal–epiphyseal fractures and are virtually always the result of abuse. Fractures of the shaft, or diaphysis, are less specific for child abuse. Transverse fractures result from a direct blow or a bending force, whereas oblique fractures are caused by rotational force. A spiral fracture of the lower extremity of a child who is not walking is usually abuse. Rib fractures in children under 2 years of age tend to be non-accidental. They may result from squeezing or from a direct blow to the chest.

■ HEAD INJURY

Injuries to the head comprise the major cause of death from abuse especially in children less than 2 years of age. Following severe intracranial injury, brain damage and mental retardation are common in the survivors. Many of the deaths result from closed head injury due to shaken infant syndrome. Shaking results in a whiplash injury that leads to tearing of the bridging vessels and laceration of the brain. The force of the injury leads to subdural hematoma, interhemispheric subarachnoid hemorrhage, and cerebral contusions. The child is usually less than 2 years of age and presents with altered level of consciousness, varying from somnolent yet irritable, to coma. There may be opisthotonic posturing, convulsions, apnea, or hypoventilation. Direct blows to the head can produce similar injuries. The cardinal feature of the shaken infant syndrome is retinal hemorrhages.

■ BURNS

Non-accidental burn injuries may be obvious. Inflicted burns such as with a cigarette, hot plate, iron, curling iron, or even an open flame produce characteristic patterns. Although burns are commonly a manifestation of abuse, it may be difficult to differentiate accidental and non-accidental burns. Accidental burns may result from some of the same hot objects. Scald burns may be from immersion or from splashing. Certain burns are classically abuse, such as the glove or stocking burn resulting from holding the hands or feet in hot water. The line of demarcation is sharp which only occurs from being held in position. Toilet training conflicts may lead to immersion in a bathtub with burns of the feet and buttocks. The cheeks of the buttock that were in contact with the bathtub may be relatively spared. The temperature of the water is important and can be measured. If the water heater produces hot water at 120°F the immersion can be for 10 minutes before full thickness burn occurs whereas if the water temperature is 150°F immersion for 5 seconds would result in a full thickness burn.

Sexual Abuse

Sexual abuse is the most under-diagnosed form of child maltreatment. It is estimated that 10 percent of children are exposed to this before the age of 18. It was defined by Kempe as "involvement of dependent, developmentally immature children and adolescents in sexual activities that they do not fully comprehend, or are unable to give informed consent, and that violate the social taboos of family roles." In the vast majority of cases of sexual abuse, the child knows the perpetrator, who may be a relative or a family friend. Children with mental retardation are at particular risk for sexual abuse because they are particularly vulnerable. Although generalizations are dangerous, teachers and sports coaches who work closely with children are in a position that sexual abuse can occur. The implication is not that people who work with children are more likely to molest children but rather that the child molester may choose an occupation that involves close contact with children.

Sexual abuse appears to have increased in the last decade, although how much is a real increase and how much is increased reporting is unclear. It is probably more true to say that there is a vast amount of sexual abuse that is not reported but that produces emotional scars in the children. The definitions include *incest*, which is physical sexual activity between family members, including non-blood-related relatives such as a stepparent or non-related siblings. *Molestation* implies inappropriate contact of a sexual nature, which ranges from touching or fondling to single or mutual masturbation. *Exhibitionism* includes indecent exposure, which is usually a male exposing the genitalia to children or female adults. *Pedophilia* is the "love of children," and does not imply a specific sexual act but preference for childhood (especially pre-pubescent) involvement in sexual acts.

Other Abuses

Abdominal trauma is important because it is the second most common cause of death (after head trauma) from child abuse. There is usually a rational history if there has been accidental trauma to the abdomen and motor vehicle or bicycling accidents are the most common causes. Victims of non-accidental abdominal trauma often present to the emergency room with an adult (usually the mother) who did not cause the trauma. The mother may be unaware of the circumstances that led to the trauma which may have been caused by the (step)father or boyfriend. The external signs may be minor and careful diagnostic and imaging studies (CAT scan or ultrasound) should be performed to define the injury. The most common non-accidental injuries include laceration of the liver, perforation of the stomach or small bowel, with splenic and renal injuries less common.

Drowning accidents are more common than intentional events. Accidental drowning tends to involve toddlers and older children in pools, hot tubs, ditches, lakes and rivers. There may be lack of supervision of the small child. The depth of water may be just a few inches. It can be difficult to distinguish accidental from non-accidental immersions in the home. Accidental immersions tend to occur at the usual bath time; there is often another child in the bathtub and there is a lack of adult supervision. Non-accidental drowning tends to occur outside the usual bath time with no other child present and there is often a history of abusive caretakers. Victims of accidental drownings tend to be 9–15 months of age and non-accidental drownings tend to occur with children 15–30 months of age. There is often delay in summoning emergency help if the drowning is intentional.

Neglect

The National Center on Child Abuse and Neglect (NCCAAN) report data of the incidence of maltreatment of children: 4.9 per 1,000 suffer physical abuse; 2.1 per 1,000 sexual abuse; and 8.1 per 1,000 physical neglect. About 2,000 children die each year from abuse and neglect and the majority of these are under 4 years of age.

Child neglect is the most common form of maltreatment and amounts to a failure to provide for the basic needs of the child. Ignorance of the needs of the child or poor parenting skills, for example failure to feed an infant every 3–4 hours, is a common cause of neglect. Poverty is a major risk factor for child neglect. Physical neglect involves failure to provide food, clothing, shelter, supervision, and education for the child. It also involves failure to provide medical care. Emotional neglect implies a failure to provide love and understanding for the child and involves also the behavior that results from alcohol or substance abuse by the parent. Medical neglect results when there is failure to follow prescribed or recommended therapies or if there is over-dosing by giving medication too much or too often. The parent may neglect to provide medical treatment for chronic conditions, for example medications for asthma or diabetes. There may be failure to seek medical care in a timely fashion.

Fetal neglect or abuse occurs when a mother exposes the fetus to alcohol or illicit drugs (most commonly cocaine). The importance of recognizing the condition lies in the fact that substance-abusing mothers are more likely to abuse the child in the future.

Munchausen Syndrome by Proxy

Munchausen syndrome by proxy (MBP) constitutes a form of child abuse wherein the perpetrator, usually the mother, presents the child for medical care with a fabricated story. Sir Roy Meadow first published "Munchausen Syndrome by Proxy—The Hinterland of Child Abuse" in 1977 in the *Lancet*. The hallmarks of MBP include the *repeated* presentations of the child for medical care. The fabrication varies from completely made-up stories to production of physical harm. Fabrication implies reporting symptoms that did not occur, such as fever, seizures, diarrhea, and so on. The perpetrator may produce actual harm, for example repeatedly suffocating the child, and claiming that the child has apnea. The principal presentations for Munchausen syndrome by proxy have been summarized by Donna Rosenberg and are listed in Table 13-3.

The child often will undergo significant medical investigation and therapy that is, of course, unnecessary. The symptoms tend to disappear when the child is separated from the perpetrator, but it must be remembered that the symptoms may be induced while the child is in the hospital. Appropriate surveillance is indicated if

**TABLE 13-3. MUNCHAUSEN SYNDROME BY PROXY:
PRESENTATIONS**

Apnea
Bleeding
Diarrhea
Fever
Rash
Seizures
SIDS
Vomiting

MBP is suspected, and the potential perpetrator should not be left alone with the child. There are many degrees of MBP ranging from multiple presentations for medical care by a mother who is having difficulty coping and may exaggerate symptoms, to the prototypical MBP perpetrator. The prototypical perpetrator acts as the caring mother who induces symptoms in the child and appears to be the savior performing heroic acts to keep her child alive. A dramatic example is the mother who suffocates her child and then performs cardiopulmonary resuscitation to revive the child.

The psychodynamics of the perpetrators of MBP are not well understood. The perpetrators deny their wrong-doing even when confronted with incontrovertible evidence of their deeds (e.g., video surveillance) and respond poorly to therapy. The child usually recovers when separated from the perpetrator although there is a significant mortality (as high as 10 percent of reported cases) and morbidity if MBP is not recognized and the child protected.

Lead Poisoning

Lead is a heavy metal that is poisonous to humans. Exposure to lead is associated with lead levels of 10–19 μg/dL and lead poisoning is greater than 19 μg/dL. Several children in Brisbane, Australia, were reported by Gibson and Turner in 1890. The children had wristdrop, footdrop, abdominal pain, vomiting, and seizures. They were able to explain that the symptoms were the result of exposure to exterior paint which had significant amounts of lead. Tetraethyl lead was first added to gasoline in 1923 and it was excluded from gasoline starting in 1982. This resulted in a significant drop in ambient lead in the atmosphere so that the exposure to lead has decreased. The geometric mean lead level in the population in 1976 was 12.8 and in 1994 had fallen to 2.3. Severe lead poisoning (> 60 µg/dL) is nearly always associated with ingestion of deteriorating lead-based paint. The older the paint the higher the concentration of lead. Other sources of lead include dust from crumbling paint, water that travels in lead pipes, glazed pottery, and soil.

Lead is well-absorbed from mucosal surfaces especially the GI tract and lungs. Children absorb a higher percentage if they are iron deficient, and they absorb more than adults. Lead distributes in the body in blood, soft tissue (brain, kidney, and liver), and bone. Most of the lead absorbed is in bone with a half-life in bone of 20 years versus 40 days for blood and soft tissues.

Presentation may be with anemia, abdominal pain, seizures, wrist or foot drop. Severe lead poisoning is associated with encephalopathy and 30 percent have residual neurologic deficits. In states that screen for lead exposure, the child may be asymptomatic. X-rays may be helpful in a child who has acutely ingested lead-containing paint chips which may show up in the abdominal film. X-rays of the knees may show lead lines which are areas of increased calcification in the proximal tibia or fibula.

■ MANAGEMENT

Screening is recommended in areas where there is a significant problem with exposure to lead. The management strategy should include evaluation of the source of the ingested lead. Deleading, removal of lead from the living unit, should be professionally done. Iron deficiency anemia is treated aggressively because iron decreases lead absorption. Oral chelation therapy is initiated with dimercaptosuccinic acid (DMSA). It is approved by the FDA for BLL > 45 µg/dL and has few side effects. There may be a significant rebound after stopping treatment. D-Penicillamine which chelates copper, mercury, and lead is a better known drug but is not approved by the FDA. It is administered orally and increases the urinary excretion of lead by 30-fold. There is potential for some side effects, including skin rashes, thrombocytopenia, neutropenia, proteinuria, or hematuria. The side effects are usually mild in children but, rarely, serious side effects may occur.

14

Ethical and Legal Issues

Ethical and legal problems may arise for clinicians, patients, and their families when children have chronic illness or disability. Advances in medical care and technology have resulted in prolonged life and raised ethical and legal questions that may need to be addressed.

Ethics

It is difficult to be dogmatic in this area where the views that are held tend to be very divergent. How does one define "a life worth living?" Who should be responsible for decision-making in life-and-death situations of children? Historically, the parents have the right to make the decisions for their children until they are old enough to make their own decisions. The age that adolescents come of age has been defined as 17 or 18 years of age but clearly many children consider that they are capable of making the right decision before this.

Culture, religion, and personal views all play a part in the decision-making process. Ethical decisions tend to be made when there is a question about the right thing to do or the correct course to follow. It tends not to be black or white, but rather gray even though some people may have opinions that are definite and often unswaying.

There is a mechanism for individuals, families and providers to deal with ethical problems related to children. The principles are different than with adults. The aim is to do good while minimizing harm. There is a standard that could be described as "in the best interest" but it is difficult to apply this to a child with a chronic illness who has pain and suffering that cannot be measured. In general, life is precious and should be saved when possible. If survival is not possible then treatments that are burdensome should not necessarily be undertaken. If survival is unlikely the decision making is more difficult.

Experimental treatment protocols or innovative procedures that may or may not benefit the child are sometimes difficult to evaluate. Clearly, the cancer treatments that have allowed improved survival should not be withheld because they are "experimental."

The standard of informed consent remains important. There needs to be disclosure, understanding, and voluntary agreement that is then acknowledged in writing. The individual who provides consent is usually the parent or legal guardian who is expected to act in the best interest of the child.

Resources allocated to support the health, development, and education of children with chronic conditions indicate the willingness of society to address the needs of this group. Unfortunately, access to rehabilitation services and long-term care facilities is limited. It is also true that home nursing and medical equipment needs are often not available for the children who need these services. This problem appears to be worsening as the impact of managed care increases. As resources become scarce, it is difficult to balance the needs of individuals against the needs of society as a whole.

Ethical decisions are made in the context of the individual and in permitting their rights to be met. The child's needs are discussed with input from the family and the providers. It is important to recognize and respect the relationship of the child and the family. The provider ensures that the information about the medical situation is understood by the patient and the family.

Decisions tend to be made using the shared model, meaning that the patient, the family, and the providers all input their information and the decisions are agreed upon. The decisions are of necessity best suited to promote the health goals and quality of life for the child. Parents should not become health professionals nor should health professionals try to act as parents. Ideally, the health professionals recommend the treatment options that have the most potential for benefit and the parents and guardians should endorse those treatments that seem the most appropriate in the circumstances. Unfortunately, it is not always this simple. There is the presumption that the parents are in the best position to represent the interests of the child and that is their clear obligation. They also must protect their child from harm. The authority of the parent is not absolute. There may be occasions when it is in the best interest of the child to remove the parents from the position of authority if it is considered morally or legally that they are not acting in the best interest of the child. The clearest examples would be if there is a significant psychiatric history that prevents a rational decision or if there has been abuse or neglect that implies that they should not be considered the advocate of the child. Health care professionals are expected to abide by the community standard of best interest. In circumstances when there is a conflict between family and health care providers, it is sometimes necessary to involve the legal system. On occasions they will appoint a surrogate decision maker who is appointed by the court and is called *guardian ad litem*.

Adolescents increasingly are involved in their health care and should be permitted involvement in the decision making. The implications of minors making decisions is that they are able to; they can comprehend the information about the medical condition and its treatment; that they are able to reason the life decisions that they might make; and that they understand the alternatives as well as the consequences of the decisions. Many children as young as 11 or 12 have the potential to participate in the process. Emancipated minors are defined as children less than 18 who have achieved a degree of independence from their family and are self-supporting financially. In most states they do not require parental decisions for medical care and may also refuse medical treatment.

Joint decisions to withhold or withdraw treatments are difficult to make. Parents may seek any possible intervention that may prolong their child's life regardless of the impact on the child's quality of life. They may also withhold permission for treatments in the desire, perhaps mistakenly, that they are relieving their child's suffering by forgoing life-sustaining interventions. In many situations there may not be a "right" answer.

Children with chronic conditions and their families tend to have an ongoing relationship with clinicians and it is likely that there has been discussion over some of these issues. With some degree of forethought it is often possible to reduce the potential conflict of ethical issues by communication. Examples might include what course of events would be acceptable for a child with cancer who was facing hospitalization to induce remission. Discussion before the hospital stay that considers some of the alternatives that might occur will permit weighing the options in advance.

Because of the emotional nature of medical decisions in life-threatening situations, it is not surprising that conflicts may arise. Some families want to know everything and question everyone. If there is a difference of opinion this may contribute to a conflict that on occasion leads to distrust. Usually an explanation can be given on the opinions and why there are often different options that can be considered. Institutional ethics boards are available to help in decision making. They are interdisciplinary committees involving medical, legal and lay personnel with ethicists who are able to provide an opinion.

■ REFUSAL OF MEDICAL CARE

Parents may refuse consent for medical care. This may be because the treatment may have serious side effects or be potentially ineffective.

Baby Doe Regulations applied to decisions involving infants under 1 year of age who were disabled. The purpose was that disabled infants should be operated upon, for example, for correction of duodenal atresia in Down syndrome. Under the Baby Doe Regulations, treatment other than "appropriate nutrition, hydration or medication" is not indicated where intervention is prolonging death rather than improving life. Examples include the irreversibly comatose infant or irreversible cessation of function of multiple organ systems.

Legal Issues

Various types of legal action include criminal, administrative law, and civil actions. Criminal actions are brought by the state against the defendant accused of crimes as defined by the state. Examples include theft, fraud, or homicide. Administrative law actions involve state agencies empowered by the legislature to investigate complaints and to take specified action. Complaints may be filed by anyone and following an investigation a hearing may result. Clinicians may be responsible for following a code of conduct specified by a regulatory board. Civil actions are used to resolve disputes between individuals or parties. Civil suits may involve personal injury, workers compensation, divorce, and malpractice complaints with the purpose of compensation of money for injuries caused.

The elements of malpractice imply that there is:

- A professional relationship
- An act or omission that results in a violation of the standard of care
- An injury that results from the action

■ DOCUMENTATION ISSUES

Any documentation that involves record keeping is liable to be used in a civil action. For this reason it is important that documentation be legible, complete, accurate, and truthful. Clinicians have the responsibility for documenting all assessments, observations, and treatments. The documents have to be dated and signed. It is sensible to document all education of caregivers. This includes education about medications and use of equipment.

It is important to remember that documentation that is reviewed in the future should be meaningful and may need to be protective to the clinician. If it is known that non-compliance, or non-adherence, has occurred this should be noted. Incident reports should be filled out if an event occurs that may have consequences. Examples include a patient falling out of bed, or a staff member accidentally being stuck by a needle, or a wrong medication being administered to a patient. These should be routed through the proper administrative channels.

Advance Directives

The purpose of advance directives is to indicate one's wishes about medical treatment when one is competent to make a decision. The Patient's Self Determination Act, which is part of the Omnibus Budget Reconciliation Act (OBRA), became effective on December 1, 1991. In order to be eligible for Medicare and Medicaid funding, health care facilities must determine at the time of admission whether the patient has an advance directive. This must then become part of the medical record.

■ LIVING WILL

This is one type of advance directive and is a written directive of a patient's wishes regarding medical treatment in the event that the patient is in a terminal condition. The living will may specify what treatments might be refused if the patient's condition is terminal. This may include mechanical ventilation, CPR, or nutritional support. There is no reason why adolescents cannot indicate their wishes in this manner.

■ PROXY

Many states have provisions wherein an agent is designated to act as the decision-maker for a patient. The agent is permitted to make decisions regarding health care, when it is deemed that the patient is unable to do so, in order to carry out the patient's wishes. Children usually do not require a proxy as it is assumed that the parent or legal guardian can make the decisions for the child or adolescent.

■ DO NOT RESUSCITATE (DNR) ORDERS

These must be signed by the physician. The physician should document in the progress notes the discussion with the family. In certain circumstances specific orders should be written or documented. This might include "no intubation."

■ MEDICAL RECORDS

In the case of a child, medical records cannot be released to a third party without the written consent of the patient or parent (or guardian). It is important for clinicians to be aware that they may not divulge confidential medical information to parties that do not have a right to the information.

Health Care Reform

The health care reforms that have occurred in the United States in the 1990s arose because of rising medical costs and the desire to reduce medical cost inflation. In 1992 the total US medical expenditures exceeded $830 billion, and they are expected to exceed $1.5 trillion in the new millennium.

Although many employers provided health insurance for their employees by 1960, the poor, the unemployed, and the elderly were without insurance. The Medicare and Medicaid programs were enacted in 1965 with the result that the largest purchaser of health care services in the United States was the federal government. In the last 40 years inflation in medical care costs has risen much faster than inflation in other areas such as food and housing.

The proposals for health care reform were to allow as much access to medical care for the largest population, while at the same time controlling costs. It is implicit that the quality of care should be maintained or improved over time. It was hoped that there should be freedom of choice of health plans and physician selection. The first of the proposals from the Clinton Administration involved managed competition. From this evolved managed care as we know it, although the impact has varied in different parts of the country.

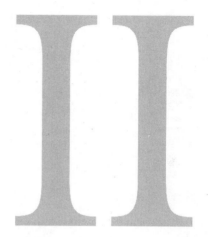

Part II

Description of Conditions

15

Chapter Fifteen

Genetic Disorders

Genetic disorders are seen when the chromosome abnormality results in a definable disorder with findings that are consistent. In many cases the result of the disorder leads to recognizable structural changes and the term *dysmorphology* is used. Congenital disorders are, by definition, present at birth. By convention, this implies genetic disorders as well as other problems including infections. Variability in genetic expression, which is known as *polymorphism*, accounts for the differences in body traits such as height, intelligence, and color of skin and hair.

Genetic Family Tree

Genetic counseling is important in the management of the conditions that will be discussed. The genetic family tree, or pedigree, is obtained with careful construction of a diagram that may span several generations. Start with the proband, then the siblings and parents, and extend as far as memory will go. It is important to inquire about miscarriages, stillbirths, and neonatal deaths, as well as deaths in infancy and childhood. Ask if there is any relationship by blood with any of the parents to try and establish consanguinity.

Causes of Genetic Disorders

Exposure of the fetus to drugs—non-prescription (including alcohol and nicotine), prescription, or illicit—and infections during the pregnancy can cause genetic disorders. Of necessity, in order to result in a genetic disorder, the exposure needs to occur early in pregnancy. Exposure to drugs or infection later in the pregnancy results in a congenital disorder. The group of disorders resulting from exposure without genetic changes is known as environmental disorders. Chromosomal abnormalities are the most important cause of miscarriage in the first trimester (3 months) of pregnancy. They account for 50 percent of early, spontaneous abortions, whereas they occur in only 0.6 percent of live births.

■ MENDELIAN INHERITANCE

Normally there are 46 chromosomes, 22 homologous pairs of autosomes, and 2 sex chromosomes that contain approximately 100,000 genes. Single gene disorders may be autosomal or X-linked. Autosomal dominant disorders are expressed in 50 percent of the offspring, but the impact varies because of different degrees of penetrance. Autosomal recessive disorders are transmitted when one abnormal gene is received in the offspring from each parent, who is called a carrier. If each parent carries the abnormal gene, the offspring may receive one of the two abnormal genes 50 percent (2 of 4) of the time, and they will be carriers of the abnormal gene. Characteristically, the carrier of the gene will have no observable effects but there may be an indirect benefit, best exemplified by protection from malaria by the carriage of the sickle cell gene. The offspring will be affected if they inherit two abnormal genes (one from each parent), which occurs in 25 percent (1 in 4) of cases. In 25 percent (also 1 in 4) of cases, no abnormal genes will be passed on. Examples of recessive disorders include cystic fibrosis, hemoglobinopathies, and most of the metabolic conditions.

X-linked disorders with recessive pattern involve carrier and non-carrier females who are normal, affected males who have symptoms of the disorder, and males who are not affected or carriers.

Down Syndrome

The original description by John Down in 1866 included the statement that a "large number of congenital idiots are typical Mongols" because of the characteristic facial appearance. It occurs in 1 in as many as 660 live births, which makes it the most common human pattern of malformation. Approximately 95 percent of all cases of Down syndrome result from an extra chromosome 21, which gives the name trisomy 21. The incidence increases with advanced maternal age, particularly over 35 years. In women 30 years of age, the incidence is 1 in 1,500 live births, whereas in women aged 40, it is about 1 in 100. Despite this, 80 percent of Down syndrome babies are born to women under 35 years of age. The chromosome abnormality is called *nondisjunction* and is not inherited. Nondisjunction occurs during the division of chromosomes and leads to the trisomy. Four to five percent of cases result from translocation of chromosomes 15 and 21 or 22. This is usually hereditary and not a result of advanced maternal age and may reoccur in future pregnancies. One to two percent demonstrate mosaicism in that some cells are normal and some are abnormal, with the physical and cognitive impairment related to the percentage of cells with abnormal chromosomes.

■ CLINICAL FEATURES

The most important features of Down syndrome are mental retardation, hypotonia, and heart disease. Death during infancy may result from complications of heart disease and pneumonia is common. Identification of Down syndrome depends on the

TABLE 15-1. MAJOR FEATURES OF DOWN SYNDROME

Head
Separated sagittal suture
Brachycephaly
Skull rounded and small
Flat occiput
Enlarged anterior fontanel
Sparse hair
Short and broad neck

Face
Flat profile
Small nose
Depressed nasal bridge
Oblique palpebral fissures
Inner epicanthal folds
Speckling of iris (Brushfield spots)

Mouth
High, arched, narrow palate
Protruding tongue; may be fissured at lip
Hypoplastic mandible
Downward curve (especially when crying)
Mouth kept open
Misaligned teeth
Delayed eruption
Periodontal disease

Ears
Small with narrow ear canal
Short pinna (vertically)
Overlapping upper helices

Chest
Short rib cage
Pectus excavatum/carinatum

Abdomen and Genitalia
Protruding
Muscles lax and flabby
   Diastasis recti
   Umbilical hernia
Small penis
Cryptorchidism
Bulbous vulva

(Continued)

TABLE 15-1. *(Continued)*

Hands and Feet
Broad and short hands
Broad and short feet
Stubby fingers
Incurved little finger (clinodactyly)
Transverse palmar (Simian) crease
Plantar crease between first and second toes
Wide space between first and second toes

Skin
Skin excess and lax
Dry, cracked, and frequent fissuring

Musculoskeletal
Hyperflexibility
Muscle weakness
Hypotonia
Atlantoaxial instability

---

presence of a number of the features rather than on a single abnormality (Table 15-1). The most identifiable features are hypotonia, inner epicanthal (eyelid) folds, slanted palpebral fissures, Simian crease (single crease across the palm), and flat face. Hypotonia is generalized and of the face results in a tendency to keep the mouth open and the tongue protruding. The joints become hyperflexible. The head has a flat occiput and there may be microcephaly. The nose tends to be small with a flat bridge. The ears tend to be small and 66 percent have hearing loss. The neck appears short. The hands have short metacarpals and there is hypoplasia of the middle phalanx of the fifth finger. There is a wide gap between first and second toes and there may be a crease extending between them. The skin is dry and hyperkeratotic and there are loose folds in the posterior neck. It is common, especially in adolescence, to have skin infections in the genital, buttock, and thigh areas. The hair tends to be soft, fine and sparse, and pubic hair is straight.

Many important congenital anomalies are associated with Down syndrome including cardiac disease, which occurs in 40 percent of cases. Endocardial cushion defect is present in 60 percent of those with cardiac disease and septal defects accounts for 28 percent. Gastrointestinal malformations are important with duodenal atresia, Hirschsprung's disease (congenital mega-colon), imperforate anus, annular pancreas, and pyloric stenosis being common. In males there are increased urogenital anomalies including micropenis, hypospadias, and cryptorchidism. Upper airway obstruction leading to sleep-disordered breathing is common. Asymptomatic atlantoaxial dislocation occurs in 12–20 percent of Down syndrome children, usually before 10 years of age, and rarely may result in spinal cord compression. Onset of bladder or bowel dysfunction or a change in walking ability may then occur.

Mental development slows with age so that while 23 percent under 3 years of age have an IQ more than 50, none have an IQ over 50 in the 3–9 year age group. Most young children with Down syndrome have an IQ 25–50, whereas the average IQ of the older patients is 24. Despite the low IQ, there are facets of Down syndrome that result in higher social performance. Babies tend to be "good" and children tend to be "happy." The children have musical tendencies and may be mischievous. About 13 percent have serious emotional problems.

Excessive weight gain, which begins after 2 years of age, may be problematic in some children. Orthopedic problems are second to cardiac problems as a cause of morbidity. Flaccid muscle tone and hyperextendable joints result in patellar subluxation, scoliosis, hip dislocation, and pes planus (flat foot). These may cause pain and difficulty walking and may require surgical intervention.

Life expectancy is reduced in Down syndrome and the major determinant is whether there is a heart defect. Premature aging also occurs, and adults are liable to develop Alzheimer's disease even in their 20s and 30s. Other complications include hypo-thyroidism, diabetes, and leukemias.

■ MANAGEMENT

The diagnosis of Down syndrome is usually made clinically in the nursery. It is recommended that chromosome analysis be performed in all cases. Genetic counseling is important with the overall recurrence rate of 1 percent. If the mother is less than 30 years of age, the probability of translocation is 6 percent, but a translocation carrier parent will only be identified in 1 case out of 3. The recurrence rate for translocation will depend on the type of translocation and the sex of the parent.

Surgical correction is available for many of the defects found in Down syndrome children. Ethical and moral dilemmas may arise, particularly if the defects are life-threatening. In addition, there are surgical procedures that may be considered to try and normalize the life of a child with Down syndrome, many of which are primarily being performed for cosmetic reasons. These include partial glossectomies, neck resections, chin and nose (silastic) implants, or ear reconstructions.

Early intervention has been shown to be beneficial in optimizing the rate of development by improving the cognitive, social, language, and motor skills. Various therapists combine to provide a program that is ideally home-based with the parents being taught the strategies. The goal is to integrate the child into the family as well as to prepare for longer term education, which may be in special or mainstream schools depending on the child and the resources available in the area.

Growth hormone has been used to increase height and muscle strength, but this is expensive and controversial. It has also been associated with increased incidence of leukemia.

■ FUTURE TREATMENTS

A number of different treatments have been suggested but so far benefit from megavitamins or other medications have not been proven. Prenatal diagnosis remains an important consideration and 3 serum markers are being used as an alternative to amniotic fluid alpha-fetoprotein in advanced maternal age screening. They are *alpha-fetoprotein, unconjugated oestriol,* and *human chorionic gonadotrophin.*

Achondroplasia and Other Bone Dysplasias

More than 100 bone dysplasias have been recognized. They are classified into 5 separate categories:

- *Osteochondrodysplasia* involves abnormal bone and/or cartilage development. This includes achondroplasia, hypochondroplasia, and osteogenesis imperfecta.
- *Dysostosis* is an abnormality of individual bones, both alone and in combination.
- *Osteolytic disorder* or resorption of bone.
- *Skeletal abnormality*, which is associated with chromosomal disorders.
- *Primary metabolic disorder* involves abnormalities of bone formation.

Achondroplasia

■ CLINICAL FEATURES

The characteristic defect of dwarfism with proximal extremity shortening is *achondroplasia*. The incidence is about 1 in 15,000. This leads to limbs that are more shortened than the trunk, but it is the large head and dysmorphic facies that are most recognizable. Inheritance is autosomal dominant with 90 percent representing a fresh gene mutation. Mutations in the gene encoding fibroblast growth factor receptor 3 located at 4p16.3 have been documented in all cases.

There is short stature with a mean adult height in males of 131 ± 5.6 cm and in females 124 ± 5.9 cm. The head is enlarged (megalocephaly) with a small foramen magnum. The forehead is prominent and there is a low nasal bridge. The fingers are of equal length and splayed and the term trident hand has been used to describe this. The vertebral bodies are small and lumbar lordosis and thoracolumbar kyphosis progress over time.

Macrocephaly may result from hydrocephalus because of the small foramen magnum. Ultrasound studies of the brain should be considered if the fontanelle size is large. Respiratory problems are common due to the small chest, and there may be upper airway obstruction and sleep-disordered breathing.

■ MANAGEMENT

Although early motor progress tends to be slow, exercises may be beneficial to reduce the spine deformity. A permanent gibbus or kyphosis may result from anterior wedging of the first two lumbar vertebrae. Complications related to spinal cord compression at the foramen magnum must be watched for although they are rare. Sudden death can occur particularly during the first year of life following cord compression.

Eventual intelligence is usually normal. Counseling may be helpful to allow integration, as opposed to isolation, into the mainstream.

■ SHORT-LIMBED DWARFISM

Short-limbed dwarfism is diagnosed with the assistance of the radiologist and the dysmorphologist. Arm span and upper-to-lower segment ratio measured from the symphysis pubis should be documented. The normal ratio for upper : lower segment is 1.7 at birth and 1.0 at about 8 years. In short-limbed dwarfism, these ratios will be increased and the arm span will be less than the height. These ratios are reversed in *short-trunk dwarfism*. Most bone dysplasias that cause dwarfism are evident at birth but sometimes the features are subtle.

Many defects are picked up by limb measurement on fetal ultrasound. Several of these conditions are lethal at, or shortly after, birth.

Arthrogryposis Multiplex Congenita

The typical form is Type I and is known as distal arthrogryposis syndrome. The most recognizable defect is a clenched hand with thumb adduction and medial overlapping of the fingers that is present at birth. There is usually a positional defect of the feet and 38 percent have hip abnormalities. Intelligence is normal. There is an autosomal dominant gene defect that has been defined but there is considerable variability. The limb deformities respond to physical therapy.

The atypical form (Type II) has (in addition to the limb deformity) cleft palate, ptosis, short stature, scoliosis, and lower intelligence. There is also a form with generalized joint contractures, hypertelorism (wide-spaced eyes), malformed ears, micrognathia (small mandible), and pulmonary hypoplasia. This is known as Pena–Shokier syndrome and has significant mortality especially in infancy.

Cleft Lip and Palate

Cleft lip results from failure of the maxillary and median nasal processes to fuse. Cleft palate is a midline fissure of the palate that results from failure of the two sides to fuse. Cleft lip may vary from a small notch to a complete cleft that extends to the base of the nose. Clefts may be unilateral or bilateral and may be associated with deformed dentition. Cleft palate alone is different etiologically from cleft lip (with and without cleft palate). It occurs in the midline and may involve the soft and hard palates.

Approximately 30 percent of patients with cleft lip and/or palate have a recognizable syndrome, about 30 percent have associated abnormalities, and 40 percent appear to have an isolated defect. The common associations include Pierre–Robin sequence and phenylhydantoin syndrome.

■ **MANAGEMENT**

The diagnostic evaluation includes obtaining a detailed history of the pregnancy, including the potential exposure to medications, drugs, or alcohol during the early pregnancy. Risk factors for clefts include fetal exposure to phenytoin and alcohol. A detailed family history is necessary to identify similar findings and provides a basis for genetic counseling. Examination is performed to define the extent of the cleft and other organ system involvement. Of particular importance are cardiac, skeletal, renal, and neurologic findings.

Work-up will require chromosome analysis and the indications for radiologic, clinical, and laboratory testing will depend on the findings on examination. Echocardiography, CAT scan or MRI, and skeletal X-rays are important to evaluate the presence of associated conditions.

Multidisciplinary team approach to management is essential. Case conferencing is important to develop a plan for the individual patient. The nature of the defect will dictate the surgical procedures that will be performed in stages. The initial lip procedure will usually be after 1 month of age and the palate at about 6 months of age. Before and after surgery, feeding problems have to be closely followed.

Fragile X Syndrome

About 25 percent of all mental retardation is X-linked with fragile X being the most common of the disorders. It is second only to Down syndrome as a genetic cause of mental retardation. It accounts for the increased male numbers with mental retardation. Fragile X is caused by an abnormal gene with a fragile site on the lower end of the long arm of the X chromosome (Xq27.3). It has been described in all ethnic groups and races with an incidence of 1 in 1,250 males. Females are affected at a rate of 1 in 2,500 and the carrier rate among females is 1 in 250. The pattern of inheritance is X-linked dominant with reduced penetrance, which means that some females exhibit the abnormality, unlike, for example, hemophilia where the carrier has no manifestations of disease.

Moderate to profound mental retardation is characteristic with IQs in the 30–55 range although mild to borderline range is possible. Hand flapping or biting (60 percent) and poor eye contact (90 percent) are associated and speech defects are common. Craniofacial anomalies can be identified in early childhood with macrocephaly, thickening of the nasal bridge, epicanthal folds, and large ears. The face appears long and thin. Prognathism (prominent jaw) may not be seen until puberty. Post-pubertal males have large testes. The most common phenotypic and behavioral features are listed in Table 15-2.

■ MANAGEMENT

There is no cure for fragile X syndrome. Medical treatment of behavior disorders including carbamazepine (Tegretol) or fluoxetine (Prozac) may be used to control temper outbursts and clonidine may reduce hyperactivity. Speech and language therapy and occupational therapy may reduce the decline of mental function. Genetic evaluation of relatives may be indicated. Life expectancy can be expected to be normal.

TABLE 15-2. CLINICAL FEATURES OF FRAGILE X SYNDROME

Physical features
Long, wide, and/or protruding ears
Long, thin face, with prominent jaw
Long palpebral fissures
Epicanthal folds
High, arched palate
Strabismus
Increased head circumference
Large testes (post-pubertal males)

Behavioral features
Mild to severe mental retardation
Speech defects
Short attention span
Hypersensitivity to taste, sounds, touch
Intolerance to change in routine
Autistic-like behaviors

Klinefelter Syndrome

The most common of all sex chromosome abnormalities is Klinefelter syndrome which affects 1 in 850 live births. The problem is the presence of additional X chromosomes resulting in 47,XXY, but there can also be 48,XXYY, 48,XXXY, etc. The degree of cognitive impairment is dependent on the number of excess sex chromosomes although the most common group have only one extra X. The disorder is not recognized until puberty when there is a failure of adolescent virilization. All patients have azospermia (no sperm in the semen), small testes, and reduced secondary sex characteristics. Gynecomastia is common and may be severe and leads to some of the behavior problems. There is a tendency toward gross motor skill difficulties, language delay, as well as behavior and learning problems.

■ MANAGEMENT

There may be some improvement with testosterone which will enhance the male pubertal changes. The gynecomastia may require surgical treatment. Counseling may be necessary for the problem of infertility.

Marfan Syndrome

This is an autosomal dominant connective tissue disorder with variability in expression. The variability means that it may be difficult to diagnose as features may be missing in individual cases. The incidence is 1–2 per 100,000 with new mutations occurring in 15–30 percent of cases. The genetic defect has been localized to 15q.

The major abnormalities that characterize Marfan syndrome include arachnodactyly (spider fingers), lens subluxation, and aortic dilatation. There is a tendency to tall stature, with long thin limbs without much subcutaneous fat. High arched palate is common. Other skeletal problems include kyphosis, scoliosis, or pectus excavatum. The lens tends to dislocate upwards, with myopia (shortsightedness) and retinal detachment also occurring.

The major morbidity is associated with necrosis of the media of the aorta that leads to aortic dilatation and incompetence. Eventually, dissection of the ascending aorta or more rarely the abdominal aorta or pulmonary artery may occur. Pulmonary abnormalities include spontaneous pneumothorax, emphysema, and an increased potential for pneumonia.

■ MANAGEMENT

Scoliosis is a major problem during the period of rapid growth and adolescence. Follow up for the early recognition of aortic dilatation is necessary. Some recommend starting beta-adrenergic blockers at the time of diagnosis as there is potential to reduce the aortic complications.

Noonan Syndrome

Noonan syndrome is also known as Turner-like syndrome. Originally reported as webbing of the neck, incomplete folding of the ears, and low posterior hairline in 1883, the features were expanded and the association with valvular pulmonic stenosis was made by Noonan and Ehmke in 1963. The features include short stature (50 percent), mental retardation (25 percent), with webbing of the neck and low posterior hairline. Facial features include epicanthal folds, low nasal bridge, low set ears, and retrognathia. There may be deformity of the chest wall including pectus excavatum, carinatum, or shield chest. The most common cardiac defect is valvular pulmonic stenosis due to a dysplastic or thickened valve. Other defects of the heart are less common including septal defects and pulmonary branch stenosis. Cryptorchidism and small penis are characteristic. Bleeding disorders occur in one-third of cases including intrinsic pathway deficiencies, Von Willebrand disease, and thrombocytopenia. Males with descended testes are fertile, as are females.

■ MANAGEMENT

This is usually a sporadic occurrence in a family and there is considerable genetic heterogeneity and the differential diagnosis includes Turner mosaicism, fetal alcohol syndrome, and fetal hydantoin. This makes it difficult to assess the recurrence risk. There is no increase in other illnesses. Management relates to the cardiac disease diagnosis and treatment.

Osteogenesis Imperfecta

Previous delineation of osteogenesis imperfecta (OI) on a clinical basis led to four types, all of which are associated with brittle bones and subsequent fractures. Type I has normal growth, blue sclera, and high-frequency hearing loss. Type II is a recessive disorder which is lethal in the newborn period with thickened bones, beaded ribs, and severe long bone deformities. Type III has progressively deforming long bones with extreme short stature and usually blue sclera. Type IV has normal sclera, some bone deformities, and variable short stature. With advances in genetics there are now more than 150 specific gene mutations associated with OI.

Type I has postnatal growth deficiency in half the cases. The hearing impairment results from otosclerosis and starts in early adulthood. Fractures are present at birth in 8 percent, 23 percent in the first year, 45 percent in preschool, and 17 percent during school years. After adolescence the incidence of fractures decreases. Scoliosis may progress during adolescence. The inheritance is autosomal dominant.

■ MANAGEMENT

Treatment of OI is supportive with exercise and physical therapy. There has been no benefit from drug therapy. Lifestyle changes are necessary because minor trauma may lead to fractures, but exercise is important to strengthen muscles and swimming is the most beneficial. Children with milder forms can participate in sports that are appropriate. Splints may be useful and surgery may be indicated to reduce deformities that interfere with standing or walking.

Prader–Willi and Angelman Syndrome

Prader–Willi is one of the microdeletion syndromes involving the segment 15q11–15q13. The deletion is in the same area as described for Angelman syndrome, but they are distinct from each other because the two conditions are so dissimilar. The phenomenon is known as genomic imprinting in that the genetic effect varies depending on whether the material passes from the father or the mother. The mother provides the deletion for the Angelman syndrome whereas it comes from the father in Prader–Willi.

Angelman syndrome is also known as the "happy puppet syndrome." First described by Angelman in 1965, the syndrome is a disorder with seizures, ataxia, inappropriate laughter, and developmental retardation. The retardation is severe with marked delay in motor and language milestones. The facies are characteristic with pale blue eyes, maxillary hypoplasia, large mouth with tongue protrusion, and wide-spaced teeth. The seizures start between 18 and 24 months of age. The ataxia and jerky arm movements led to the term "happy puppet." Most Angelman syndrome individuals are incapable of independent living.

Prader–Willi was first described 40 years ago, although it is possible that the "fat and red-faced boy in a state of somnolency" in Charles Dickins' *The Pickwick Papers* may have been the first description. The mother may note reduced fetal movement, and hypotonia may be severe in infancy. Mental deficiency in infancy appears more severe because of the hypotonia. Obesity starts to be problematic between 6 months and 6 years of age, and there is excessive caloric intake and binge eating with reduced activity. Mental retardation is mild in 63 percent, moderate in 31 percent, and severe in the remainder.

Mean adult height in males is 155 cm and females 147 cm. Hands and feet tend to be excessively small and there is small penis and cryptorchidism. There is hypogonadism because of hypogonadotropism.

■ MANAGEMENT

Life expectancy in Prader–Willi is reduced because of the complications of obesity. It is possible to control the calorie intake but it requires cooperation of the family. Very strict habits to limit the intake are necessary.

Turner Syndrome

The incidence of Turner syndrome is 1 : 2,500 newborn females. It is a disorder where there is one X chromosome and the sex chromosome from the father tends to be missing. The majority of pregnancies with 45X0 conceptions result in pregnancy loss due to fetal hydrops. This is somewhat surprising because the majority of survivors with X0 have a relatively mild phenotype. The lymphedema becomes less during infancy. At birth there is edema especially of the dorsum of the feet, and there is excess skin of the neck leading to the webbed appearance. The features of Turner syndrome include short stature, broad chest with wide-spaced nipples, ovarian dysgenesis, and delayed development.

■ MANAGEMENT

When puberty is anticipated, replacement therapy with estrogens should be instituted to induce maturation of the breasts, labia, vagina, uterus, and fallopian tubes. Although there may be improvement in linear growth during the first year of hormonal therapy, predicted stature will not be achieved. Growth hormone therapy has not been shown to be beneficial. Gonadal tumors are increased in the presence of mosaicism involving the Y chromosome, and it is recommended that streak gonads be removed in patients with evidence of virilization or a Y-containing line.

Williams Syndrome

Most cases appear to be sporadic but there have been parent-to-child transmissions. There is a deletion of one elastin allele which has been shown to be present in both sporadic and familial forms. The original description by Williams in 1961 included four unrelated children who had mental deficiency, abnormal facies, and supravalvular aortic stenosis. The average IQ has been 56 and ranges from 41–80. There is mild growth deficiency, neurologic deficits, and microcephaly. The voice tends to be hoarse and the children tend to be outgoing and friendly. The facial features include blue eyes, short palpebral fissures, anteverted nares, long filtrum, prominent lips with an open mouth.

The most common cardiac defect is supravalvular aortic stenosis, but peripheral branch pulmonic stenosis or pulmonic valve stenosis and septal defects may occur. Renal anomalies include renal artery stenosis and nephrocalcinosis as well as urethral and bladder problems.

■ MANAGEMENT

Sudden death has occurred and this is more likely associated with administration of general anesthesia. Various medical complications are associated with this syndrome as well as psychosocial problems.

16

Metabolic Disorders

Inborn errors of metabolism are genetic disorders, almost all being autosomal recessive, that interfere with function at the metabolic level. Most of the disorders, and there are more than 400 described, are enzyme defects that result in biochemical changes. The classification of the metabolic disorders keeps on updating as the knowledge base increases. Although they are very diverse, many share characteristics but the diagnostic dilemma arises because the proof often lies in complicated and expensive biochemical analysis. Table 16-1 provides a concise approach to classification of metabolic disorders.

The presentation of metabolic disorders is most commonly an acute or chronic encephalopathy. Many of them produce clinically recognizable features, such as Hurler's syndrome where the facies are recognizable, and many produce organ system dysfunction, especially liver and kidney, that suggest a metabolic disorder.

Encephalopathy may present in many ways. Acute encephalopathy, as a presentation, often occurs in the newborn period, but can occur at any time. It results from inborn errors of small diffusible particles that accumulate in toxic amounts in the brain because of the enzyme defect. After a period of time to accumulate the toxic substance, the symptoms develop. For example, a baby may be discharged from the nursery only to return with poor feeding, vomiting, seizures, and an acidosis, which is

TABLE 16-1. CLASSIFICATION OF METABOLIC DISORDERS

Diseases of small diffusible molecules
Amino acid disorders (e.g., maple syrup urine disease)
Organic acid disorders (e.g., methylmalonic aciduria)
Fatty acid oxidation defects (e.g., medium-chain acyl-CoA dehydrogenase [MCAD] deficiency)
Hyperammonemias (e.g., ornithine transcarbamylase deficiency)
Lactate and mitochondrial disorders (e.g., cytochrome oxidase deficiency)
Encephalopathy with seizures (e.g., non-ketotic hyperglycinemia)

Diseases of organelles
Mitochondrial disorders:
Electron transport chain defects (e.g., cytochrome c oxidase deficiency)
Defects of pyruvate metabolism (e.g., pyruvate dehydrogenase deficiency)
Lysosomal storage disorders:
Mucopolysaccharidoses (e.g., Hurler disease)
Gangliosidoses (e.g., GM2 gangliosidosis)
Sphingolipidoses (e.g., Gaucher disease)
Leukodystrophies (e.g., metachromatic leukodystrophy)

Liver disease
Defects of carbohydrate metabolism (e.g., galactosemia)
Defects of amino acid metabolism (e.g., tyrosinemia)
Defects of metal transport (e.g., Wilson disease)
Defects of protease inhibitors (e.g., α_1-antitrypsin deficiency)

Muscle disease
Skeletal: Acute rhabdomyolysis (e.g., muscle phosphorylase deficiency),
        Chronic myopathy (e.g., mitochondrial electron transport chain defects)
Cardiac: Lysosomal storage disorders (e.g., Pompe disease)

Renal disease
Lysosomal storage disorder (e.g., cystinosis)
Enzyme defect (e.g., oxalosis)
Defective transport (e.g., cystinuria)

Miscellaneous
Defects of gluconeogenesis (e.g., glucose-6-phosphatase deficiency)
Lysosomal storage disorders (e.g., Gaucher disease)
Enzymopathies (e.g., Lesch–Nyhan syndrome)
Teratogenic metabolites (e.g., maternal phenylketonuria)
Defects of lipoprotein metabolism (e.g., familial hypercholesterolemia)

the clue to the metabolic disorder. If the disorder is not recognized for what it is, and not treated, it may progress rapidly to death. The small molecule diseases may be caused by amino acids, organic acids, fatty acids, or hyperammonemia.

Inborn errors of metabolism may also present as chronic encephalopathic disorders, with a slowly progressive problem that is accompanied by deterioration in mental and neurologic function. They may be caused by a milder form of small molecule disease which may be a less severe enzymatic dysfunction than that producing the acute encephalopathy. Phenylketonuria and homocystinuria are examples of this. Diseases of organelles result in impaired mitochondrial function, which may cause acute or chronic disease, and lysosomal storage diseases and peroxismal disorders, which produce chronic disease. Metabolic disorders of hepatocellular function may also present in the newborn period and also lead to chronic conditions.

Neonatal Screening

Screening for metabolic and genetic disorders is recommended for early diagnosis in the hope that intervention can alter the natural history. Phenylketonuria (PKU) is screened in the newborn period in the United States and in more than 30 countries throughout the world. There is not any universal law that dictates who screens for which condition, and most programs are established by states and voluntary guidelines. Metabolic disorders are screened in the newborn period, and many states also screen for hypothyroidism and galactosemia.

Phenylketonuria

The liver enzyme *phenylalanine hydroxylase*, which converts phenylalanine to tyrosine, is absent in phenylketonuria (PKU). This results in accumulation of phenylalanine in the blood. One of the byproducts is phenylpyruvic acid, which produces the characteristic musty smell of the urine. The severe classic form is phenylketonuria, which results from excessive amounts of phenylketones in the urine. The excess phenylalanine and the reduced amount of neurotransmitters dopamine and tryptophan lead to the mental retardation. The mental retardation precedes the finding of metabolites in the urine and is progressive unless treatment is initiated. The lack of tyrosine means that melanin, epinephrine, and thyroxine are not able to be produced in adequate amounts.

The diagnosis is made by the Guthrie test which measures serum phenylalanine levels greater than 4 mg/dL compared to the normal less than 2 mg/dL. The Guthrie test is a bacterial inhibition assay that is performed on a spot of blood. It is usually done shortly after birth and after the newborn has ingested enough protein to get a build-up of phenylalanine. With early discharge from the nursery, it is possible for the test to be performed before there has been enough protein intake to achieve the abnormal levels. If a test is administered before adequate feeding is established or if the baby is less than 24 hours of age, then the test must be repeated within 2 weeks.

■ CLINICAL FEATURES

PKU is inherited as an autosomal recessive disorder with a prevalence of 1 in 10–15,000 Caucasian live births and a carrier rate of 1 in 50. It is very rare in African, Asian, and Jewish populations. The lack of melanin results in many of the phenotypic findings, which include blond hair, blue eyes, and fair skin that is susceptible to various skin disorders including eczema. The clinical effects of PKU are secondary to the neurotoxic metabolites, which result in severe intellectual impairment and seizures with behavior changes, especially aggression.

■ MANAGEMENT

Treatment is initiated as soon as possible and is based on reducing the intake of phenylalanine to safe levels. It cannot be eliminated because it is an essential amino acid and at the same time there has to be an adequate caloric intake to avoid growth retardation. The diet is calculated to provide 20–30 mg of phenylalanine per kilogram per day in order to achieve phenylalanine levels between 2 and 8 mg/dL. If the level is less than 2 mg/dL, growth retardation is likely and levels greater than 10 mg/dL tend to result in mental retardation.

During infancy, one of the special milk substitutes should be used. They include Lofenalac (Mead Johnson & Co.), Pro-Phree, or Phenex (Ross Laboratories). They contain treated casein hydrolysate which has 0.4 percent phenylalanine and are supplemented with amino acids, vitamins, and minerals. Breast feeding may be possible although phenylalanine levels need to be measured and milk substitute supplementation may be necessary if growth is not adequate. Introduction of solid foods should not be a problem.

The sweetener aspartame (tradename Equal, by NutraSweet) is converted to phenylalanine in the body and so must be avoided by the PKU patient. Diet soft drinks contain only small amounts of aspartame and can be included in the overall diet plan.

Patients with PKU who desire to get pregnant need to restrict intake prior to the pregnancy because exposure to phenylalanine levels greater than 20 mg/dL are associated with fetal damage. The risk of a PKU mother having a baby with PKU is 1 in 120.

Parents of children with PKU have to provide a safe upbringing, which involves education of relatives, friends, and the school that the child has specific dietary needs that have to be adhered to strictly. In addition, the parents as carriers of the gene have the potential to have future affected children. The families tend to have emotional problems because of the difficulty of controlling the diets of ambulatory children and the realization that even small amounts of regular foods may cause mental retardation.

■ PROGNOSIS

The goal of early diagnosis is to initiate early dietary treatment. Even with optimal care, it is not always possible to prevent neurologic impairment which may be evident as language delay or behavior disorder. The recommendation is to continue the dietary restrictions for life, although there are adult patients who seem to tolerate a fairly normal diet.

Cystinosis and Cystinuria

Cystinosis is a lysosomal storage disease caused by an abnormality in the transport protein that mediates cystine efflux from the lysosome. Accumulation of cystine in most tissues results, but the dominant effect is in the renal tubules resulting in renal parenchymal destruction that gradually leads to renal failure. The condition presents in the first year with failure to thrive, dehydration, and electrolyte problems. Eye problems result from deposition of cystine crystals in the cornea and retina. The diagnosis is confirmed by leukocyte cystine content.

Cystinuria occurs in 1/7,000 births and is caused by impaired renal transport of cystine, ornithine, arginine, and lysine. The problem results from the low solubility of cystine, which leads to renal stones. The stones tend to be multiple and result in infection and progressive renal failure.

■ MANAGEMENT

The electrolyte problems of cystinosis need to be corrected initially. Cystinosis is treated with cysteamine, which reduces the intracellular accumulation of cystine. If it is started early, it delays the onset of renal failure and improves growth. Cysteamine eyedrops can clear cystine crystals from the cornea. Renal failure can be treated by kidney transplant, but the effects of cystine deposition in other tissues may not be prevented. This may lead to hypothyroidism, diabetes mellitus, liver, or CNS disease.

Cystinuria is treated by alkalinization of the urine and increased fluid intake to reduce the solubility of the cystine.

Familial Hypercholesterolemia

Hyperlipidemia means excessive lipids (fats) and hypercholesterolemia is a specific term implying excess cholesterol in the blood. Their importance lies in the role they play in the development of atherosclerosis and subsequent cardiovascular disease.

Low-density lipoproteins (LDL) contain high concentrations of cholesterol and low triglyceride and moderate protein levels. LDL is the major carrier of cholesterol for cellular metabolism. Elevated LDL is a strong risk factor for heart disease. High-density lipoproteins (HDL) contain very low levels of triglycerides, small amounts of cholesterol, and high levels of protein. HDL transports free cholesterol to the liver. High levels of HDL are considered protective for heart disease.

Screening children for hypercholesterolemia is controversial and opinions vary from recommending universal testing to only checking selective high-risk populations. The importance relates to the potential for treatment. Familial hypercholesterolemia is an autosomal dominant disorder with a heterozygote frequency of 1/500, which means that it is one of the commonest mendelian defects. It is caused by mutations in the LDL receptor that take up LDL cholesterol from the extracellular fluid. The cholesterol and LDL levels are elevated.

Homozygotes may present with xanthomas (depositions of cholesterol) at birth and all patients have them by 4 years of age. The earliest documented heart attack occurred at 18 months of age, and most do not survive beyond 30 years of age. Xanthomas appear in the Achilles tendon, the extensor tendons of the hand, and the extensor surface of the elbows and knees. Around the eye they are called xanthelasma and in the edge of the cornea it is called arcus senilis, appearing as a white-gray line around the iris.

Heterozygotes also have xanthomas that tend to appear in the second decade and myocardial infarction may occur in their 30s and 40s. Heterozygotes may be confirmed by assay of LDL function in cultured skin fibroblasts. Treatment is by restricting dietary cholesterol, by enhancing bile acid excretion with cholestyramine, or by inhibiting cholesterol biosynthesis with specific medications such as lovastatin or provastatin.

Galactosemia

This rare autosomal recessive disorder occurs 1 in 50,000 live births. There is an absence of galactose-1-phosphate uridine transferase, which is one of the enzymes involved in the conversion of galactose to glucose. Infants may present with gram-negative sepsis before there is suspicion of a metabolic disorder and neonatal screening for the disorder is recommended. Lactose, the main carbohydrate in milk, contains glucose and galactose and normally the galactose is converted to glucose in the liver. Another enzyme deficiency, galactokinase, results in cataracts because galactose is converted to galactitol, a sugar to which the lens is impermeable. This also occurs in classical galactosemia, but the accumulation of galactose and galactose-1-phosphate results in cirrhosis of the liver and mental retardation in addition. In the kidney, there is renal tubular dysfunction that leads to inhibition of amino acid transport. Ovarian dysfunction occurs in 80 percent of females.

Symptoms of galactosemia present within days or weeks after birth. There is reluctance to feed followed by vomiting and failure to thrive. Jaundice, hepatomegaly, and other evidence of liver disease develop. The cataracts form over weeks or months. Mental retardation is evident usually in the second 6 months of life. The diagnosis is suspected if there are reducing substances in the urine, although their absence does not exclude the diagnosis.

Management is by excluding galactose and lactose from the diet. Despite this, the mental retardation may still develop and the ovarian dysfunction seems independent of treatment. The galactose-free diet should be continued, probably for life.

Gaucher Disease

This is the most common lysosomal storage disease and is a deficiency of glucocerebrosidase. The common form is non-neuronopathic and the clinical features are the result of accumulation of glucocerebrosides in the reticuloendothelial system. The clinical features are variable and include hepatosplenomegaly, pancytopenia, and degenerative bone changes usually with onset in adolescence or early adulthood. Often the initial complaint is abdominal swelling and the splenic enlargement tends to be more than the liver enlargement. Hypersplenism results in anemia and thrombocytopenia. Bone and joint pain and swelling may be early manifestations and pathological fractures may be found. This is sometimes called adult Gaucher's despite the onset in many cases in childhood. It is 30 times more common in Ashkenazi Jews with a reported incidence in this group of about 1/2,500 births.

There is an acute severe neuronal form that affects infants who have strabismus, trismus, and opisthotonos with seizures that leads to early death. The infant type is much rarer than the adult type, which does not have neurologic features. In both types there is the presence of foamy lipid-laden "Gaucher" cells, but the diagnosis should be confirmed by enzyme assay of leukocytes or fibroblasts.

Treatment is with a chemically modified form of glucocerebrosidase with varied results. Bone marrow transplantation has been used with success in the non-neuronopathic form.

Glycogen Storage Disease

The most common of the defects of gluconeogenesis is glucose-6-phosphatase deficiency, which is Von Gierke disease or Type I glycogen storage disease. The incidence is 1 in 100,000 to 400,000. When patients present in the newborn period, there is symptomatic hypoglycemia and pronounced hepatomegaly, but only mild ketosis. If the presentation is later in the first year, there is an enlarged liver, hypoglycemia, failure to thrive, and a doll-like face (full-cheeked, rounded face). The diagnosis is suspected on the basis of the hepatomegaly, which may be massive, and the increased lactate level, hyperlipidemia, and hypercholestero-lemia. The hypoglycemia results in increased mobilization of fat, and, when glucagon is given, the response is further elevation of lactate rather than hyperglycemia. Growth is usually normal at first and then falls off in the first few months. Mental development is normal unless damaged from hypoglycemia. The hypoglycemia tends to be severe, with levels of 15 mg/dL being common. Diagnosis is by enzyme assay of liver biopsy tissue.

The treatment is with frequent feedings and correction of hypoglycemia and acidosis. The diet should contain 60 percent glucose with avoidance of galactose and fructose as they do not improve the glucose levels. Raw cornstarch may be the most useful source of slow-release glucose and become the primary source of carbohydrate. With good metabolic control, the growth improves and the biochemical abnormalities can be minimized. Uric acid may be elevated and allopurinol may be indicated and hepatomas may occur in adulthood.

Krabbe Disease

This is Krabbe leukodystrophy, also known as global cell leuko-dystrophy (GLD). The leukodystrophies are genetic disorders with progressive degeneration of the white matter of the brain. The defect causes symptoms that start at 3–6 months of age with generalized irritability and crying, fever, stiffness of the limbs, seizures, and unexplained vomiting. Babies are asymptomatic at birth and when the symptoms appear there is progressive mental and motor development deterioration. When children are about 2 years of age, they may be decerebrate and blind and in a persistent vegetative state. Treatment is supportive.

Maple Syrup Urine Disease

This disorder is a defect of branched chain amino acids with keto-aciduria. The branched chain amino acids are leucine, isoleucine, and valine. The name derives from the characteristic smell of the urine. Infants are normal at birth and 3–5 days later develop symptoms of feeding difficulty, irregular respirations, and severe hypoglycemia. There is progression to seizures, opisthotonus (arching of the back), and generalized rigidity. Death occurs rapidly in a matter of 2–4 weeks. It is an autosomal recessive disorder and there is a milder variation with intermittent symptoms.

Increased amounts of the three amino acids are found in the urine and plasma. Treatment involves limitation of these in the diet. Despite treatment, brain damage is often present before therapy is started, although if the diagnosis is anticipated because of a previously affected sibling, it may be possible to achieve a normal IQ.

Mucopolysaccharidosis

▪ I. HURLER SYNDROME

Hurler described the syndrome in 1919, and it has also been called *gargoylism*. This autosomal recessive disorder results in accumulation of mucopolysaccharides and increased amounts of dermatan sulfate and heparan sulfate in the urine. The gene has been mapped to 4p16.3.

Hurler syndrome is associated with initial rapid growth followed after a few months by failure so that the achievable height is less than 110 cm. There is significant mental retardation so that the progression fails to advance beyond 2–5 years. There is scaphocephalic macrocephaly with frontal prominence, coarse facial features with thick lips, low nasal bridge, and hypertelorism (wide-spaced eyes). The tongue is large and teeth are small and misaligned. Corneas tend to be cloudy.

There are considerable skeletal deformities including claw hand, flared rib cage, and short neck and spinal deformities including kyphosis and thoracolumbar gibbus. During the first year, the changes in the face, the large head, limited hip mobility, and respiratory tract infections occur. Profuse nasal discharge results from the deformed pharynx, which tends to be blocked by lymphoid tissue. There may be upper airway obstruction with sleep disordered breathing. Death usually occurs in childhood with survival beyond 10 years of age being rare. There is only supportive treatment, which may include spinal surgery.

Scheie syndrome is essentially the same as Hurler syndrome with little or no impairment of intelligence. The onset is slower with onset after 5 years of age and the diagnosis being made between 10 and 20 years of age.

■ II. HUNTER SYNDROME

Hunter syndrome was first described in 1917. Hunter syndrome is a sex-linked recessive disorder characterized by coarse facies, clear corneas, dysostis, dementia, hepatosplenomegaly, and sensineural deafness. The enzyme defect is iduronate sulfatase and the accumulated substance is dermatan sulfate. The gene has been mapped to Xq27-q28 and there is a broad variability of expression because of different mutations in the same gene. There is a mild and a severe form based on the age of onset and severity of neurologic involvement and rate of deterioration.

The severe form may lead to death before 15 years of age. Growth decline starts at 1–4 years of age with an adult height that is 120–150 cm. The juvenile severe form has mental and neurologic dysfunction that starts between the ages of 2 and 5, and tends to progress to severe mental retardation. Cardiac and respiratory complications may be significant with valvular and ischemic heart disease and airway anomalies that lead to upper and middle airway (trachea) obstruction.

The mild type has been associated with maintenance of intelligence and survival to the fifth and sixth decade. Hearing loss and joints that are stiff are characteristic.

■ III. SANFILIPPO SYNDROME

This most commonly identified mucopolysaccharidosis disorder was first recognized in 1963. It is an autosomal recessive condition with Sanfilippo A being 'a defect of heparan N-sulfatase and Sanfilippo B, C, and D being other enzyme defects, all of which have excess heparan sulfate in the urine. All four types have an identical clinical phenotype. The onset is early in childhood with initially accelerated growth followed by slow growth. There is deterioration of mental functioning as well as gait, speech, and behavior. The facies are characteristic with coarse features, saddle nose, prominent eyebrows, and poor dentition.

Management

The early features of the disorder include frequent upper respiratory infections and sleep disturbance which precede the mental retardation. The mental retardation tends to be severe and the behavior problems difficult to control. Survival of 10–20 years is usual, with death from pneumonia.

■ IV. MORQUIO SYNDROME

Morquio described the condition in 1919, and it was recognized as a mucopolysaccharidosis in 1963. There are two forms (A is severe and B is mild) secondary to different enzyme defects. The disorder is autosomal recessive and the genetic defects and enzyme deficiencies of the two forms have been identified and heterozygotes can be identified. There is considerable heterogeneity probably secondary to different mutations.

   The onset is between 1 and 3 years of age with flaring of the lower rib cage, prominent sternum, and frequent upper respiratory infections. Growth limitation becomes severe with cessation during childhood so that the adult stature is 82–115 cm. There is mild coarseness of facial features, wide-spaced teeth, and at 5–10 years of age corneal cloudiness can be seen by slit lamp. There are considerable skeletal abnormalities, including vertebral anomalies, that may result in severe kyphosis and may lead to spinal cord compression and respiratory insufficiency. The long bones tend to be curved and irregular and knock knees and short stubby hands are common. There may be hearing loss. The severe form is associated with death before 20 years of age from spinal, respiratory, or cardiac problems. The mild form has longer survival. Mental retardation is not a feature of either form.

Niemann–Pick Disease

Niemann–Pick disease is a sphingomyelin lipidosis with a deficiency in most cases of sphingomyelinase. Type A is the "classical" form and begins shortly after birth with hepatosplenomegaly and failure to thrive with neurologic impairment. Retinal cherry red spot may occur and blindness from macular degeneration. Death tends to occur by 2 years of age. Type B tends to be milder without the neurologic degeneration so that long-term survival is possible. Type C is the most common with motor and intellectual handicaps appearing in late infancy. The visceral abnormalities are milder and survival to 3–6 years of age is usual.

The diagnostic feature is the examination of the bone marrow which shows foam cells. There is no treatment but splenectomy may be indicated if there is hypersplenism.

17

Chapter Seventeen

Endocrine Disorders

Endocrinology is the science of hormones, which are the substances that integrate and coordinate the metabolic functions of the body. The classic definition of endocrinology is that specialized glands secrete hormones into the circulation and effect a response at a distance from the origin. More recently, this definition has been extended to include the regulation of cell function by chemical messengers that are secreted by other cells. The adrenal and thyroid glands fit both descriptions but, for example, certain neurosecretions or cardiac secretory cells that control renal function fit the newer description. The endocrine system regulates the metabolic and homeostatic functions of the cell. It regulates growth and development and reproduction. It regulates fluid and electrolyte balance and the response to stress. The endocrine system is closely linked to the nervous system so that neurotransmitters such as norepinephrine circulate in blood as hormones. The hypothalamus helps to integrate the two systems. Disease results if there is an upset in the balance of function or feedback mechanism as well as a problem with end-organ responsiveness. The diseases tend to be a function of excess or of deficiency of the hormone. The causes of abnormal function are variable and include genetic abnormalities, infectious agents, immunologic disorders, and glandular damage by toxins.

Hormones exert their effect by interacting with specific receptors at target cells. They exert their influence in embryogenesis directing the process of differentiation of cells. There is a great diversity in hormonal response resulting in modulation of metabolism and growth throughout life. The functioning of the hormonal system is based on a negative feedback system.

The endocrine system comprises the pituitary gland, which consists of the anterior adenohypophysis and the posterior neurohypophysis. The anterior pituitary secretes somatotropic

TABLE 17-1. GLANDS, HORMONES, AND THEIR EFFECTS

Anterior pituitary	
Growth hormone (GH)	Promotes growth
Thyroid-stimulating hormone (TSH)	Stimulates thyroid secretion
Adrenocorticotropic hormone (ACTH)	Stimulates adrenal cortex to secrete glucocorticoids and androgens
Gonadotropins	
Follicle-stimulating hormone (FSH) ⎫	Stimulate gonads to produce sex hormones and germ
Luteinizing hormone (LH) ⎭	cells
Prolactin	Stimulates milk secretion
Melanocyte-stimulating hormone (MSH)	Increases skin pigmentation
Posterior pituitary	
Antidiuretic hormone (ADH)	Causes reabsorption of water by kidneys
Oxytocin	Causes uterus to contract
Thyroid gland	
Thyroid hormones	Controls metabolic rate and growth
Thyrocalcitonin	Regulates bone ossification
Parathyroid glands	
Parathyroid hormone (PTH)	Regulates calcium
Adrenal cortex	
Aldosterone	Regulates sodium
Sex hormones	Influences sexual organs and secondary sex characteristics
Glucocorticoids	Promotes host defense and suppresses inflammation
Adrenal medulla	
Catecholamines (epinephrine, norepinephrine)	Stimulates sympathetic response and increases blood pressure
Pancreas	
Insulin	Lowers blood glucose
Glucagon	Raises blood glucose
Somatostatin	Inhibits insulin and glucagon secretion
Ovaries	
Estrogen	Stimulates ova
	Controls female secondary sex characteristics
Progesterone	Prepares uterus for fertilization
Testes	
Testosterone	Stimulates spermatogenesis
	Controls male secondary sex characteristics

hormone (STH), growth hormone (GH), thyrotropin or thyroid-stimulating hormone (TSH), adrenocorticotropic hormone (ACTH), melanocyte-stimulating hormone (MSH), and the gonadotropins. The gonadotropins are follicle-stimulating hormone (FSH), luteinizing hormone (LH), and prolactin. The posterior pituitary secretes antidiuretic hormone (ADH) and oxytocin.

The thyroid gland secretes thyroxine (T4), triiodothyronine (T3), and thyrocalcitonin. The parathyroid secretes parathyroid hormone (PTH) also known as parathormone. The adrenal gland comprises the cortex, which secretes mineralocorticoids (aldosterone), sex hormones (androgens, estrogens, and progesterone), and glucocorticoids (cortisol and corticosterone). The adrenal medulla is the central part of the gland and secretes epinephrine and norepinephrine.

The islets of Langerhans of the pancreas secrete insulin (beta cells), glucagon (alpha cells), and somatostatin. It is the exocrine component of the pancreas that secretes pancreatic enzymes and bicarbonate. The ovaries secrete estrogen and progesterone and the testes secrete testosterone. The glands, hormones, and effects are shown in Table 17-1.

Most endocrine disorders are chronic and many present in childhood.

Adrenal Gland Defects

■ ADRENAL INSUFFICIENCY

Addison's Disease

Addison's disease is chronic adreno-cortical insufficiency, which is rare in children. It results from destruction of the adrenal cortex, the usual reason being tumor or tuberculosis, although in many cases no cause is found. It may result from hypopituitarism with ACTH deficiency. Presentation may be gradual and does not occur until 90 percent of the gland has become non-functional. The symptoms of chronic insufficiency include weakness and irritability. There are skin pigment changes with darkening of scars, creases, and at pressure points especially the elbows and knees. There may be weight loss and symptoms of hypoglycemia. The signs of chronic deficiency may be over-shadowed by the onset of acute adrenal insufficiency which may be precipitated by stress or infection. These same signs may occur if there is abrupt discontinuation of steroid therapy that has been chronic (even as short as a few weeks).

The symptoms of acute insufficiency are headache and abdominal pain, nausea and vomiting, and diarrhea. The signs are those of shock and include low blood pressure with weak pulse, shallow respirations, cold clammy skin, and altered level of consciousness.

Management

Adrenal insufficiency results in hyponatremia (low sodium), hypochloremia (low chloride), hyperkalemia (high potassium), and hypoglycemia (low sugar). Diagnosis is made by measuring functional cortisol reserve. Tests include cortisol measurement and ACTH stimulation. Treatment involves replacement of glucocorticoids (cortisol) and mineralocorticoids (aldosterone). Long-term management may often be achieved by oral steroids and supplemental salt. During periods of stress, the steroid dose must be increased 3–4 times the baseline therapy.

Congenital Adrenal Hyperplasia

The adrenal glands are situated adjacent to the upper pole to the kidneys. They function to synthesize the hormones cortisol, aldosterone, and androgens. Cortisone and aldosterone are involved with the regulation of glucose, salt, and water in the body, and androgens are involved with sexual development. They are produced in the outer cortex and epinephrine (adrenaline) is produced by the inner medulla.

Congenital adrenal hyperplasia (CAH) results from deficiency of one of the enzymes involved in the production of cortisol or aldosterone. Almost all cases of CAH are autosomal recessive disorders. The most common defect (90–95 percent) is 21-hydroxylase deficiency, which causes a reduction in cortisol production. The hypothalamus secretes corticotropin-releasing factor (CRF), which in turn causes the pituitary to release ACTH, which stimulates the adrenals to produce cortisol. If there is no cortisol, the feedback to the hypothalamic–pituitary–adrenal axis is not turned off so that ACTH is secreted, which stimulates the adrenals and causes a build-up of precursors and hypertrophy of the adrenals. The results of 21-hydroxylase deficiency include salt-losing CAH, in which both cortisol and aldosterone are blocked and there is excessive sodium loss by the kidneys. Presentation is often with non-specific signs, including failure to thrive, lethargy, vomiting, and dehydration. The clue to the diagnosis is the high serum potassium and low serum sodium usually with low glucose. The adrenal insufficiency may be associated with rapid deterioration and, if not recognized, death.

In the non-salt-losing form, the problem is virilization. The male may be difficult to diagnose because the penis may only be slightly larger with mildly increased genital pigmentation. Females will demonstrate physical findings at birth that vary from mild clitoral enlargement to ambiguous genitalia. The latter occurs with severe virilization such that they may be mistaken for males with no palpable gonads (testes) or with a micropenis and hypospadias (urethra at the base of the phallus). The commonest cause of ambiguous genitalia is CAH.

Children with non-salt-losing CAH may not be diagnosed because their only effect may be cortisol deficiency, resulting in an inability to handle minor illness or stress.

Management

The diagnosis is based on identification of the enzyme defect. Treatment of shock and hypoglycemia is most urgent. Cortisol can be replaced with hydrocortisone, and in salt-losing CAH, replacement of aldosterone with fludrocortisone acetate (Florinef) is necessary. The baseline dose of hydrocortisone needs to be increased at times of stress or illness. Parents need to be aware that if the dose of the medication is vomited more than once, then injectable hydrocortisone must be given. Salt supplementation is often indicated to replace excessive salt losses. Many females with CAH have severe enough virilization that surgical treatment of external genitalia is indicated, usually before 2 years of age.

Caretakers, including school personnel, need to be aware of the rapidity of onset of adrenal insufficiency and the need for rapid intervention. There is acceleration of bone growth by androgens so that a 5-year-old child may resemble an 8–10-year-old in size. Unfortunately, there may be early closure of the growth plates, which results in significant shortness of ultimate height. If CAH is appropriately controlled, there is potential for normal puberty and advice from the endocrinologist is beneficial in achieving control of CAH. Precocious puberty may be a problem for the school-age child. If untreated, males have potential for impaired testicular development or benign tumors and girls may not progress to breast development or menarche.

Cushing Syndrome

The clinical features result from excessive serum cortisol and conventionally the term is applied to all forms of glucocorticoid excess. Cushing syndrome is sometimes used to specifically mean cortisol oversecretion by adrenal tumor but it should not only imply this etiology. Iatrogenic Cushing syndrome is used to describe the symptoms resulting from the effects of high-dose long-term use of ACTH or glucocorticoids. Cushing disease may result from pituitary overproduction of ACTH, which usually results from a pituitary adenoma.

All forms of Cushing syndrome are very rare in children except the iatrogenic form. They are also rare in adults although those cases may well have their onset in adolescence. The importance of recognition of the clinical manifestations lies in the recognition of the signs of excessive use of steroid. Table 17-2

TABLE 17-2. FEATURES OF CUSHING SYNDROME

Growth:	Impaired linear growth
	Retardation of skeletal maturation
Habitus:	Fat pads on neck and back "buffalo hump"
	Muscular wasting
	Truncal obesity, thin legs (centripetal fat distribution)
Facies:	Rounded "moon" face, plethoric
Skin:	Thin skin, easily bruises
	Wide red striae on abdomen and thighs
	Acne
	Poor wound healing
	Hirsutism (excessive body hair)
Metabolic:	Insulin resistance, hyperglycemia
	Hypertension
	Osteoporosis
	Hypokalemia and alkalosis
	Hypercalciuria—renal calculi
Other:	Muscle weakness
	Fatigue
	Depression
	Increased susceptibility to infection
	Compression fractures of vertebrae
	Kyphosis
	Amenorrhea
	Impotence

lists the most important clinical findings associated with Cushing syndrome.

Diabetes Mellitus

The word *diabetes* comes from the Greek word for "siphon," which relates to the thirst and increased urination that come from the increased amount of sugar excreted by the kidneys, and *mellitus* is from the Latin word for "sweet," for the sweet urine.

Hyperglycemia (high blood sugar) results from a number of causes. Diabetes that is caused by a deficiency of insulin is described as type I or insulin-dependent diabetes (IDDM). If the cause is resistance to insulin, it is referred to as type II and formerly was called adult-onset (or maturity-onset) diabetes. Ninety-seven percent of children with diabetes have type I diabetes. The cause of diabetes is not completely understood and appears to be multifactorial. There is an autoimmune destruction of the beta cells of the pancreas that occurs over years. There is a genetic component in that there is a 5 percent chance of first-degree relatives of a patient with IDDM to develop diabetes. There is an increased risk conferred by genes in the class II region of the HLA locus. The onset of diabetes is often related in time to a traumatic, infectious, or stressful incident. The clinical symptoms tend to appear when 80–90 percent of the beta cells of the pancreas have been destroyed. Early in the evolution, positive serum antibodies directed against cellular antigens, including islet antigens and insulin itself, may be detected. Type II diabetes is non-insulin-dependent (NIDDM) and the onset tends to be after age 40. The problem involves resistance to insulin or defective secretion of insulin in response to glucose. Many patients will require daily insulin despite the name. Type II diabetes has a greater risk for genetic transmission and adolescent onset is associated with autosomal dominant inheritance. The term applied is maturity onset diabetes of youth (MODY).

Insulin is required for gluconeogenesis and glucogenolysis, glucose entry into tissues, and control of both fat and protein synthesis and lysis. Insulin deficiency results in hyperglycemia, depletion of liver glycogen stores, release of free fatty acids, and breakdown of muscle. Insulin deficiency results in glucagon excess, which leads to hepatic production of ketones, which leads to ketoacidosis. Dehydration ensues and is often associated with vomiting and an inability to keep up with the kidney losses.

The mean age of onset of type I diabetes is 11 years in girls and 12.5 years in boys. Below age 5, the diagnosis is more common in boys, whereas from 5–10 years of age the diagnosis is more commonly made in girls. The prevalence rate in children and adolescents is about 2 per 1,000 children below the age of 18 years.

■ CLINICAL FEATURES

Under usual circumstances when the serum glucose level is greater than 180 mg/dL, the filtered glucose load exceeds the capacity of the renal tubules to reabsorb the glucose. Polyuria results from the osmotic diuresis that occurs when glucose spills over into the urine. The renal tubular threshold is lowered in the presence of infection.

When the blood sugar is high, the osmolarity is increased and that results in the brain being confused into thinking that there is dehydration and so thirst results. The kidneys diurese because of the high sugar and then there is a vicious cycle of thirst and urination which is called polydipsia and polyuria. On occasions, this may be very severe, but it could be mild particularly if there is only spilling of sugar after a large meal. Because of the inability of glucose to enter the cell, protein is broken down and converted to glucose by the liver. Fat and protein stores become depleted as the body attempts to meet its energy needs. When insulin is absent, which results in inability to utilize glucose, fat is broken down into fatty acids and ketones result. Ketoacidosis is a feature of type I diabetes. On occasions, the child is found to have glucose in the urine on routine testing or during an acute illness. Blood sugar needs to be measured to ensure that the blood sugar is high and that it is not just renal glycosuria. Most children will have symptoms related to the high blood sugar and insulin deficiency. Polydipsia and polyuria may be accompanied by nocturia and enuresis may occur in a child who was previously toilet-trained. Weight loss occurs despite a good appetite and there is tiredness and lethargy. If the symptoms are not recognized there may be progression to ketoacidosis. This progression may take weeks or months or may be rapid, especially in small children. The symptoms of ketoacidosis include dehydration, nausea, vomiting, and altered mental state that may progress to coma. There is weight loss and weakness and difficulty in breathing. Kussmaul breathing, with deep and labored respirations, is classical, and acetone may be smelled on the breath.

The importance of early recognition of diabetic ketoacidosis is that there is potential mortality even with appropriate treatment. Persistent vomiting and lethargy in a small child must be recognized as possibly being caused by diabetic ketoacidosis.

■ MANAGEMENT

The diagnosis is suggested by a fasting blood sugar greater than 120 mg/dL, random sugar greater than 200 mg/dL, and glycosuria. Ketoacidosis is suggested by blood glucose more than 300 mg/dL with acidosis, glycosuria, and ketonuria.

Treatment of diabetic ketoacidosis (DKA) involves lowering the blood sugar and correction of acidosis and electrolyte abnormalities. The initial management includes evaluation of airway and circulation, which may be compromised to the extent that resuscitation and critical care are necessary. Patients may present with more than 20 percent dehydration which needs to be aggressively corrected. The initial fluid resuscitation includes normal saline 10–20 mL/kg. It may be difficult to assess the degree of dehydration clinically. The continued output of urine, because of the osmotic diuresis, is different from other causes of dehydration that result in oliguria. Insulin should be given and a continuous infusion of insulin may be started. The goal is to lower the glucose level by 50–100 mg/dL per hour. Electrolyte abnormalities must be corrected, especially hypokalemia, secondary to total body depletion of potassium.

It is important to be aware of the potential for cerebral edema which may be difficult to prevent. It is probably related to the flux of water into the brain related to changes in salt and glucose concentrations. The typical presentation is 6–12 hours after initiation of treatment with acute neurologic deterioration. Symptoms include headache, lethargy, seizures, incontinence, and pupil changes. There may be signs of raised intracranial pressure including decreasing heart rate with increasing blood pressure. Treatment involves the use of mannitol although it is not always effective in preventing neurologic devastation.

Long-term management of diabetes is a real challenge to the patient, the family, and the caregivers. The goals are to achieve normal growth and development, both physical and mental; to achieve normal glucose levels without producing hypo- or hyperglycemia; and to reduce the complications and morbidity associated with diabetes. This is achieved by monitoring blood glucose, by administering insulin, and by maintaining a good program of nutrition and exercise. There has to be considerable education and support from the health care team.

The insulin regimen varies with age and can usually be managed with two injections per day. Insulin is short acting (regular) or intermediate acting (NPH or lente). Duration of action is shown in Table 17-3. The dose of insulin should be documented and a correlation made between the diet, the glucose level, and the response to a particular dose of insulin. Current recommendations include checking blood glucose at least 4 times a day. Older children should be taught as much self-care as possible. Learning to give the insulin injections is often a source of stress for the family and child. Children usually master the techniques of testing and giving injections fairly quickly.

Children with diabetes should be seen regularly, every 3 months, to check height and weight, pubertal development, and blood pressure and to survey complications. Measurement of HbA1C (pronounced hemoglobin A-one-C, or glycosylated hemoglobin) provides a measure of the amount of heme protein to which glucose has been non-enzymatically linked and reflects the average blood sugar during the life span of the red cell. Levels over 10 percent indicate poor control with 8–10 percent indicating fair control.

TABLE 17-3. TYPES OF INSULIN

	Onset	Peak	Duration
Regular	0.5 h	2–4 h	6–16 h
NPH*	1–2 h	4–8 h	14–24 h
Ultralente	4–6 h	10–14 h	24–36 h

*NPH = neutral protamine Hagedorn.

Hyperglycemia may become worse with infection or stress, and if untreated, ketoacidosis may result. If an excess of insulin is given, there is danger of an acute and rapid fall in blood sugar. The symptoms of hypoglycemia need to be known by all who are close to the patient, including school personnel and babysitters, and a treatment plan needs to be in place. The symptoms include sweating, tachycardia, confusion and anxiety, which if not recognized may progress to loss of consciousness and seizures.

■ LONG-TERM COMPLICATIONS

As time goes on, the complications characteristic of diabetes tend to develop especially when the control has not been optimal. The manifestations that are most common include retinopathy, nephropathy, neuropathy, and cardiovascular disease. The rate of development varies but close surveillance should start 5 years after diagnosis. With good control, it may be possible to delay complications for 20 or more years. If control is poor, complications may be evident in as little as 2–3 years.

■ FUTURE

Transplantation or implantation of pancreatic tissue has been successful in controlling blood sugar. There are newer insulin preparations that are available with less variability in action. Lispro is an insulin analog that has an onset in 10 minutes with 2-hour duration and may be available for pediatric use.

Growth Disorders

■ SHORT STATURE

By definition, 3 percent of children are below the third percentile. However, not all 3 percent need endocrine work-up because in most cases the cause is genetic or from delayed physiologic maturation. Adequate nutrition is important for linear growth. Chronic illness may reduce appetite, which may limit growth, but some chronic illnesses are associated with growth retardation for unknown reasons. Glucocorticoids may initially stimulate growth and increase appetite but in the long term they are associated with growth velocity reduction and premature epiphyseal closure (which limits final height). Some causes of short stature are listed in Table 17-4.

Initial management should include a few months' observation to document the growth velocity. If there is delayed puberty, androgens may be indicated. The use of growth hormone (GH) remains controversial. GH provocation should be performed if no other cause for growth deficiency is evident. Two studies are indicated because the response is variable. Injections may be prescribed 2–3 times per week for growth-hormone-deficient children and the best results tend to be seen in the first year of treatment. GH is approved for use in the United States for growth hormone deficiency, for chronic renal failure, and for girls with Turner syndrome.

TABLE 17-4. CAUSES OF SHORT STATURE

Disproportionate short stature
Osteochondrodysplasia
Rickets

Proportionate short stature
Genetic short stature
Constitutional delay
Intrauterine growth retardation
Dysmorphic syndromes
Growth hormone deficiency or unresponsiveness
Hypothyroidism

Systemic diseases
Inflammatory bowel disease
Chronic liver disease
Cystic fibrosis
Severe asthma
Chronic heart failure
Cyanotic heart disease
Chronic renal failure
Renal tubular acidosis
Immunodeficiency
Metabolic disorders
CNS impairment

Parathyroid Dysfunction

The parathyroid glands secrete parathormone, which is involved in calcium homeostasis. Along with vitamin D, parathormone increases the amount of calcium and phosphate that is removed from bone, increases absorption of calcium and the excretion of phosphate by the kidneys, and increases calcium absorption from the gut.

Autoimmune hypoparathyroidism usually accompanies multiple gland failures and may be familial. Pseudohypoparathyroidism involves failure of end-organ responsiveness despite excess production of parathormone.

Calcium and phosphorus are essential for normal growth of bone and their concentrations are maintained by interaction between bone, intestine, and kidneys. The hormones involved are vitamin D, parathormone, and calcitonin. A decrease in serum calcium results in secretion of parathormone. Parathormone decreases renal calcium excretion and increases phosphorus excretion. Release of calcium from the bone is stimulated by 125-(OH)2D with parathormone.

Rickets results when there is insufficient calcium and phosphorus for mineralization of bone. The most common form of rickets is vitamin D deficiency, which results from inadequate intake often with the additional effect of lack of sunlight. It is much less common in countries which have fortification of milk and food with vitamin D. The effect of limited availability of calcium and phosphorus to the bones results in palpable enlargements at the growing ends of bones, especially the wrists and ankles. The costochondral junctions are classically involved producing the rickety rosary. Bowing of the tibia and femur result from weight bearing.

Pituitary Disorders

The pituitary gland is also called the hypophysis and is considered the master gland because of its role in regulating other glands. In fact, the pituitary is under the control of the hypothalamus and releasing factors from the latter result in the secretion of seven hormones by the anterior pituitary. These hormones control the secretion of the endocrine glands which regulate growth and sexual function of the body. Abnormalities of excess or deficient hormone secretion result in specific clinical conditions.

Deficient secretion of (GH) or somatotropin may result from developmental defects or destructive lesions, including tumor, trauma, vascular disease, or other metabolic disorder.

Jacob–Creutzfeldt disease is a rare complication of cadaver-derived human growth hormone that does not occur with synthetic human recombinant growth hormone. It is thought that the condition results from a slow-growing virus-like particle.

Hypersecretion of growth hormone results in giantism, the commonest cause being a pituitary tumor. If the hypersecretion occurs after the growing epiphyses have closed, then enlargement of the skull and face occurs in a lateral direction producing the condition known as acromegaly.

■ DIABETES INSIPIDUS (DI)

The principal antidiuretic hormone is arginine vasopressin (AVP). It is produced in the hypothalamus and the termination of neurons in the posterior pituitary is the site of AVP secretion. AVP regulates water balance by increasing permeability to water in the renal tubules by enhancing absorption. The secretion of AVP is regulated by changes in plasma osmolarity.

There are two main forms of diabetes insipidus: neurogenic and nephrogenic. Neurogenic DI is the principal disorder of the posterior pituitary and results from reduced secretion of anti-diuretic hormone (ADH). Nephrogenic DI is a rare X-linked genetic disorder that affects the renal tubules which are unresponsive to ADH. Acquired nephrogenic DI occurs with some primary renal diseases, hypokalemia and hypercalcemia, and sickle cell disease. The causes of neurogenic DI include primary idiopathic or familial or secondary. The secondary causes are from trauma, tumor, granuloma, infections, or vascular anomalies in the region of the posterior pituitary.

The effects of reduced ADH secretion are polyuria and polydipsia. The other important cause of polydipsia is urinary excretion of osmotic substances, especially glucose. The management of neurogenic DI is vasopressin replacement. This can be by nasal spray, or intramuscular or subcutaneous injection of aqueous vasopressin. The aqueous form is known as DDAVP which is 1-deamino-8D-arginine vasopressin. Nephrogenic diabetes insipidus is managed with hydrochlorothiazide, with or without the diuretic amiloride.

With significant free water loss, hypernatremia is a major hazard and water replacement should be achieved slowly. Rapid correction can result in cerebral edema and seizures. The potential for this complication can be reduced by replacing the free water deficit using the following formula:

$$0.6(\text{body weight in kilograms})(1 - 140/(\text{serum sodium}))$$

Correction of mild hypernatremia can be achieved with hypotonic intravenous or oral replacement but, if the serum sodium is above about 160 mEq/L, normal saline should be used initially to reduce the potential of cerebral edema.

Sexual Maturation Disorders

Puberty is the transition from childhood to adulthood with physical, physiologic, and mental changes that progress in response to hormonal change. The physical changes result from increase in gonadal sex steroid concentrations which are produced in response to the pituitary gonadotrophins, luteinizing hormone (LH), and follicle stimulating hormone (FSH).

■ AMBIGUOUS GENITALIA

Ambiguous genitalia includes masculinized female, which is female pseudohermaphroditism. The management includes assignment of the female sex. Surgical correction may be indicated. Male pseudohermaphroditism is incompletely masculinized male. The true hermaphrodite has both testes and ovary

■ DELAYED PUBERTY

In males, the definition of delayed puberty is a failure of testicular enlargement by 14 years of age. The female definition is lack of breast development by 13 years of age. Constitutional delay in growth is the most common cause of delayed puberty and is a normal variant. There tends to be a family history of delayed puberty and there may be delayed bone age but there is no endocrine abnormality. Hypogonadotropic hypogonadism is caused by various CNS disorders and hypergonadotrophic hypogonadism is caused by deficient gonadal function.

The approach to diagnosis is initiated by measuring basal gonadotrophins LH (luteinizing hormone) and FSH (follicle-stimulating hormone).

■ PRECOCIOUS PUBERTY

Precocious puberty is considered if there is advanced sexual maturation before the age of 9 years in boys or 8 years in girls. It may result from abnormalities of the gonad, the adrenal gland, or the hypothalamic–pituitary gonadal (HPG) axis. True (or complete) precocious puberty results when there is premature activation of the HPG axis with secretion of sex hormones and the development of secondary sexual characteristics. Precocious pseudopuberty (or incomplete) occurs when there is no over-production of gonadotropin. This usually results from overproduction of sex hormones, either by a tumor of the ovary or testis, hyperplasia or tumor of the adrenal gland, or exogenous sources of androgens or estrogens.

Management of precocious pseudopuberty is directed toward the cause. Management of true precocious puberty is with monthly injections of a synthetic analog of luteinizing hormone-releasing hormone which regulates pituitary secretions. The injections should be continued until it is age-appropriate for puberty to resume.

Thyroid Gland Dysfunction

The thyroid gland secretes the thyroid hormones, thyroxine (T4) and triiodothyronine (T3), as well as thyrocalcitonin. The thyroid hormones (TH) are regulated by thyroid-stimulating hormone (TSH) from the anterior pituitary. TH regulates the rate of metabolism and alterations of thyroid function alter growth and metabolism. Excess or deficiency results from a defect in the thyroid gland, abnormal TSH secretion, or thyroid-releasing factor, which originates in the hypothalamus. Thyrocalcitonin has effects that are opposite to parathormone so that it decreases calcium levels and promotes calcium deposition in bone.

■ HYPOTHYROIDISM

Hypothyroidism may be congenital or acquired and results from deficiency of TH. Congenital hypothyroidism occurs in 1 per 4,000 live births and is diagnosed by neonatal screening of blood spot T4. The importance of early diagnosis relates to the effect of neurologic function if there is a delay. The severe deficiency results in the condition previously called *cretinism* and, if treatment is delayed, permanent mental retardation results. There can be a mild deficiency of TH that does not produce significant hypothyroidism for months or years. If the deficiency is after 2–3 years of age, the effect on cerebral function is less because of brain maturation.

The symptoms of hypothyroidism vary depending upon the age. At birth there may be post-term (>42 weeks) delivery of a large baby (>4 kg, 8.8 lb), with a wide posterior fontanelle, hypothermia, lethargy, edema, vomiting, delayed passage of meconium, and feeding difficulties. In the first few months of life, the findings include umbilical hernia, large tongue, lethargy, constipation, and dry mottled skin. The older child shows growth failure with weight gain and the signs of myxedema. The features of myxedema include dry thickened skin, wide puffy eyes, broad short upturned nose with large protruding tongue. The hair is dry, soft and brittle, and the dentition is delayed.

The treatment is lifetime replacement of thyroid hormone. Thyroid hormone levels should be checked at intervals and growth and bone age followed carefully.

■ LYMPHOCYTIC THYROIDITIS

Goiter means enlargement of the thyroid gland. Congenital enlargement is usually the result of iodides or antithyroid drugs given to the mother during pregnancy. Acquired goiter may result from iodine deficiency or increased secretion of TSH, from tumor, or from inflammatory processes. It is common during adolescence when it is usually caused by lymphocytic thyroiditis.

Lymphocytic thyroiditis (Hashimoto's thyroiditis) is the most common cause of hypothyroidism in children and adolescents and was probably the cause of "adolescent goiter." The condition is also known as juvenile autoimmune thyroiditis and is often discovered because of the enlarged thyroid rather than complaint of symptoms of abnormal thyroid function. Thyroid enlargement tends to be soft and symmetrical. If the gland is nodular or hard, it is important to exclude a tumor. Initially, the thyroid function tests may be normal, but with time the T4 tends to decrease and the TSH to increase. It is not unusual for the function to return to normal in a few years, even without treatment. When the diagnosis is made, it is usual to treat with thyroid hormone and the swelling quickly resolves. Surgery is not indicated.

■ HYPERTHYROIDISM

Hyperthyroidism (Graves disease) is caused by increased secretion of a thyroid-stimulating immunoglobulin for unknown reason. It is 5 times more common in females than males. It may occur at birth from transmission of the immunoglobulin from the mother causing a temporary hyperthyroidism, but the peak incidence is between 12 and 14 years of age. The diagnosis is made by elevated serum T3 and T4 with depressed TSH levels. The symptoms include weight loss despite voracious appetite, restlessness and irritability, and heat intolerance. Physical signs include exophthalmos, goiter, tremor, and tachycardia.

Thyrotoxicosis used to be the medical name for Graves disease, but now the term is used for a sudden secretion of thyroid hormone resulting in a thyroid "crisis," or "storm." This is more commonly seen in adults but it can be precipitated in adolescents by surgery or infection or if antithyroid medications are stopped. This can be a life-threatening episode of severe irritability with palpitations and heart failure. Treatment is with beta-adrenergic antagonists (e.g., propranolol) in addition to antithyroid drugs.

The treatment for hyperthyroidism includes drugs that interfere with thyroid synthesis or surgery to remove part of the thyroid gland. The condition can also be treated with radioactive iodine (except in potentially child-bearing patients). The commonly prescribed drugs include propylthiouracil and methimazole.

18
Chapter Eighteen

Allergy and Immunology Disorders

The function of our immune system is to distinguish self from nonself and to protect us from external factors, such as infections and toxins, and internal factors including tumors and autoimmunity. If the immune system is not working properly, a wide spectrum of clinical disease, both mild and severe, may result. This includes mild atopic disease, crippling rheumatoid arthritis, severe immunodeficiency, and cancer.

In mammals, the primary lymphoid organs are the thymus and bone marrow and the secondary lymphoid organs are the lymph nodes (and gut-associated lymphoid tissue) and the spleen. The thymus produces T lymphocytes and is the site of T lymphocyte differentiation as well as the regulation of immune function by secretion of hormones that are essential for T cell-mediated immunity. The bone marrow is the origin of all cells of the immune system and is the site of production of B lymphocytes which are the antibody-producing cells.

Lymph nodes are interconnected organs of the immune system that attempt to localize and prevent the spread of infection. Lymph nodes have an inner medulla which is the primary T cell area and B cells are primarily in the outer cortex. The spleen filters and processes antigens from the blood. Gut-associated lymphoid tissue includes the tonsils and Peyer's patches in the small intestine.

Lymphocytes are responsible for the initial specific recognition of an antigen. About 10–15 percent of lymphocytes are B lymphocytes and 70–80 percent are T lymphocytes, the remainder being called null cells. Phenotypic identification of B and T lymphocytes is achieved using monoclonal antibodies which react with individual cell surface molecules or antigens. B lymphocytes are coated with surface membrane-bound immunoglobulin and they produce antibody. T cells are involved with cell-mediated immune response such as delayed (type IV) hypersensitivity, graft rejection, and immune surveillance of neoplastic cells. T cells are subdivided into CD4, which are helper cells, and CD8, which are suppressor (cytotoxic) cells. Null cells include natural killer (NK) cells which have the capability of destroying cells without the involvement of antibody.

The bone marrow produces the blood cells which include erythrocytes (red cells), phagocytes (white cells), and megakaryocytes (platelet precursor). The phagocytes are polymorphonuclear leukocytes (polys or polymorphs), eosinophils and basophils, and monocyte-macrophages. The immature polymorphs are known as "bands" and the mature form as "segs" (segmented polymorphs). Eosinophils play a central role in allergy, in the inflammatory response of asthma, and in host defense against parasites. Macrophages are derived from monocytes and have important roles in immune defense. They are involved in chemotaxis (cell movement), phagocytosis (antigen engulfment), and processing and presentation of antigen so that it can be recognized by the T lymphocyte.

Basophils and mast cells release the mediators of immediate hypersensitivity which affect the inflammatory response. These include histamine, leukotrienes, prostaglandins, and other substances that are involved in the immune response.

An allergen possesses the ability to stimulate an antibody response (immunogenicity) as well as the ability to react to preformed antibody (reactivity). Allergy is an immunopathologic process wherein specific IgE (reaginic) antibodies mediate a hyperactive immune response against an antigen (type I immediate hypersensitivity). In pediatric practice, the common allergic conditions include allergic rhinitis, atopic dermatitis (eczema), and asthma.

Antibodies are immunoglobulins that combine with antigens to initiate the humoral response. Circulating immunoglobulins have unique specificity for one particular antigenic structure. There are five types of immunoglobulin: IgG, IgA, IgM, IgD, and IgE. IgG is primarily involved in the secondary or recall immune response. Four subclasses (IgG1–4) have separate functions in the immune process. IgG crosses the placenta and so plays an important role in protecting the newborn from infection during the first few months. IgM is the major part of the early antibody response, particularly in response to non-protein bacterial antigens. IgA is the primary immunoglobulin of mucosal surfaces and exocrine gland secretion. IgD is not well understood. IgE is normally present in very low quantities and is elevated principally in allergic disorders. Deficiency of the immunoglobulins (excluding IgE) results in altered response to infection.

Cell-mediated immunity consists of different phenomena than antibody-mediated immunity. T lymphocytes do not recognize antigens directly but do so after the antigen is processed and presented on the surface of an antigen-presenting cell with a cell surface glycoprotein that is coded for by the major histocompatability complex (MHC) gene. CD4 (T-helper) cells play an

TABLE 18-1. CLASSIFICATION OF IMMUNODEFICIENCY DISORDERS

Immunoglobulin deficiency (IgG) (B-lymphocyte abnormality)
    Hypogammaglobulinemia
        (a) Congenital
        (b) Acquired
        (c) Common variable hypogammaglobulinemia
Selective immunoglobulin immunodeficiency (B-lymphocyte abnormality)
    IgG subclass deficiency
    IgA deficiency
    IgM deficiency
Cell-mediated immunodeficiency (T-lymphocyte abnormality)
    DiGeorge syndrome
    Common variable cell-mediated immunodeficiency
Antibody and cell-mediated immunodeficiency (B- and T-lymphocyte abnormality)
    Severe combined immunodeficiency
    Ataxia-telangiectasia
    Wiskott–Aldrich syndrome

TABLE 18-2. COMMON OPPORTUNISTIC INFECTIONS

Bacterial
  Pneumococcus
  Staphylococcus aureus (both coagulase positive and negative)
  Pseudomonas aeruginosa
  Mycobacterium avium intracellulare

Viral
  Varicella
  Herpes simplex
  Epstein–Barr
  Hepatitis A, B, and C
  Cytomegalovirus
  Cryptococcus
  Respiratory syncytial virus

Fungal
  Aspergillus species
  Candida albicans and non-*albicans*
  Mucor
  Cryptococcus neoformans

Protozoa
  Pneumocystis carinii
  Toxoplasma gondii

important role in helping B cells to produce antibody by generating stimulating cytokines, such as interleukin-2 (IL-2). The CD4-positive cells are stimulated by interacting with antigen in the context of MHC class II molecules on antigen presenting cells. Cytotoxic T cells play an essential role in fighting infection that involves targeting and killing cells infected with viruses. This recognition process involves CD8+ cells interacting with viral antigen in MHC class I. Classification of immunodeficiency disorders is shown in Table 18-1 and opportunistic infections, which are more common in immunodeficiency states, are listed in Table 18-2.

Asthma

The cause of asthma remains unclear and genetic and environmental factors are considered to be important. The definition has been extensively debated but the common threads are consistent. It is a condition associated with reactive airways and reversible airway obstruction that is associated with inflammation. The three components of this definition are agreed to by most, but this does not make the diagnosis specific because there are other conditions that fit the criteria.

Wheezing can be defined as the sounds generated by air passing through airways that are narrowed. The cardinal feature of asthma is that the obstruction tends to be more prominent on expiration. In addition, the airway obstruction is dynamic and not fixed but it is related to both bronchoconstriction and airway inflammation. The feature that makes asthma different from other conditions that cause wheezing is the response to stimuli. There are many different triggers for the asthmatic reaction (Table 18-3).

The early phase response occurs within a few minutes of exposure to the stimulus. An antigen binds to IgE which leads to mast cell degranulation with release of mediators that result in bronchoconstriction as well as initiating the inflammatory response. The early response can spontaneously resolve within 60–90 minutes and will respond to $beta_2$ (adrenergic) bronchodilators. The late phase response starts 3–6 hours later and tends to last until 8–12 hours after exposure. This is presumed to be the inflammatory phase which is less responsive to bronchodilators and needs anti-inflammatory treatment to reverse. Most commonly there will be a dual response with combined early and late reactions. The severity of the response will dictate the treatment that is needed.

TABLE 18-3. TRIGGERS FOR THE ASTHMATIC RESPONSE

Exercise
Viral infection
Animals with fur
Domestic dust mites (in mattresses, pillows, upholstered furniture, carpets)
Smoke (tobacco, wood)
Pollen and other inhaled allergens
Changes in temperature, especially cold air
Strong emotional expression (laughing or crying hard)
Aerosol chemicals
Foods

■ CLINICAL FEATURES

The incidence of asthma is not known, partly because the criteria for diagnosis are not strict, and it is a clinical impression that leads most physicians to apply the label "asthma." A history of wheezing at some time during childhood can be obtained in 30–60 percent of children under 17 years of age. Recurrent or persistent wheezing occurs in about 20 percent of children and most studies that report a prevalence rate for the diagnosis of asthma in children fall in the range of 2–15 percent. The rates for asthma are increasing and it is thought that this is a real increase in number, in addition to the heightened awareness of making the diagnosis and collecting data. There clearly has been a rise in morbidity and mortality of childhood asthma in the last 20 years. The sex difference shows that until puberty it is more common in boys than girls (2 : 1.5). It is also more common in certain geographic areas (e.g., the southern and western United States), in urban areas, and in the African-American population. Asthma is the most common pediatric chronic respiratory disorder. It is a major cause of school absenteeism. It costs at least $2 billion per year to diagnose, to treat, and to prevent asthma in children.

Many young children wheeze in association with upper respiratory infections (URIs). The first time they wheeze commonly follows infection with respiratory syncytial virus (RSV) and, in the future, wheezing accompanies URIs. Children with asthma have symptoms of coughing, wheezing, and shortness of breath during an acute episode that is brought on by the triggers that have been mentioned. The severity of the disease relates to the degree of hyper-responsiveness of the airways.

Various techniques to diagnose reactive airway disease have been validated in the research laboratory and the clinically useful tests include exercise and inhalation challenges. The simplest exercise test is to run fast enough to get the heart rate to about 70 percent of the maximum for 6 minutes and measure the peak flow or FEV1 (forced expired volume in 1 second) at the end of the exercise. If there is a 15 percent (some use 20 percent) fall in pulmonary function, the test implies exercise-induced bronchoconstriction which is supportive of the diagnosis of asthma. Free-range running or the treadmill are reliable triggers for the asthmatic response, the bicycle is less consistent, and swimming usually does not result in bronchoconstriction. The standard inhalation test is the methacholine challenge when increasing doses of methacholine are inhaled, and the asthmatic patient will respond by wheezing or fall in pulmonary function with relatively small doses of the drug. A further indication of reversibility is the rise in PEF or FEV1 that follows inhalation of a beta$_2$-agonist.

The physical signs of asthma include acute as well as chronic findings. Listening to the chest during the acute episode will reveal high-pitched wheezes that tend to be bilateral and on inspiration as well as expiration. Expiration will be prolonged and the degree of distress will be related to the amount of airway obstruction either from bronchoconstriction or airway inflammation. If there is significant air trapping, the chest may assume a barrel shape. A better indication of the severity of wheezing is to assess the air movement by concentrating on the breath sounds. If there is reasonable air entry, there is less of a problem than if it is severely diminished or even absent. Very quiet (or even absent) breath sounds may indicate life-threatening airway obstruction.

The differential diagnosis for asthma is extensive and the adage applies "all that wheezes is not asthma." Asthma is very common, but there are many other causes of wheezing that may need to be diagnosed or treated differently (Table 18-4). The young child who presents with wheezing and cough with URIs may have bronchiolitis and this can be recurrent. Chronic air trapping in young children results in hyperinflation with a deformity of the chest that is called pigeon chest or pectus carinatum. Clubbing of the fingers does not occur in uncomplicated asthma and suggests another diagnosis, for example cystic fibrosis.

The history of persistent or recurrent coughing or wheezing in a child who has a family history of allergy or asthma is suspicious for asthma. The wheezing responds to bronchodilator therapy. It is usual for symptoms to be worse at night and to wake the child.

TABLE 18-4. CAUSES OF WHEEZING IN CHILDREN

Aspiration (GE reflux, foreign body)
Asthma
Congenital
   Laryngo-tracheo-broncho-malacia
   Vascular ring
   Tracheoesophageal fistula
   Bronchogenic cyst
Bronchopulmonary dysplasia
Ciliary dyskinesia
Cystic fibrosis
Gastroesophageal reflux
Heart failure
Hypersensitivity pneumonitis
Immunodeficiency
Tuberculosis
Viral infection
   Laryngotracheobronchitis (croup)
   Bronchiolitis

■ MANAGEMENT

The goals of therapy are to prevent the symptoms of asthma that interfere with daily living and to restore normal lung function. Table 18-5 indicates classification of severity. The National Asthma Education and Prevention Program (1997) presents guidelines for management of asthma in adults and children and is an excellent resource for the practitioner. A written plan for the family is most useful and the approach is individualized for each patient.

Management of asthma includes treatment of the asthma attack as well as measures to reduce the number and severity of attacks. The objectives are to reduce the symptoms to the level that results in the ability to lead as normal a life as possible in spite of asthma.

The diagnostic work up includes identification of the triggers that make the symptoms worse or bring on an attack of asthma. The first approach to management then becomes avoidance of the triggers as much as is reasonable (Table 18-6). This does not mean isolation from society, but there are many sensible steps that can be taken. It makes sense to avoid tobacco smoke and to

TABLE 18-5. CLASSIFICATION OF SEVERITY: CLINICAL FEATURES BEFORE TREATMENT

	Symptoms	Nighttime symptoms	PEF
Step 4: Severe persistent	Continuous Limited physical activity	Frequent	≤60% predicted Variability >30%
Step 3: Moderate persistent	Daily Use β_2-agonist daily. Attacks affect activity	>1 time a week	>60% to <80% predicted Variability >30%
Step 2: Mild persistent	≥1 time a week but <1 time a day	>2 times a month	≥80% predicted Variability 20–30%
Step 1: Intermittent	<1 time a week Asymptomatic and normal PEF between attacks	≤2 times a month	≥80% predicted Variability <20%

avoid exercising outside when air pollution is heavy. If there is sensitivity to foods containing sulfites, they should be avoided. Annual influenza vaccine is recommended for children with persistent asthma (unless there is egg protein allergy).

TABLE 18-6. ENVIRONMENTAL CONTROL AND ALLERGEN AVOIDANCE

Dust mite allergens
Wash bed linens and blankets once a week in hot water and dry in a hot dryer or the sun. Encase pillows and mattresses in air-tight covers. Remove carpets, especially in sleeping rooms. Use vinyl, leather, or plain wooden furniture instead of fabric-upholstered furniture. Do not have stuffed animal toys.

Tobacco smoke (whether the patient smokes or breathes in the smoke from others)
Stay away from tobacco smoke. Patients and parents should not smoke.

Allergens from animals with fur
Remove animals from the home, or at least from the sleeping area.

Cockroach allergen
Clean the home thoroughly and often. Use pesticide spray—but make sure the patient is not at home when spraying occurs.

Outdoor pollens and mold
Close windows and doors and remain indoors when pollen and mold counts are highest.

Indoor mold
Reduce dampness in the home; clean any damp areas frequently.

Reduction of exposure to inhalant allergens can go a long way to reducing symptoms. Perennial indoor allergens should be identified by skin testing or by RAST (radio-allergo-sorbent test). The advantage of skin tests is reduced cost and immediate results. The RAST is a blood test to measure specific IgE so that it quantifies the presence of a specific allergen. The advantages of the RAST are that it can be used for children with widespread eczema and there is no risk of systemic reaction.

The peak flow meter provides a useful objective measure of the degree of airway obstruction and helps in the evaluation of treatment. When children are seen in the clinic or doctor's office, they should bring a diary of symptoms, of medication taken, and of the peak flows. The peak flow is not used to diagnose asthma but rather to help in treatment, particularly in the child who does not have an awareness of the severity of obstruction until it becomes severe. The timing will vary so that most will recommend a peak flow measurement before the morning medications and, if it is below 80 percent of the desired, additional readings would be taken. If there are symptoms at other times, the PF can be repeated and also after treatment to evaluate improvement. Usually, the best of three readings is recorded.

It is important to be aware that hyperventilation can be a trigger for an asthmatic attack and multiple peak flows, one after another, may actually result in more airway obstruction. No more than three tries should be done at any time. Repeatedly blowing in the hopes of achieving a better PF may lead to bronchoconstriction that will be associated with falling numbers.

A stepwise approach to medications is based on the classification of severity of asthma (Table 18-7). It is usual to initiate therapy at a higher level and reduce therapy gradually when symptoms reach minimum control. Medications are either quick-relief or long-term control. Quick-relief medications include $beta_2$-adrenergics, anticholinergics, and systemic steroids. Long-term control medications include corticosteroids (especially inhaled), mast cell inhibitors, long-acting $beta_2$-adrenergics, methylxanthines, and leukotriene modifiers.

Intermittent asthma is treated with intermittent $beta_2$-adrenergics when needed. If they are needed more than twice a week, the next step should be taken. Mild persistent is treated with inhaled corticosteroids or a mast cell inhibitor for long-term control and $beta_2$-adrenergics for treatment of symptoms. Moderate persistent asthma is treated with more aggressive anti-inflammatory medications and with more regular quick-relief medications. Severe persistent asthma is treated with the similar

TABLE 18-7(a). STEPS FOR TREATMENT: INFANTS AND YOUNG CHILDREN (5 YEARS AND YOUNGER)

	Long-term preventive	Quick-relief
Step 4: Severe persistent	Daily medication: **Inhaled corticosteroid** —MDI with spacer and face mask >1 mg daily or —nebulized budesonide >1 mg bid —If needed, add oral steroids, lowest possible dose on an alternate-day, early morning schedule	Inhaled short-acting bronchodilator: **inhaled** β_2**-agonist** or ipratropium bromide, or β_2-agonist tablets or syrup as needed for symptoms, not to exceed 3–4 times in one day.
Step 3: Moderate persistent	Daily medication: **Inhaled corticosteroid** —MDI with spacer and face mask 400–800 mcg daily or —nebulized budesonide ≤1 mg bid	Inhaled short-acting bronchodilator: **inhaled** β_2**-agonist** or ipratropium bromide, or β_2-agonist tablets or syrup as needed for symptoms, not to exceed 3–4 times in one day.
Step 2: Mild persistent	Daily medication: Either **inhaled corticosteroid** (200–400 mcg) or cromoglycate (use MDI with a spacer and face mask or use a nebulizer)	Inhaled short-acting bronchodilator: **inhaled** β_2**-agonist** or ipratropium bromide, or β_2-agonist tablets or syrup as needed for symptoms, not to exceed 3-4 times in one day.
Step 1: Intermittent	None needed.	Inhaled short-acting bronchodilator: **inhaled** β_2**-agonist** or ipratropium bromide, as needed for symptoms, but not more than three times a week. Intensity of treatment will depend on severity of attack.

Preferred treatments are in bold. Patient education is essential at every step.

TABLE 18-7(b). STEPS FOR TREATMENT: ADULTS AND CHILDREN OVER 5 YEARS OLD

	Long-term preventive	Quick-relief
Step 4: Severe persistent	Daily medications: **Inhaled corticosteroid**, 800–2,000 mcg or more, and long-acting bronchodilator: either **long-acting inhaled β_2-agonist** and/or sustained-release theophylline, and/or long-acting β_2-agonist tablets or syrup, and corticosteroid tablets or syrup long term.	Short-acting bronchodilator: **inhaled β_2-agonist** as needed for symptoms.
Step 3: Moderate persistent	Daily medications: **Inhaled corticosteroid**, ≥ 500 mcg AND, if needed, long-acting bronchodilator: either **long-acting inhaled β_2-agonist**, sustained-release theophylline, or long-acting β_2-agonist tablets or syrup. (Long-acting inhaled β_2-agonist may provide more effective symptom control when added to low-medium dose steroid compared to increasing the steroid dose). Consider adding anti-leukotriene, especially for aspirin-sensitive patients and for preventing exercise-induced bronchospasm.	Short-acting bronchodilator: **inhaled β_2-agonist** as needed for symptoms, not to exceed 3–4 times in one day.
Step 2: Mild persistent	Daily medication: Either **inhaled corticosteroid**, 200–500 mcg, or cromoglycate or nedocromil or sustained release theophylline. Anti-leukotrienes may be considered, but their position in therapy has not been fully established.	Short-acting bronchodilator: **inhaled β_2-agonist** as needed for symptoms, not to exceed 3–4 times in one day.
Step 1: Intermittent	None needed.	Short-acting bronchodilator: **inhaled β_2-agonist** as needed for symptoms, but less than once a week. Intensity of treatment will depend on severity of attack. Inhaled β_2-agonist or cromoglycate before exercise or exposure to allergen.

approach as moderate asthma, with combinations of medications that include potentially all the groups and may require systemic corticosteroids intermittently.

The route of treatment for asthma medications also increases the options that are available. Under 2 years of age, small-volume nebulizer (SVN) is probably the most effective. The alternative that can be tried is the MDI with spacer and face mask which requires a careful technique to achieve good results. The 5-year-old should be able to achieve good results with the MDI and spacer and the nebulizer becomes the alternative. There are many new devices that are coming into the marketplace with promises of improved deposition of drug in the lower airway. These include breath-activated MDIs which have potential of 35 percent of the dose reaching the lower airways, compared to 10–15 percent, which is the more usual deposition from nebulizer or MDI.

The complications of asthma include status asthmaticus which can be defined as asthma that is not responding to treatment. There can be bacterial and viral infections that may produce bronchitis, bronchiolitis, or pneumonia. Because the secretions are thick, obstruction of airways may lead to segmental consolidation (atelectasis). This may result in chest X-ray findings that are similar to those of pneumonia. The differentiation between pneumonia and atelectasis is clinical rather than radiological. Pneumothorax, which is air in the pleural cavity, or pneumomediastinum, which is air in the mediastinum, are more common during an acute episode of wheezing. They present with chest pain, usually with worsening respiratory difficulty. If the pneumothorax is enlarging or associated with increased distress, it may be necessary to insert a chest tube until the airleak resolves.

The natural history of asthma is variable and not predictable. It cannot be cured, but it can be controlled. The symptoms can improve, worsen, or stay the same over time. Children with mild asthma tend to have a reduction in symptoms during adolescence. It is difficult to predict the course of an individual child and it is better not to make prognostic statements about "growing out of asthma," because many children have persisting symptoms to adulthood.

The number of children who die from asthma is increasing and the reason for the increase is not known. Various factors and behaviors have been identified in population studies. The dominant themes are delay in seeking treatment and this may be from failure to realize that the child is severely distressed as well as the fact that the deterioration can be extremely rapid. The high mortality rate may be related to poor compliance in following the prescribed treatment, which has many facets including denial, depression, lack of education (about asthma), overuse of rescue medications, as well as a reluctance to seek medical care.

Eczema

Eczema means "to boil over" and applies to the changes in the skin rather than to a specific disorder. The pattern refers to spongiosis which is intracellular edema as well as pruritis, erythematous papules, and vesiculation. The term eczema tends to be used by people to describe what is medically known as atopic dermatitis (AD). AD is one variant of pruritic eczema that is associated with allergies.

AD is the cutaneous component of immediate hyper-sensitivity, although the role of IgE in this disorder is unclear. Elevation of IgE is usual but the level does not parallel the skin involvement. There are often coexisting allergic respiratory symptoms, either allergic rhinitis or asthma or both. It occurs in all age groups but especially in children. It affects 30 percent of the pediatric population and accounts for one-third of pediatric dermatologist visits.

■ CLINICAL FEATURES

Infantile eczema starts between 2 and 6 months of age and usually resolves spontaneously by 3 years of age. Childhood eczema may follow infantile eczema and tends to start by 5 years of age. Adolescent eczema begins about 12 years of age and lasts for a few years or indefinitely. There is a strong family association and if one parent is atopic there is a 60 percent chance that the child will be affected; if both parents are atopic there is an 80 percent chance.

The infantile form tends to be generalized with involvement of the cheeks, scalp, trunk, and the extensor surface of the arms and legs. The childhood form involves principally the flexures including neck, antecubital, wrist, popliteal, and ankles. The adolescent form affects the face, neck, hands and feet, and elbows and knees.

The most consistent symptom is itching, which is due to excessive amounts of histamine. The itching produces excoriation and secondary infection is common in severe forms. There is excessive dryness of the skin. Active lesions may be generalized (over a large area) or localized (limited to small patches). The appearance starts with erythema, followed by edema (spongiosis), excoriations, weeping, bleeding, and secondary infection. Chronic changes lead to lichenification (thickening), with fissuring, scaling, and hyperpigmentation.

Associated findings include "allergic shiners," which are dark rings around the eyes, and "atopic pleats" of the lower eyelids (Dennie-Morgan lines). There may be increased linear markings of the palms and keratosis pilaris (follicular plugs) which produce thickened skin of the extensor surface of the upper arms and knees and on the cheeks (often mistaken for acne).

■ MANAGEMENT

This is a chronic disorder with no cure but it tends to improve with time and eventually resolves. Management is directed at relieving itching, at reducing inflammation in the skin, and at preventing and treating infection. The itching relates in part to dry skin and there are different approaches to management that appear contradictory. The wet method involves frequent (up to 4 times daily) bathing with application of lubricants to trap moisture in the skin. Hypoallergenic or very mild soap or none at all are used and the emollients are applied while the skin is still wet. Various emollients containing, for example, petrolatum or lanolin can be tried. Oils added to the bathwater and oilated oatmeal baths may be soothing especially at bedtime. The dry method involves cleaning the skin with a non-lipid, hydrophilic agent such as Cetaphil.

Moderate or severe pruritis may benefit from a mild antihistamine such as hydroxyzine (Atarax) or diphenhydramine (Benadryl). Occasionally, flare-ups may require topical corticosteroids to reduce the inflammation. Judicious use of topical steroids is appropriate. Awareness of the different potency of the many preparations that are available is necessary. Percutaneous absorption of steroids can occur in high enough amounts to produce systemic side effects if a large area is treated for a long period of time with steroids. Bacterial infection, particularly with *Staphylococcus aureus*, must be watched for and treated with oral antibiotics.

Severe Combined Immunodeficiency Disease

There is absence of both humoral and cell-mediated immunity in severe combined immunodeficiency disease (SCID). The defect in X-linked SCID has been identified as a mutation in the gene for the IL-2 receptor gamma chain. Approximately half of the patients with the autosomal recessive form of SCID have a deficiency of the enzyme *adenosine deaminase* (ADA) which results in metabolites that are toxic to the lymphocyte. This form is also known as Swiss-type lymphopenic aggamaglobulinemia.

■ CLINICAL FEATURES

Infants with SCID present with severe infections by 3–6 months of age. The infections tend to be serious, recurrent, and with unusual organisms. Frequently, the first indication is infection with an opportunistic organism such as *Pneumocystis carinii* or cytomegalovirus. The diagnosis is made on the basis of the history of recurrent infections and the presence of lymphopenia. For the first few months of life, there may be immunoglobulins present from the mother. The infections tend to be difficult to eradicate and there are frequent re-infections with the same or different organisms. Chronic respiratory infections are common and failure to thrive is frequently associated with SCID.

■ MANAGEMENT

Treatment is identification and therapy for the infection. The definitive treatment is a histocompatible bone-marrow transplant from a sibling. Ninety percent survival may result if performed early and before there has been severe infection. Alternatively, if there is not a sibling donor a haploidentical, for example a parent, bone-marrow transplant is performed after depleting the bone marrow of mature T cells. Infants with enzyme deficiencies may receive replacement therapy and gene therapy may be an option for ADA deficiency.

Infants with SCID should not receive live-virus vaccines and all patients must receive irradiated blood products to prevent fatal graft-versus-host disease.

Ataxia-Telangiectasia (AT)

This is an autosomal recessive disorder with cerebellar ataxia, oculocutaneous telangiectasia, recurrent sinus and pulmonary infections with variable immunodeficiency. The immunodeficiency involves both humoral and cell-mediated immunity. The defect has recently been discovered in a gene on chromosome 11q22-23 which encodes a phosphatidylinositol-3-kinase protein that seems to be involved in DNA repair.

Patients with AT present as early as infancy and up to 6 years of age with progressive cerebellar ataxia and telangiectasia. The immune deficiency is a later event and there is considerable variation. Diabetes mellitus may develop. There is an increased risk of various neoplasms especially lymphomas. Gonadal dysgenesis occurs frequently. The confirmatory laboratory study is elevation of serum alpha-fetoprotein.

■ MANAGEMENT

There is no treatment for the neurologic or skin manifestations. The infections should be aggressively treated and prophylactic trimethoprim-sulfamethoxazole is beneficial. Appropriate surveillance for malignancy is necessary. Many patients survive to adulthood.

Chediak–Higashi Syndrome

This is a rare autosomal recessive disorder with recurrent infections with pyogenic organisms, especially staphylococcus and streptococcus, as well as gram-negative bacteria and fungi. There are giant cytoplasmic granules in the granulocytes (white cells) with abnormal phagocyte chemotaxis, meaning that white cells do not get mobilized to fight infection. The diagnosis is made by identification of these granules.

In addition, there is partial albinism with dilution of skin and hair color. There is a high incidence of lymphoma.

■ MANAGEMENT

The treatment is supportive and anti-infective agents are used to treat acute infections. There have been successful reports of improvement with bone marrow transplant.

Chronic Granulomatous Disease

Chronic granulomatous disease (CGD) represents a group of patients with disorders of neutrophil and monocyte oxidative metabolism. It is rare, occurring in about 1 in 1 million individuals. The common form is X-linked recessive and there is also an autosomal recessive form (15 percent). Leukocytes from patients with CGD have severely diminished hydrogen peroxide production. Patients present with recurrent infections with catalase-positive microorganisms which destroy their own hydrogen peroxide. This results in infections especially with

Staphylococcus aureus, Escherichia coli, Serratia marcescens, Nocardia, Aspergillus, and *Candida albicans.* When patients become infected, there is often an extensive inflammatory reaction and healing is slow even with the appropriate antibiotic. Chronic inflammation of the nose is common and granulomas are frequent and may cause obstruction in the gastrointestinal and genitourinary tracts. Impaired killing of intracellular microorganisms by macrophages leads to persistent cell-mediated immunity and granuloma formation.

■ MANAGEMENT

Treatment is supportive and long-term and prophylactic antibiotics may be indicated. Surgical drainage of abscesses may be required in the lung, liver, and bones.

Chronic Mucocutaneous Candidiasis

Infection with *Candida albicans* is an almost universal condition in severe deficiencies of cell-mediated immunity. The syndrome of chronic mucocutaneous candidiasis is different because this is the only major manifestation of immunodeficiency. The infection remains local and systemic infection with *Candida* or other fungal agents does not occur, nor is there susceptibility to other bacterial or viral infections.

The infection occurs in the skin, mucous membranes, and nails. There is a family history in 20 percent of cases but the cause is unclear and no uniform immunologic defects have been described. About half the patients have an associated endocrinopathy, including Addison's disease, hypothyroidism, hyperparathyroidism, or diabetes mellitus.

■ MANAGEMENT

The response to antifungal agents is variable. Fluconazole and ketoconazole have been tried with some success. Surgical treatment of the nail infection may be necessary.

Chronic Urticaria

This is a disorder of unknown etiology in which the urticaria persists for more than 6 weeks. Urticaria is the formation of wheals which are elevations of the skin with erythema and edema. Acutely they are caused by ingestion of drugs or foods (especially shellfish) to which the body reacts. Chronic urticaria is not mediated through IgE. It is important because it may indicate an underlying medical problem including lymphoma, systemic lupus erythematosis, primary or metastatic cancer, intestinal parasites, acute hepatitis, systemic vasculitis, or dermatomyositis. It can also occur as a result of taking aspirin or non-steroidal anti-inflammatory medications.

Common Variable Immunodeficiency

Primary immunodeficiencies may be either congenital or acquired and are classified by mode of inheritance and whether the defect involves T cells, B cells, or both. The World Health Organization places the majority of immunodeficiency diseases in a category called common varied immunodeficiency (CVI). It is a heterogeneous group of disorders without a unifying pathogenesis. The disease is frequently caused by an intrinsic B-cell defect and abnormalities of cytokines or T–B cell interaction have been described.

Most patients are well during early childhood with recurrent infections developing during the second or third decades of life. The most common manifestations are sinopulmonary infections because of pyogenic bacteria. In addition, chronic diarrhea due to *Giardia lamblia* is frequently seen. There may be autoimmune hemolytic anemia and thrombocytopenia. Physical examination reveals lymphadenopathy, tonsillar hypertrophy, and splenomegaly in 25 percent of cases. Laboratory evaluation reveals hypogammaglobulinemia with normal T-cell function.

Malignant neoplasms, including non-Hodgkin lymphoma, thymoma, and gastric adenocarcinoma, occur in about 10 percent of patients. The incidence of neoplasms increases with age.

Treatment of the infections needs to be aggressive and intravenous immunoglobulins are given to normalize gammaglobulin levels.

Cow's Milk Protein Allergy

This is the most common food allergy in children. The other foods that commonly produce a food allergy are peanuts, egg, soy, wheat, and nuts. Cow's milk allergy may present as colic, vomiting or diarrhea, or eczema. There may be anemia secondary to blood loss in the stools. There may be respiratory symptoms including rhinitis, wheezing, or cough. There may be sleeplessness in an otherwise healthy infant.

The diagnosis is suspected from the history and treatment is based on removal of the offending allergen. Usually switching to a soy-based formula is beneficial, but in 15–20 percent of cases the allergy is also to soy-milk protein.

DiGeorge Syndrome

22q11 deletion syndromes include the velocardiofacial syndrome (VCFS), DiGeorge syndrome, and conotruncal face syndrome. The velocardiofacial syndrome is the commonest syndrome associated with cleft palate with an incidence of 1 in 5,000. There are several instances of VCFS and DiGeorge syndrome occurring in the same family and it is likely that they correspond to opposite ends (mild versus severe) of the same syndrome. DiGeorge syndrome has more serious heart defects and a higher incidence of thymic and parathyroid hypoplasia.

DiGeorge syndrome has thymic hypoplasia, congenital tetany, abnormal facies, and an increased susceptibility to infection and heart disease. Immunodeficiency varies from mild to severe with low levels of T3 lymphocytes. Lymphocyte counts may be near normal but all the lymphocytes are B lymphocytes. Many patients present with congenital heart disease or hypocalcemia (tetany). The heart disease tends to involve the aortic arch and great vessels; interrupted aortic arch is the most common defect.

Patients with severe immunodeficiency have benefited from thymic transplants and human leukocyte antigen (HLA)-identical bone-marrow transplantation. The bone marrow cannot be depleted of T cells because the success depends on the presence of mature T cells.

Hyper-IgE (Job's) Syndrome

This is a rare disorder with recurrent staphylococcal skin infections, dermatitis, and very elevated serum IgE levels. The cause is unknown and the presentation is in middle childhood with skin and lung infections. The lung infections are associated with abscess formation and pneumatoceles. The skin infection is similar to infected eczema. Laboratory studies include elevated eosinophil count. Treatment is antistaphylococcal antibiotics for prophylaxis as well as to treat acute and chronic infection. Intravenous immunoglobulins may be beneficial.

Selective IgA Deficiency

This is the most common immunodeficiency occurring in 1 in 500 patients. There is deficiency of IgA1 and IgA2 in both serum and mucous secretions. Many adults with isolated IgA deficiency do not have much problem with infection. Some patients develop precipitating antibodies to IgA and may have severe anaphylactic reactions when they receive a blood transfusion. Patients with IgA deficiency tend to have increased respiratory infections and some develop bronchiectasis or diarrhea.

The incidence of asthma in IgA-deficient patients is increased and atopic patients are 20–40 times more likely to have IgA deficiency. Although there are familial cases, no specific pattern of inheritance has been defined. Treatment of IgA deficiency is symptomatic and there is no specific replacement. Patients should be screened for the development of IgA antibodies and ideally receive blood from IgA-deficient donors.

Wiskott–Aldrich Syndrome

This is an X-linked recessive disorder with thrombocytopenia, eczema, and T- and B-cell immunodeficiency affecting males. At birth, the problem is bleeding because of the thrombocytopenia. With time, the bleeding problem improves and there are progressive problems with recurrent infections and eczema. Eczema tends to be allergic in nature and infection is common. Recurrent respiratory infections and otitis media are characteristic. Chronic infection of the eye with herpes simplex may result in chronic keratitis and loss of vision. The immunoglobulins usually show low IgM, normal IgG and IgA, with elevated IgE. Although B-cell lymphocyte numbers are normal, there is an inability to make antibodies to polysaccharide antigens normally. T cells are diminished and do not function normally.

There is a 10 percent incidence of leukemia or lymphoma. Death may occur from bleeding, infection, or malignancy during childhood. There has been some success with bone marrow transplantation.

19

Chapter Nineteen

Infectious Diseases

Infectious diseases are a most important part of acute care pediatrics. Many of the chronic illnesses described in this book are risk factors for acute infections that increase the morbidity and mortality of the illnesses. Chronic infectious disorders are less common but acquired immunodeficiency syndrome (AIDS) and tuberculosis are major health care problems worldwide. Hepatitis is increasing in its significance as a cause of chronic ill health.

Acquired Immunodeficiency Syndrome

In 1981, there were a number of reports of clusters of homosexual men with *Pneumocystis carinii* pneumonia. This pneumonia is rare in normally immune individuals and the patients subsequently developed other unusual complications. A pattern developed and the Centers for Disease Control (CDC) named the new epidemic "acquired immunodeficiency syndrome," and the criteria for diagnosis were based on the presence of a number of illnesses that tend not to be seen without immune compromise. In 1983, researchers identified the virus that causes AIDS and it was initially called HTLV-III and is now named human immunodeficiency virus type 1 (HIV-1). There is an HIV-2 that is common in West Africa and rare in the United States and elsewhere. The first cases in children were reported in 1982.

Worldwide, it is estimated that there are more than 1 million children infected with HIV with over a quarter of a million in Africa alone.

■ PATHOPHYSIOLOGY

The HIV virus is an RNA cytopathic human retrovirus that infects CD4+ T-helper lymphocytes and eventually destroys the cells. The virus integrates into the target cell genome and the virus genome is copied when the cell replicates with the result that the virus persists in infected persons for life. The commonly infected cells include T-helper lymphocytes, macrophages, monocytes, and glial cells. Reduction in the number of these and other immunologic cells results in an impairment of the ability of the body to protect against infection.

The virus has been isolated from blood and other body fluids, including semen, vaginal secretions, saliva, tears, urine, and breast milk. The routes of transmission that have been described include blood or blood products, and this includes intravenous drug needles that have been in contact with HIV-positive blood, and intimate sexual contact with semen and vaginal secretions, as well as through breast milk. Casual contact does not result in transmission of the virus. High-risk factors for HIV in children are shown in Table 19-1.

The perinatal transmission of HIV accounts for the majority (90 percent) of pediatric cases. Infection occurs in utero by vertical transmission through the placenta, during delivery by exposure to infected maternal blood and vaginal secretions, and by feeding infected breast milk. The rate of transmission from infected mothers to their babies is reported to be 14–30 percent but the rate can be definitely lowered by giving zidovudine (AZT) to the mother (after 14 weeks gestation), intravenously during delivery, and to the newborn baby for 6 weeks. Many children became infected in the early years of the AIDS epidemic, when they received contaminated blood and blood products. This was espe-

TABLE 19-1. RISK FACTORS FOR HIV IN CHILDREN

Maternal factors
Intravenous drug use
Maternal promiscuity
Diagnosis of AIDS in mother
Haitian or sub-Saharan African origin

High-risk adolescents
Intravenous drug abusers
Sexual partners of risk-group
Sexually active homosexual males
Bisexual males
Disadvantaged, out-of-school youth, especially females

cially true of the hemophilia population. Children who are sexually abused by HIV-positive individuals are at risk for infection. The average 10-year delay between infection and the development of AIDS means that adolescent behavior, which may include intravenous drug use and unprotected sex, results in many cases in the young adult population.

■ CLINICAL FEATURES

Perinatal HIV infection is usually clinically silent at birth but the incubation period is shorter than in adults. During the incubation period, there is immune dysregulation especially with regard to B-cell function. Hypergammaglobulinemia with production of non-functional antibodies often starts at 3–6 months of age. There is an inability to respond to new antigens with immunoglobulin production and, with no prior antigen exposure, there is a resulting increase in bacterial infections. Depletion of CD4 lymphocytes is commonly a later finding. Infants and children may have normal numbers of total lymphocytes and 15 percent of patients with pediatric AIDS may have a normal ratio of CD4 to CD8 lymphocytes.

The Centers for Disease Control and Prevention and the American Academy of Pediatrics have outlined the clinical manifestations for AIDS in children and adolescents. The infection is different in children compared to adults with more failure to thrive (FTT) and central nervous system involvement (Table 19-2). The presentation in infants is often non-specific with fever, hepato-megaly, and splenomegaly, generalized lymphadenopathy, and diarrhea being common. Chronic candidiasis and parotitis are conditions that are seen more commonly in infected rather than normal infants. About 20 percent of infants present with immune compromise and AIDS, often with *Pneumocystis carinii* pneumo-nia (PCP) or a serious bacterial infection. Twenty-five percent of children are "rapid progressors" with onset of symptoms by 1 year of age and 75 percent are "slow progressors" with symptom onset at 4–6 years of age.

PCP is the most common infection occurring in one-third of infants and children. The median age for presentation is 9 months. Presentation is with fever, cough, tachypnea, hypoxia, and

TABLE 19-2. FEATURES OF AIDS IN CHILDREN AND ADULTS

More common in children
Recurrent severe bacterial infections
Lymphoid interstitial pneumonitis
Oral candidiasis
Parotitis
Failure to thrive
Encephalopathy leading to developmental delay

Common in children and adults
Opportunistic infections
Chronic diarrhea
Chronic fevers
Weight loss
Diffuse lymphadenopathy
Hepatosplenomegaly
Chronic eczema
Renal disease
Cardiomyopathy

More common in adults
Disseminated fungal infections
Toxoplasmosis
Cryptococcal disease
Neoplasms

crackles. It is important to make the diagnosis, usually by bronchoscopy and bronchoalveolar lavage (BAL), so that treatment can be initiated early. Preventive treatment with oral trimethoprim-sulfamethoxazole is effective.

Lymphoid interstitial pneumonitis (LIP) is a chronic interstitial infiltration of the lungs that is seen in 20 percent of children. Lymphocytic infiltration shown on lung biopsy is confirmation. It is associated with generalized lymphadenopathy and salivary gland enlargement. LIP as the presentation of HIV infection is associated with a better prognosis.

Recurrent bacterial infections comprise one of the diagnostic criteria including two or more episodes of sepsis, pneumonia, meningitis, bone or joint infection, or deep abscess. Infection with *Streptococcus pneumoniae,* group A Streptococcus and *Haemophilus influenzae* type b are common. Otitis media, sinusitis, and pneumonia may recur with these organisms. With time, infection with *Staphylococcus aureus* and *Pseudomonas aeruginosa* are common. Disseminated infection with *Mycobacterium avium* complex is seen in about 10 percent of cases. Cytomegalovirus infection and varicella infections are common and may be atypical.

Up to 60 percent of children with HIV infection have signs and symptoms of central nervous system involvement. There is considerable variation with one-third having a progressive encephalopathy with loss of milestones and significant cognitive and motor deficits. There may be mild developmental delay and cerebral imaging may reveal atrophy, white matter abnormalities, and/or cerebral calcifications.

Cancers are less common in children than adults but they do occur. Non-Hodgkin lymphoma is the most common tumor and smooth muscle tumors (leiomyomas and leiomyosarcomas) are associated with HIV infection in children. Kaposi's sarcoma is very rare in children.

■ DIAGNOSIS

Laboratory findings include progressive loss of cell-mediated immunity. The initial lymphocyte count may be normal but lymphopenia develops with reduction of T-helper CD4+ lymphocytes. The T-suppressor CD8+ lymphocytes increase until the later stages of the disease when they decrease. The normal ratio of CD4+ to CD8+ decreases, however this is a non-specific finding as it also occurs with cytomegalovirus and Ebstein-Barr virus infection and other acute viral infections. Anergy to skin test antigens is common including mumps, candida, trichophyton, tetanus, and tuberculin (PPD, purified protein derivative).

Diagnostic testing for HIV infection is by serum antibody tests except in children younger than 18 months in whom passively acquired maternal antibody may be present. Enzyme-linked immunosorbent assays (ELISA) are used most widely to screen for HIV antibody to HIV. A single positive ELISA is repeated and, if positive, Western blot for HIV-specific antibody is the confirmation. Children born to mothers with HIV infection passively acquire maternal IgG antibody. The ELISA may be reactive for 18 months so that detection of the virus or virus product is necessary to confirm HIV infection. The preferred tests are HIV culture and the detection of HIV genomic sequences by PCR. Using these techniques, the diagnosis of HIV infection can be made in 96 percent of cases by 1 month of age and definitely by 4 months of age.

■ MANAGEMENT

This includes early diagnosis, general and specific treatment, and preventative measures. Early diagnosis implies an aggressive approach to testing for the virus in high-risk individuals. It is important for the primary care provider to participate in the care of the children with HIV infection and their family in conjunction with the specialists who will be necessary for management of the case. Strategies for diagnosis and treatment of HIV infection are rapidly changing and it may be beneficial to enroll in research protocols and clinical trials.

Antiretroviral therapy for children with HIV infection must be coordinated by specialists who are experienced in treating this condition. Treatment will depend upon virology, immunology, and clinical findings and will vary with the classification of infection. Antiretroviral therapy is indicated for HIV-infected children with moderate to severe immunocompromise and in those with symptoms and signs of disease. Data concerning the asymptomatic child is less than adults but antiretroviral therapy is recommended under 1 year of age to reduce the viral load. Oral zidovudine (AZT, ZDV, azidothymidine) given in combination with a nucleoside analogue reverse transcriptase inhibitor plus a protease inhibitor is the treatment strategy of choice at the time of writing. Intolerance and side effects may lead to a change in dosage or medication. Monitoring the effect of therapy with CD4 cell counts and quantitative plasma HIV RNA is necessary.

Prevention of opportunistic infection is an important part of management and protocols have been established for children and adolescents. PCP prophylaxis is recommended for all children who have had PCP infection and those with less than 15 percent CD4. It is also recommended for all children born to women with HIV infection and should be started at 4–6 weeks of age and continued at least until 1 year. If the infant is negative after 4 months of age, however, it can be stopped. The usual prophylaxis is trimethoprim-sulfamethoxazole given twice a day for 3 days a week, usually Monday, Wednesday, and Friday.

Children with HIV infection and a positive (5 mm) PPD without evidence of active disease (or prior antituberculous therapy) should receive isoniazid for 12 months. Rifampin should be considered as an alternative if there is a high risk for isoniazid resistance. Clarithromycin (Biaxin) or azithromycin (Zithromax) are recommended for prevention of *Mycobacterium avium* complex. Blood cultures should be taken prior to treatment and if positive 3 or more drugs should be used for treatment.

Patients with hypogammaglobulinemia may benefit from intravenous immunoglobulin (IVIG), which has been shown to reduce the incidence (but not the overall mortality) of serious bacterial infections by 25 percent. Recommendations for active and passive immunization are discussed in Chapter 2 and in the Red Book (2000).

■ PREVENTION

Prevention of the spread of HIV infection is an enormous public health issue. Reduction of perinatal HIV transmission by zidovudine therapy of selected HIV-infected pregnant women and their newborns has been very successful. Oral zidovudine during pregnancy, intravenous during delivery and 6 weeks of treatment of the newborn resulted in a reduction of the perinatal transmission from 25 percent in untreated women to 8 percent in treated women. HIV counseling and testing is recommended for all pregnancies. Women with HIV infection should not breast feed their infant unless they are in countries where the risk of malnutrition and infection from bottle feeding resulting in death is greater than the risk of HIV infection. Health care workers must observe appropriate precautions to reduce the risk of acquiring HIV infection, which will include reducing exposure to blood and other body fluids that may contain the virus.

Adolescents need to receive education that high-risk behaviors related to illicit drugs and unprotected sex makes them vulnerable to the acquisition of HIV. Children with HIV infection should be allowed to attend school and there are guidelines that allow safe integration of the child with HIV into school and community. The American Academy of Pediatrics, Task Force of Pediatric AIDS, is a very important resource for further information.

Support services are available in each community and the clinician needs to know which resources are available and how to access them.

■ PROGNOSIS

The prognosis for pediatric HIV infection and disease has improved as a result of early diagnosis and aggressive treatment.

Unfortunately, it is almost always a terminal disease with hope for future breakthroughs in care.

Tuberculosis

Tuberculosis has increased in incidence in the last decade, at a time when there had been hope that it may be possible to eradicate the disease. It causes considerable morbidity and mortality around the world. Tuberculosis is caused by *Mycobacterium tuberculosis* which is an acid-fast bacillus. Some cases of tuberculosis are caused by *Mycobacterium bovis* which is the cause of bovine tuberculosis. This is rare in countries where there are strict regulations concerning pasteurization of milk because it is transmitted by drinking milk from an infected cow.

The tubercle bacillus is transmitted from person to person by respiratory droplet. An infected adult coughs or sneezes and large numbers of bacilli, usually from a cavity in the lung, are expelled into the air. The susceptible individual inhales the bacilli into the lung which reach the alveoli where they multiply. A primary complex develops at the site and the regional lymph node draining that site. Necrosis of the central part of the lesion or lymph node is called caseation. If the lesion heals, calcification results. At some time in the future there may be spread of bacilli, especially from the lymph nodes, to other areas of the body.

■ PATHOPHYSIOLOGY

The most important concept in understanding tuberculosis is that exposure refers to a patient who has had recent contact with a person who has contagious pulmonary tuberculosis. At the time, the patient has a negative tuberculin skin test and no abnormality on physical examination or chest X-ray. After exposure, some patients will have conversion of the skin test and some will not. Patients who do have conversion of the skin test but who have no physical findings or symptoms of disease and whose chest X-ray is normal or has evidence of a granuloma or calcification in the lung or lymph node (implying old primary complex) are described as having tuberculosis infection. Tuberculosis disease is defined as a person who has signs, symptoms, and X-ray findings of infection with *M. tuberculosis* that may be in the lungs or elsewhere.

The incubation period from the time of acquisition of the tubercle bacilli to the development of a positive skin test is from 2–12 weeks with the median time of 3–4 weeks. The risk of developing disease is highest during the 6 months following infection and remains high for 2 years. The progression from infection to disease may be delayed for several years. The vast majority of cases of infection become dormant, even when untreated, and never progress to disease in the healthy patient. If for any reason a patient becomes immune compromised, then disease is much more likely to result.

■ TESTING

The only reliable test to diagnose tuberculous infection in the asymptomatic individual is the skin test. The Mantoux test is 5 tuberculin units (TU) of purified protein derivative (PPD) that is administered intradermally. It is recommended that this be the only method of skin testing for TB. Alternative doses of PPD, which have ranged from 1 to 250 TU, have not been standardized. The multiple puncture tests have not been proved reliable with unacceptable levels of false-positive and false-negative results. The definitions of the interpretation are shown in Table 19-3. The size of the induration that is palpable is the basis of the measurement. Mantoux test results must be read by experienced health care professionals as it has been clearly shown that untrained personnel are unreliable in interpretation of the findings. The test must be read within the time frame of 48–72 hours.

The negative Mantoux test is not an absolute indication of absence of disease. There are many situations where the skin test is negative despite culture-proven disease. A small population (10 percent) does not react to 5 TU of PPD and young age, poor nutrition, and intercurrent illness may suppress the response. The

TABLE 19-3. DEFINITIONS OF POSITIVE MANTOUX SKIN TEST

5 TU of PPD results in children read at 48–72 hours after placement

Induration >5 mm
Children in close contact with known or suspected infectious cases of tuberculosis
  ` Households with active or previously active tuberculosis
Children suspected to have tuberculosis
  Chest X-ray consistent with active or previously active tuberculosis
  Clinical evidence of tuberculosis
Children receiving immunosuppressive therapy or with immunosuppressive condition including HIV
  infection

Induration >10 mm
Children at increased risk of disseminated disease
  Young age: <4 years of age
  Other medical risk factors, including Hodgkin's disease, lymphoma, diabetes mellitus, chronic renal
  failure, or malnutrition
Children with increased environmental exposure to tuberculosis
  Born, or whose parents were born, in high-prevalence regions of the world
  Frequently exposed to adults who are HIV-infected, homeless, users of illicit drugs, residents of
    nursing homes, incarcerated or institutionalized persons, and migrant farm workers
  Travel and exposure to high-prevalence regions of the world

Induration >15 mm
Children >4 years of age without any risk factors

Note: These definitions apply regardless of previous BCG vaccination.

most common causes include HIV infection, disseminated TB, immunosuppression, and viral infections, notably measles, varicella, and influenza. If anergy to skin testing is suspected, it is reasonable to test with alternate antigens, for example tetanus or candida, but it is not necessary, nor reliable, in the otherwise healthy individual who has a negative PPD. Patients with tuberculosis disease should be tested for HIV infection. The indications for widespread tuberculin testing should be focused on populations at risk. Routine testing of populations, for example schools that are in low-risk areas, has a very poor yield and is not recommended.

The diagnosis is confirmed by culture of tubercle bacilli. The usual source is from sputum, which may be induced, or early morning gastric aspirate. Depending on the site of infection, pleural fluid, urine, bone marrow aspiration, CSF or biopsy specimen, including lymph node, may provide the diagnosis. If a child with suspected pulmonary TB cannot produce sputum, early morning gastric aspirates are recommended. This is done by passing a nasogastric tube on waking and before ambulation or feeding. Three aspirates should be taken for smear and culture.

M. tuberculosis is slow growing and it may be 10 weeks before the organism is isolated. Identification by PCR (polymerase chain reaction) and other genetic (DNA fingerprinting) methods are expensive and performed more in the research laboratory than the clinical setting, although hopefully this will change in the future.

Transmission of tubercle bacilli is almost always airborne and skin, mouth, and mucous membranes have rarely been the route. Transplacental transmission or exposure to infected amniotic fluid can lead to fetal infection.

Tuberculosis tends to affect low-income urban communities where there are problems with overcrowding and the incidence has increased in association with HIV infection. Specific groups with high rates of infection include first-generation immigrants from areas with high incidence of TB, Native Americans including Alaskan natives, the homeless, and residents of correctional institutions.

■ **CLINICAL FEATURES**

Primary Tuberculosis

Primary tuberculosis is the disease produced by initial infection with tubercle bacilli and includes the primary complex of parenchymal lesion and regional lymph node. The incubation period is 2–8 weeks with negative tuberculin test. Most infected children and adolescents are asymptomatic when the tuberculin test is found to be positive. The primary complex of infection is not visible on chest X-ray and in most cases does not progress to disease. Early clinical manifestations occurring 1–6 months after the initial infection tend to be non-specific and include fever, weight loss, cough, and/or night sweats.

Progressive Primary Tuberculosis

There may be rapid local progression with the development of lobar pneumonia or bronchopneumonia. Cough and fever are usual and there may be sputum production and hemoptysis. Chest X-ray may show a cavitary lesion. Involvement of the bronchial wall by an enlarging adjacent lymph node may cause compression and segmental or lobar atelectasis or collapse. In infants, this commonly involves the right upper lobe and, in children, the right middle lobe. Endobronchial lesions develop if the lymph node erodes into the wall of the bronchus and then infectious caseous material can disseminate to other segments of the lungs.

Unilateral pleural effusion is a common finding in the adolescent or young adult (5–35 percent) and is an extension of a subpleural tuberculous focus. The effusion may be large enough to cause respiratory distress. The fluid tends to be non-hemorrhagic, lymphocytic, and tubercle bacilli can be cultured in 50 percent of cases.

Post-Primary Tuberculosis

This is also called adult-type or reinfection tuberculosis. It represents infection that results from tubercle bacilli that have been dormant. If the source is the lungs or regional lymph node, chronic pulmonary disease tends to localize to the lungs because of the sensitization to tuberculin that reduces spread. The disease tends to be in the upper lobes and to be cavitory. There is usually cough, sputum production, hemoptysis, and weight loss.

Hematogenous spread results when there is passage of tubercle bacilli from lymph nodes into blood and dissemination occurs to other areas. Miliary tuberculosis is an early complication of primary tuberculosis, mostly affecting infants and young children and occurring within 6 weeks after onset. There is massive invasion of the bloodstream by tubercle bacilli from a caseating focus that erodes into the blood stream. The tubercle bacilli lodge in small capillaries and form tubercles of uniform size. The X-ray appearance of generalized mottling is characteristic. It is usual for the child to appear ill with few pulmonary signs initially. There may be enlargement of the liver and spleen and lymph nodes (50 percent). Meningitis occurs in about one-third of patients. The tuberculin test may be negative (anergy). Diagnosis may be made from liver biopsy or bone marrow in suspected cases. The prognosis is good if the child is not moribund when treatment is started.

Extrapulmonary Tuberculosis

Tuberculous meningitis is an early complication of primary tuberculosis affecting children under 5 years of age occurring in the first 12 months of illness. A metastatic caseous lesion develops in the cerebral cortex from hematogenous spread. It spreads to involve the meninges and then infects the subarachnoid space. Involvement of the meninges around the brainstem results in paresis of the third and sixth cranial nerves and hydrocephalus is common. The onset is insidious with fever and intermittent vomiting. As the illness progresses, apathy and lethargy are the dominant symptoms. The course of the illness tends to be 1–2 weeks of normal neurologic signs followed by sudden onset of drowsiness and nuchal rigidity. Neurologic signs may be present. The final phase is coma, opisthotonus (arching), decerebrate rigidity, and signs of increased intracranial pressure. If treatment is not started until the later stages, the prognosis is poor.

Diagnosis of tuberculous meningitis involves examination of cerebrospinal fluid (CSF). The CSF findings include white count 10–350 cells/μL which are mostly lymphocytes except in the early stages when polymorphonuclear leukocytes may dominate. CSF protein is elevated and tubercle bacilli cultured in 50 percent of cases.

Skeletal tuberculosis usually appears a year or more after the primary infection. The most common site is the spine (Pott disease) and the vertebral body undergoes progressive destruction. Vertebral collapse may occur leading to kyphotic deformity that is called a gibbus. Paravertebral abscesses are seen in 75 percent of cases of Pott disease.

Urinary-tract disease follows hematogenous spread of the tubercle bacilli to the renal cortex. This complication tends to occur 4 years after initial infection. Caseous necrosis destroys the renal parenchyma and the infection may spread to the bladder and, in males, to the prostate and epididymis. Pyuria, from which no bacteria are cultured, and hematuria suggest the diagnosis.

■ MANAGEMENT

The tubercle bacillus is slow growing and is susceptible to treatment only when multiplying. Antituberculous drugs arrest the progression of tuberculosis arresting the complications of primary disease. Treatment of already caseous or granulomatous lesions is slow. Isoniazid is bactericidal and rapidly absorbed and penetrates well into body fluids. The drug is well tolerated in children and adolescents and hepatitis is unusual in this group and pyridoxine does not need to be given (except with dietary or nutritional deficiencies). Rifampin is metabolized by the liver and alters the metabolism of many drugs. It may produce orange urine, sweat and tears, discolor soft contact lenses, and render oral contraceptives ineffective. Pyrazinamide is well tolerated by children. Ethambutol is bacteriostatic at doses of 15 mg/kg per day and bactericidal above 25 mg/kg per day. It is associated with optic neuritis and monitoring for visual fields and red–green color discrimination is difficult in young children. It is important in reducing the development of resistance.

Treatment of tuberculous (active) disease requires a 6-month regimen consisting of isoniazid, rifampin, and pyrazinamide for the first 2 months and isoniazid and rifampin for the remaining 4 months. Extrapulmonary tuberculosis often will require a longer regimen. The major problem limiting successful treatment is non-compliance so that directly observed therapy (DOT) is strongly advocated. This means that a health care worker or trained third party who is not a relative or friend is present to ensure that the medication is taken as prescribed.

If initial drug resistance is suspected, which is based on the community rates of resistance, then a fourth drug should be added until susceptibility studies of the organism are available.

Chemotherapy for tuberculous infection (preventive therapy) is isoniazid daily. After the first month, it may be acceptable to give isoniazid twice a week for a total of at least 6 months. Patients with HIV infection or other immunocompromising conditions should be treated for 12 months. DOT should also be considered for preventive therapy if non-adherence is likely.

Coccidioidomycosis

Coccidioides immitis is a dimorphic fungus that is found in the soil and endemic in the southwestern United States, northern Mexico, and parts of Central and South America. The infection is also known as "valley fever," taking the name from the San Joaquin Valley in California. Individuals are infected by inhalation of fungal elements in the atmosphere that lead to a primary infection after an incubation period of 10–16 days. It is more common in patients who are immunocompromised. The primary infection may be asymptomatic or may resemble influenza with cough, fever, and chest pain. There may be a rash or arthralgia. Dissemination occurs to skin, bones and joints, central nervous system, and lungs. *C. immitis* reaches the CNS by hematogenous spread from the lungs or more rarely from direct extension from the skull or spine. Symptoms of coccidioidal meningitis tend to develop within a few weeks of the primary infection. The patient develops a headache and there is progression of neurological signs and symptoms. The progression is variable and may become a chronic disorder with personality change and tiredness accompanying the headaches. There may be development of hydrocephalus.

CSF examination reveals increased white cells, predominantly lymphocytes, but eosinophils may be suggestive, with elevation of protein. It is difficult to isolate the organism from the CSF. Immunodiagnosis is by skin testing that should be read at 36 hours and greater than 5 mm implies exposure to *C. immitis*. IgM precipitin test becomes positive in the first weeks after infection but reverts to negative after 6 months. Complement fixation (IgG) becomes positive at 2–3 months and remains so for months or years.

Amphotericin B had been the mainstay of therapy for many years until the azoles have been available. The side effects, while less in children than adults, are significant and the CNS penetration is inadequate. Ketaconazole has been approved for use in cocidioidomycosis and fluconazole and itraconazole have been used successfully.

Cryptococcosis

Infection is thought to be caused by inhalation of the fungus *Cryptococcus neoformans* into the lungs. The infection in the lungs is mild or asymptomatic and resolves. Silent hematogenous spread to the brain leads to clusters of the fungi in the perivascular areas of cortical gray matter. Spread may occur to bones and joints, heart, skin, and mucous membranes. The majority of patients have meningoencephalitis at the time of diagnosis. The symptoms include headache, nausea, and dizziness. Signs of increased intracranial pressure appear after weeks or months. Without treatment, coma ensues and death from respiratory failure. Skin infection usually occurs on the face.

Cryptococcal infection occurs in 5–10 percent of adults with AIDS but is less common in HIV-infected children. It is seen in patients with malignant lymphoma, Hodgkin's disease, leukemia, diabetes, and during corticosteroid therapy. Treatment is with amphotericin B in combination with oral flucytosine. Patients with

HIV who have completed initial therapy for cryptococcosis should remain on fluconazole for life.

Cytomegalovirus

Cytomegalovirus (CMV) is a DNA virus that is a member of the herpesvirus group. Infection may be transferred horizontally from patient to patient and vertically from mother to fetus or infant. Spread of CMV may be from saliva or sexual transmission and has been well-documented in households and child-care centers. Seropositive individuals have CMV in their leukocytes and it can be transmitted by blood transfusion and by transplantation of tissue. CMV may be reactivated in individuals who are immunocompromised.

CMV is associated with a broad range of clinical syndromes. Congenital infection may present with hepatosplenomegaly, jaundice, petechial rash, microcephaly, chorioretinitis, and cerebral calcifications. Twenty percent of these infants die within 2 years and 90 percent of the remainder will have auditory or CNS deficits. Perinatally acquired infection (during birth or from breast milk) may be associated with interstitial pneumonia.

Acquired CMV is usually not apparent although cough or petechial rash with enlargement of the liver and/or spleen may occur. There may be a mononucleosis-like infection with malaise and fevers and headache. The symptoms may persist for months.

CMV can be a major problem in the immunocompromised patient, particularly organ transplant recipients. It may also be a problem for the patient with HIV infection and is a frequent contributing cause of death. Syndromes include fever, leukopenia, hepatitis, pneumonia, colitis, retinitis, nephritis, and encephalitis.

Treatment is unsatisfactory and may need to be prolonged. There are two drugs approved for CMV disease: guanciclovir and foscarnet.

Hepatitis ....

Hepatitis is a viral disease that is usually self-limiting and uncomplicated but chronic hepatitis and cirrhosis may result. There are 5 distinctive types of hepatitis and chronic disease occurs following hepatitis B, C, and D viral infection (Table 19-4). Even though hepatitis A does not become chronic, it is described in some detail because it may affect children with chronic illness, especially in institutional and day care settings.

Hepatitis A is an acute, self-limiting illness that results from person-to-person fecal-oral transmission. Hepatitis A virus (HAV) is an RNA virus classified as a member of the picornavirus (enterovirus) group. It tends to occur in outbreaks in selected populations who are exposed to contaminated water or food but in many cases (44 percent) the cause may not be found. The incubation period is 15–50 days with the average being 25–30 days. The highest titers of viral shedding occur in the 1–2 weeks before the illness becomes symptomatic and so patients are unaware that they are contagious. The highest rates of infection have occurred in children aged 6–14 years of age and there is a high household attack rate (10–20 percent). Viral shedding becomes minimal within a week of the appearance of jaundice.

The illness tends to be fever, malaise, jaundice, anorexia, and nausea that lasts for a few weeks. Infants and preschool children

TABLE 19-4. FEATURES OF HEPATITIS A, B, AND C

	Type A	Type B	Type C
Transmission	Fecal-oral	Parenteral, sexual, perinatal	Parenteral, sexual, perinatal
Incubation	15–50 days	50–180 days	1–5 months
Onset	Usually rapid	More insidious	Usually insidious
Fever	Common and early	Less frequent	Less frequent
Anorexia	Common	Mild to moderate	Mild to moderate
Nausea	Common	Less common	Mild to moderate
Rash	Rare	Macular, common	Sometimes
Jaundice	Usual (except preschool age)	Present	25 percent
Chronic disease	No	Varies with age	65–70 percent of cases

have a non-specific illness without jaundice. Fulminant hepatitis A is rare. Immune globulin administered intramuscularly within 2 weeks of exposure is 80–90 percent effective in preventing symptomatic infection. It is indicated for household and sexual contacts and child care center staff.

Hepatitis B virus (HBV) causes a wide spectrum of illness. HBV is a DNA hepadenovirus and is transmitted through blood or body fluids including wound exudates, semen, cervical secretions, and saliva that are HBsAg-positive (sAg = surface antigen). The HBV-chronic carrier who is HBsAg-positive for 6 months (or with IgM anti-HBc-negative meaning surface antigen positive but IgM core negative which implies previous infection) is the primary reservoir for infection.

Transmission is rare from transfused blood because of screening and viral inactivation of blood products. The modes of transmission include sharing or reusing contaminated needles, exposure to blood or body fluids through mucous membranes or non-intact skin, and homosexual or heterosexual activity. Chronic liver disease is a significant risk particularly for infants with HBV infection who have a 90 percent risk versus 5–10 percent of adults. There may be vertical transmission from mother to infant in the perinatal period and there can be horizontal transmission from mother to child during the first several years of life. Most infections result from injectable drug abuse, heterosexual activity with multiple partners and homosexual activity so that adolescents or adults are at greatest risk.

Hepatitis C virus (HCV) produces signs and symptoms that are similar to HAV and HBV. Acute disease tends to be mild and children are often asymptomatic. Jaundice occurs in 25 percent of cases and elevations of liver enzymes tend to be less than with HBV infection. The major problem is that 65 to 70 percent of patients develop chronic hepatitis and 20 percent develop cirrhosis. HCV is an RNA virus and the prevalence of infection in the general population in the United States is estimated to be 1.8 percent. In children, the seroprevalence rate is 0.2 percent less than 12 years of age and 0.4 percent for ages 13–19 years.

Infection is spread primarily by parenteral exposure to blood and blood products from HCV-infected individuals. The highest rate of seroprevalence is in the users of injectable drugs and the patients with hemophilia who have received multiple transfusions. Interferon-alpha is the only treatment currently available for chronic HCV infection in adults but less than 20 percent have a sustained response. Primary hepatocellular carcinoma has not been reported in children but occurs with increasing age in adolescents and adults.

Histoplasmosis

Histoplasma capsulatum is found principally in soil around pigeon lofts and chicken houses. It is endemic in the central and eastern United States, especially the Mississippi and Ohio River valleys. The fungus enters the body through skin, mucous membrane, respiratory, or intestinal tract. The initial lesion in the lung is similar to the granuloma of tuberculosis and involves the regional lymph node. Chronic pulmonary histoplasmosis is rare in children. There is considerable clinical variation. Acute disseminated histoplasmosis is most frequent in immunocompromised hosts, including HIV infected, and children under 2 years of age. Symptoms include fever, cough, hepatosplenomegaly, pneumonitis, skin lesions, and diarrhea. Chronic disseminated histoplasmosis is unusual in children.

Culture of bone marrow, blood, sputum, and material from lesions can be cultured, requiring 2–6 weeks. Treatment is not necessary for simple pulmonary infection. Chronic disseminated infection should be treated with amphotericin B for at least 6 weeks.

Congenital Infections

TORCHS is an acronym for *Toxoplasmosis, Rubella, Cyto-megalovirus, Herpes,* and *Syphilis,* all of which can potentially cause congenital infections. The letter *O* stands for *Other* viral infections that also can affect the fetus.

■ TOXOPLASMOSIS

Toxoplasma gondii is a protozoan parasite and the predominant host for toxoplasmosis is cats. It is transmitted to humans after eating uncooked meat from intermediate hosts, including pigs, sheep, and cattle. It also can be acquired from the soil or from cat litter, and congenital infection results if the mother has the primary infection during pregnancy. Most human infections acquired after birth are asymptomatic.

Acute neonatal toxoplasmosis may result in a severe infection with jaundice, maculopapular rash, thrombocytopenic purpura, and hepatosplenomegaly. Seizures, opisthotonus, and chorio-retinitis occur and these babies usually die within the first month. Survivors can be expected to have partial or complete blindness and severe mental retardation. Occasionally, the onset of symptoms is delayed with intracranial calcifications, chorio-retinitis, and hydrocephalus.

Although acquired toxoplasmosis is usually asymptomatic, there is a rare fulminant form with rash, myocarditis, encephalitis, and myositis that may be fatal. The most common clinical presentation is chronic lymphadenopathy with an infectious mono-nucleosis-like picture. The diagnosis may be difficult and most commonly is a measure of IgG-specific antibody which peaks 1–2 months after infection and remains elevated indefinitely.

Treatment, when indicated, is with pyrimethamine and sulfadiazine. Folinic acid is supplemented to avoid hematologic toxic effects.

20

Chapter Twenty

Pulmonary Disease

The chest functions as bellows, moving air in and out of the lungs. Oxygen is inhaled and absorbed and carbon dioxide is excreted and breathed out. The major muscles of respiration are the diaphragm (which separates the chest from the abdomen) and the chest wall muscles called intercostals. At birth, the chest wall is very compliant and the ribs are flexible, being comprised more of cartilage than bone. The lungs mature until about 8 years of age when they increase in size until growth ceases in adolescence. Babies breathe about 25–35 times a minute, children breath 20–30, adolescents 15–29, and adults 12–15 times a minute. When breathing is difficult, the term used is *dyspnea*. It can be recognized as tachypnea which is an increase in the rate above normal for age. There may be increased work of breathing which is seen as retractions of the chest wall and use of accessory muscles of respiration. Noisy breathing may also indicate distress. Stridor, a high-pitched sound on inspiration, is a sign of upper airway obstruction and wheezing occurs with lower airway obstruction.

Apnea is defined as cessation of breathing and is central in origin if there is no respiratory effort. Obstructive apnea occurs when there is chest wall movement but no airflow because of obstruction in the airway. This obstruction is usually in the upper airway which includes the nose, mouth, pharynx, and larynx. Apnea is often a mixture of central and obstructive and the duration is defined as 20 seconds for premature babies, 15 seconds for infants, and 10 seconds for adults. Bradycardia means low heart rate and is less than 100 beats per minute for newborns, 80 for infants, 60 for children, and 40 for adults.

Chronic lung disease is a major cause of disability and death for all ages. Many adult respiratory illnesses start in childhood. Genetic mechanisms are important in many lung diseases, including cystic fibrosis, immunologic disorders, and probably asthma. Environmental factors, including exposure to cigarette smoke and air pollution, and bacterial and viral infections contribute to the development and progression of lung disease. Fifty percent of deaths of children less than 5 years of age in developing countries are caused by acute respiratory infections and they are the commonest cause of death in children worldwide. Children with chronic illness are potentially more susceptible to respiratory illness than their well counterparts.

The morbidity and mortality associated with smoking is enormous and remains a major public health issue. When it is realized that 90 percent of adult smokers start during their teenage years, reducing teenage smoking would have a major impact on adult health.

Lung disease is evaluated by chest X-ray, pulmonary function testing, and blood gases. Chest X-ray will indicate the presence of hyperinflation that occurs with obstructive disorders and parenchymal (lung tissue) changes that may be acute or chronic. CAT scan or MRI may be helpful to define lung and mediastinal abnormalities. Pulmonary function tests are useful to define the normal versus abnormal respiratory function. It can differentiate obstructive versus restrictive lung disease and allow change in lung function over time and treatment response to be followed. The most useful test is the flow–volume curve which measures forced vital capacity (FVC), the amount that is able to be exhaled completely after a full inspiration. The amount breathed out in the first second is called the forced expired volume in 1 second (FEV1). The test can be performed by most 5-6-year-old children. The management of asthma will often include following daily peak flow measurements which are useful to measure the degree of airway obstruction and to help with treatment decisions.

Bronchoscopy is the visualization of the airway. Initially the technique was performed using a rigid metal tube passed through the mouth and it still is used to evaluate the large airways and to remove foreign bodies. Flexible bronchoscopy is usually performed through the nose (or through an endotracheal tube) and allows a dynamic look at the airway. The patient can breathe around the tube so general anesthesia may not be necessary. The flexible scope is composed of fiberoptics which allow visualization of the airway and there is a channel for suctioning in all but the smallest scopes. This permits sampling of the secretions of the lower airway which is called bronchoalveolar lavage (BAL). Aspiration of secretions may be therapeutic as well as diagnostic. Therapeutic indications include suctioning of mucus plugs that obstruct the airways. Diagnostic includes collection of airway secretions for bacterial or viral culture and to identify cells that are causing disease (e.g., tuberculosis, phagocytic cells, or lipid-laden macrophages).

Lung disease can be restrictive or obstructive. Restrictive disease implies that there is less lung volume which may be from a reduced amount of lung tissue or from an inability of the lungs to expand fully. Obstructive lung disease results from narrowed airways most commonly because of constriction of the bronchi and smaller airways.

Cystic Fibrosis

Cystic fibrosis (CF) was suggested by a European physician who stated about 150 years ago that "The child will soon die, whose brow tastes salty when kissed." Recent history relates to the landmark report in 1938 by Dorothy Andersen, who linked together the chronic lung infection and cystic changes in the pancreas. For a long time the condition was known as fibrocystic disease of the pancreas. The other early-recognized feature was thick mucus from exocrine glands that led to the term *mucoviscidosis*. The sweat defect was recognized during the summer heatwave in New York in 1949, when several children with CF developed heat stroke. Almost 20 years ago the chloride channel was noted to function abnormally both in the sweat gland and the respiratory mucosa.

In 1989, the CF gene was discovered by groups of researchers in Michigan and Toronto. The CF gene was located on the long arm of chromosome 7 which encodes a protein product called cystic fibrosis transmembrane conductance regulator (CFTR). The most common mutation is the deletion of 3 base pairs that code for phenylalanine and is known as the ΔF508. This mutation is responsible for 70 percent of the CF genes, approximately half being homozygous 508/508 and half heterozygous 508/other. CF is an autosomal recessive disorder that requires one CF gene from each parent to be transmitted so that the CF patient has two CF genes. The remaining CF genes (amounting to 30 percent of all CF genes) that have been identified number over 900. The genotype–phenotype relationship is more complicated than it first seemed. Homozygosity of ΔF508 is associated with pancreatic insufficiency in almost all cases.

■ **DESCRIPTION**

CF is a recessive disorder so that the CF patient receives 1 CF gene from each parent. The incidence in Caucasians is 1 in 2,000–3,000 live births with the heterozygote or carrier rate of 1 in 20–25. Numbers for other populations are not completely known but the best estimate is 1 in 11,000 Hispanic live births and 1 in 17,000 African-American. The Hawaiian, or Polynesian, incidence is 1 in 90,000 and it is even rarer in the Asian, or Oriental, population. There are about 30,000 children and adults with CF in North America with a median age of about 15 years of age. The median survival is now over 30 years of age.

■ CLINICAL FEATURES

The diagnosis of CF is made if there is elevation of sweat chloride >60 mEq/L, since most people without CF have sweat chloride about 20 mEq/L. The diagnosis is accompanied by clinical symptoms of chronic pulmonary disease and, in more than 90 percent of cases, pancreatic insufficiency. All CF patients will have 2 CF genes although some patients with 2 CF genes may only manifest congenital bilateral absence of the vas deferens (CBAVD).

CF is a disorder of epithelial surfaces that affects the sweat glands, the respiratory system, gastrointestinal system, and reproductive organs. There are no primary clinical effects of the nervous system or kidneys.

The sweat gland in CF has reduced reabsorption of chloride, resulting in the high salt content of sweat. Patients are prone to heat exhaustion particularly if they exercise in hot weather. During infancy, sweat losses may result in hypochloremia. There may be salt crystals on the skin with excessive sweating and skin rash may result.

The lungs appear to be normal at birth. Mucus hypersecretion occurs early and inflammation and infection often appear before clinical symptoms are evident. There is mucus plugging and airway obstruction that is associated with infection and a vicious cycle of infection and inflammation that leads to chronic lung disease. The end result is bronchiectasis and hyperinflation. Chronic pulmonary disease accounts for more than 90 percent of the mortality from CF. The symptoms include cough and expectoration of sputum with crackles and wheezing that are worse with exacerbations. Pulmonary function testing is useful to follow the course of disease.

The characteristic of CF is the presence of *Pseudomonas aeruginosa* in the pulmonary secretions. The term *colonization* is used to describe the persistence of the organism in the sputum. Younger patients (40 percent) tend to have *Staphylococcus aureus* which may be present in the older patient (20 percent) unless antistaphylococcal antibiotics are taken. More recently there has been increasing colonization with *Burkholderia cepacia* and *Aspergillus fumigatus*. The presence of atypical mycobacteria and *Stenotrophomonas maltophilia* is also increasing but the long-term significance of these organisms is not known.

The upper airways are also involved so that pansinusitis is a consistent feature. The radiographic findings are usually more obvious than the clinical symptoms. The frontal sinuses do not develop and the remaining sinuses become filled with mucoid secretions. Nasal polyps are common with symptoms of nasal obstruction. The presence of pansinusitis or nasal polyps is an indication to perform a sweat test and normal sinuses in childhood would make the diagnosis of CF unlikely.

Approximately 90 percent of patients with CF have exocrine pancreatic insufficiency, although it is only present in about 50 percent at birth. Meconium ileus is GI obstruction secondary to thick meconium. It may result in dilated bowel loops evident on fetal ultrasound. Small bowel obstruction may result in perforation of the ileum in utero. After birth, there may be delayed passage of meconium and abdominal distension.

Pancreatic insufficiency causes steatorrhea and malabsorption which leads to failure to thrive. Even when the dominant presenting symptoms are pulmonary, an inability to gain weight is often a clue to the diagnosis of CF. The pancreatic insufficiency results from thick secretions with failure of exocrine function of the pancreas. There is a lack of enzymes for digestion and absorption of fats, carbohydrates, and protein. There is difficulty absorbing fat-soluble vitamins. During adolescence and adulthood, fibrosis of the pancreas results in glucose intolerance and CF-related diabetes mellitus in about 20 percent of adult patients.

Rectal prolapse may occur in the first few years and can be a presenting symptom. It tends to improve when pancreatic enzymes are instituted and may recur if enzymes are not taken. If there is intestinal obstruction later, it is called meconium ileus equivalent which can occur at any age. The present term is DIOS (distal intestinal obstruction syndrome).

Intrahepatic cholestasis results in micronodular biliary fibrosis which is more commonly focal. In about 2 percent of cases, there is multilobular cirrhosis with portal hypertension and hypersplenism. Abnormal gall bladder anatomy may lead to gall stones that may necessitate cholecystectomy.

There is some reduction in fertility of females because the cervical mucus, which is also thick, results in a potential barrier to sperm. Males with CF have thick secretions in the testes with resultant obstructive azospermia and 98 percent are sterile. The sperm can be aspirated from the epididymis so that in-vitro fertilization is possible. If there is significant malnutrition, puberty tends to be delayed in both males and females.

Presentations of CF at various ages are shown in Table 20-1.

■ MANAGEMENT

The approach to management of CF is multidisciplinary with the recommendation that care is coordinated or provided by a CF Center accredited by the CF Foundation. Pulmonary management is designed to reduce the rate of the inevitable decline in lung function that occurs over time. Treatment includes measures to improve airway clearance of thick and infected pulmonary secretions as well as antibiotics to control infection. Many patients receive oral antibiotics that are treating *S. aureus* or *H. influenzae* including a semisynthetic penicillin, trimethoprim-sulfamethoxazole, or a cephalosporin. The dominant organism in older children and adults is *P. aeruginosa*, which is found in the sputum, and the decision to treat is based on clinical findings. If there is deterioration from the baseline condition, the term *pulmonary exacerbation* is used. This usually means that there are increased symptoms (Table 20-2). Many exacerbations result from community acquired infection and it is often difficult to decide how aggressive to be. Upper respiratory infections in children are very common and not all colds need a change in antibiotic treatment. Treatment of a pulmonary exacerbation usually implies treating *P. aeruginosa* which limits the choice of antibiotics. The only oral antibiotics with anti-pseudomonal properties are the quinolones, the aerosol antibiotics commonly prescribed are tobramycin or colimycin, and various intravenous antibiotics.

TABLE 20-1. PRESENTATIONS THAT SUGGEST CYSTIC FIBROSIS AT DIFFERENT AGES

All ages
Family history of CF or persistent pulmonary infections
Chronic or recurrent respiratory symptoms (especially wheezing)
Staphylococcus aureus or *Pseudomonas aeruginosa* isolated from respiratory secretions
Hypochloremic metabolic alkalosis

Newborn
Meconium ileus
Prolonged jaundice

Infants
Persistent infiltrates or hyperinflation on chest X-ray
Failure to thrive
Peripheral edema (anasarca)
Hypoalbuminemia
Chronic diarrhea (loose, oily or smelly stools)
Rectal prolapse
Abdominal distension or protuberance
Salty-tasting skin

Childhood
Nasal polyps
Chronic sinusitis
Clubbing of the fingers
Steatorrhea
Rectal prolapse
Distal intestinal obstruction syndrome (DIOS)

Adolescence and adulthood
Allergic bronchopulmonary aspergillosis
Chronic pansinusitis/nasal polyposis
Hemoptysis
Pancreatitis (acute or chronic)
Portal hypertension (cirrhosis)
Delayed puberty
Infertility (males—azoospermia)

The combination of a beta-lactam (e.g., ceftazidime) and an aminoglycoside (e.g., tobramycin) is the most commonly prescribed treatment of pseudomonas infections. The choice of antibiotic should be adjusted on the basis of sputum culture results. The duration of the intravenous antibiotics averages 13 days. The decision to provide treatment in the hospital or at home depends on the medical circumstances as well as the home situation.

TABLE 20-2. FEATURES OF CYSTIC FIBROSIS
EXACERBATION

Increased cough
Increased sputum production
Darker thicker sputum (clear → yellow → green)
Hemoptysis
New or more crackles or wheezes on auscultation
Anorexia
Weight loss
Fever
10% drop in PFTs
Increased tiredness
Increased shortness of breath on exertion

Airway clearance techniques (ACTs) include traditional postural drainage, percussion, and vibration. Percussion is performed manually with cupped hands or by machine. It is usually taught to the caregivers soon after the diagnosis of CF is made. Preventive therapy is recommended for patients with significant pulmonary symptoms. Alternative ACTs are varied and efficacy is probably more dependent on how enthusiastically the techniques are utilized. Autogenic drainage was popularized in Europe by Dr Chevalier and involves controlled breathing maneuvers. Positive expiratory pressure (PEP), intrapulmonary ventilation, therapy vest, and Flutter valve are all techniques that have been shown to help mobilize thick pulmonary secretions. Exercise is recommended as an important maintenance therapy.

The patient with CF has increased calorie needs because of several factors, including maldigestion, malabsorption, and chronic lung infection. Pancreatic insufficiency is managed with replacement pancreatic enzymes with the dosage calculated on the amount of lipase. There are several strengths of capsules and the amount of lipase per meal is usually in the range of 1,000–2,000 units per kg per meal. In many patients, the efficiency of the enzymes is improved with supplemental antacids or inhibitors of gastric secretion which are useful because of the lack of neutralizing pancreatic bicarbonate secretion. In addition, fat-soluble vitamins (A, D, E, and K) should be supplemented.

Human recombinant DNase (Pulmozyme) alters the viscosity of CF sputum. The viscoelastic properties of infected sputum are the result of increased amounts of extracellular DNA from the nuclear material of white blood cells. DNase hydrolyzes extracellular DNA and is delivered to the airway by aerosol. There is improvement in pulmonary function and reduction of the incidence of pulmonary infection.

High-dose aerosol tobramycin has been shown to reduce the amount of pseudomonas in the sputum and to improve pulmonary function. A newer preparation (TOBI) of 300 mg tobramycin inhaled twice daily for alternate months has been shown to improve lung function and to reduce the need for intravenous antibiotics.

■ COMPLICATIONS

Glucose intolerance is more common with increasing age because of deficiency of insulin as a result of fibrosis of the pancreas. Approximately 20 percent of adults with CF require insulin. Dietary considerations are different from classical diabetes mellitus because of the nutritional requirements of the patient with CF.

The major morbidity and mortality of CF relates to the progression of lung infection. Pneumothorax may require placement of a chest tube and has a tendency to recur. Hemoptysis is a common symptom. Streaking of the sputum with blood often indicates worsening infection and responds to antibiotic therapy. Massive hemoptysis is defined as greater than 300 cc of blood that is coughed up. It results from bronchial artery hemorrhage that may require embolization of the vessels because they arise from the aorta.

Eventually cor pulmonale, or right-sided heart failure secondary to lung disease, may result from chronic hypoxia and pulmonary hypertension. It may not be recognized because peripheral edema is a late sign in cor pulmonale caused by CF and the electrocardiogram may not indicate right ventricular hypertrophy. The echocardiogram is used to diagnose pulmonary hypertension and cor pulmonale.

Respiratory failure is the most common cause of death in CF. The progression of lung infection usually is not amenable to improvement with mechanical ventilation and usually the decision is made not to start ventilatory support for terminal lung disease. Experience has shown that it is rare to be able to wean off mechanical ventilation in this situation. Ventilatory support can be considered if there is an acute deterioration that has potential for recovery or if endotracheal intubation is used for a surgical procedure.

When the lung disease is so severe that survival for more than 2 years is unlikely, lung transplantation is considered. The waiting list for donor organ lungs is 1–3 years for most programs. It is usual to discuss the possibility of transplantation when the FEV1 is consistently less than 30 percent when the patient is stable. The procedure performed in the United States is bilateral sequential single lung transplantation. Both lungs have to be removed because of the infection. One-year survival following transplantation is about 90 percent. Most transplantation involves cadaver lungs but living lobar transplantation has also been successful.

■ THE FUTURE

When the CF gene was discovered in 1989, it was hoped that there would be an ability to successfully correct the basic defect by gene therapy. It has been possible to deliver a normal CFTR gene into the CF epithelial cell using a viral or liposomal vector. The expression of the gene has not yet achieved the levels necessary to alter significantly the course of the disease. Many therapeutic possibilities are under investigation to correct the basic defect in CF.

Bronchopulmonary Dysplasia

The condition was first described by Northway in 1967 in a review of premature infants who required mechanical ventilation and high oxygen concentrations to treat respiratory distress syndrome (RDS). They reported radiologic progression of the chest X-ray that was consistent among the group of patients. Stage I was the same as RDS lasting 2–3 days; stage II showed opacification of the lung fields (white-out) that occurred between 4 and 10 days. Stage II tends not to be seen unless there is pulmonary edema or pulmonary hemorrhage. Stage III lasted from 10–20 days and was characterized by small round cystic lesions and stage IV showed hyperinflation and scarring. They also correlated the pathological findings and suggested the relationship between high inspired oxygen concentrations and positive pressure ventilation and the subsequent lung damage.

The definition that is most used involves infants who require assisted ventilation in the newborn period for a variety of causes including extreme prematurity, RDS, meconium aspiration, pneumonia, and heart failure. If at 28 days there is a requirement for supplemental oxygen and there are typical chest X-ray findings, the infant may be classified as meeting the criteria for BPD. This tends to include a large number of premature infants without much lung disease who required low concentrations of oxygen and so some authors restrict the definition to include only those prematures who still required oxygen at 36 weeks post-conceptional age.

The incidence of BPD has declined since the introduction of surfactant for the treatment of RDS. Increasing numbers of extremely premature infants, some of whom will develop BPD, are surviving because of improvement in neonatal care. The incidence of BPD is not known because the definition is not agreed among authors. One report of the incidence of BPD in infants with birthweight between 1,000 and 1,500 g who required intubation and survived for 30 days was 25 percent. With birthweight between 700 and 1,000 g it was 70 percent and with birthweight less than

700 g it was 100 percent (using the definition of requiring oxygen at 30 days of age).

■ CLINICAL FEATURES

The clinical condition results from injury to the immature lung. There is pulmonary fibrosis, increased lung water, and hyper-inflation. This results in hyperreactive airways with obstruction that results in wheezing and impaired gas exchange. The more severe patients have hypoxia, CO_2 retention, increased work of breathing, and retractions. Increased calorie requirements and reduced intake lead to growth failure.

Complications common to infants with BPD include apnea, tracheomalacia and bronchomalacia, and pulmonary hypertension. In addition, there may be neurologic consequences of a difficult neonatal course including cerebral palsy.

■ MANAGEMENT

The most important strategy in treatment of BPD is avoidance of hypoxia. It is necessary to achieve adequate tissue oxygenation to improve growth and to reduce the potential of pulmonary hypertension developing. The goal is to achieve arterial oxygen tension of 60 mm Hg or oxygen saturation of 92 percent for most of the day and night. Prolonged desaturation during sleep may result in pulmonary hypertension. It is important not to withhold oxygen because the complications of hypoxia are significant and the risk of retinopathy of prematurity is minimal at this stage. Oxygen may be delivered by mask or nasal cannula and children with a tracheostomy tube can use a collar. When symptoms improve, growth occurs, and the patient can achieve oxygen saturation in the mid-90s, then oxygen can be weaned.

Additional treatment with bronchodilators and/or diuretics will be indicated for infants who have symptomatic airway obstruction. Fluid restriction may be indicated. Diuretics reduce lung water and improve airway resistance. The use of oral or intravenous corticosteroids remains controversial as they have been shown to help weaning from the ventilator but have not been shown to alter the long-term outcome. Inhaled steroids are prescribed by many clinicians.

Home oxygen and home ventilation have been widely used for the management of BPD and require a commitment from the family. Home nursing may be critical to successful outcome.

Long-term follow-up studies of BPD have shown that there is persistence of pulmonary function abnormalities of airway obstruction and hyperreactivity for many years.

Congenital Central Hypoventilation Syndrome

Congenital central hypoventilation syndrome (CCHS), also called Ondine's curse, is a rare condition with marked depression of respiratory drive during sleep. This results in apnea during sleep without any demonstrable cause. There is no neurologic, cardiac, or pulmonary abnormality to explain the apnea and hypoventilation. There is an association with Hirschsprung's disease and neural tumors. During the awake time, ventilation is clinically normal in the majority of patients but some hypoventilate also when awake.

Central hypoventilation (defined as arterial carbon dioxide greater than 45 Torr) occurs in many conditions, most notably morbid obesity (Pickwickian syndrome) and the Arnold–Chiari malformation which is a brainstem abnormality.

■ MANAGEMENT

Many of the patients with CCHS will require tracheostomy and assisted ventilation while asleep. Phrenic nerve pacing has been successful in some children.

Immotile Cilia Syndrome ....

The original description was based on the observation in 1933 by Kartagener that some children had chronic sinusitis, bronchiectasis, and situs inversus (dextrocardia, with the liver and spleen inverted). In the 1970s, ultrastructure of the sperm tails of infertile men was demonstrated to be associated with immotility of the flagella. Ciliary dyskinesia is a better description than immotile cilia syndrome because the cilia show disorganized rather than absent motion, but the latter term is more widely used.

The syndrome is an autosomal recessive disorder with an incidence of approximately 1 : 16,000. The patients with Kartagener's syndrome have an incidence of 1 : 32,000 because half of the patients with immotile cilia syndrome have situs inversus and half of them have normal placement of the heart and abdominal organs.

The severity of involvement of the sinuses and lungs is variable. The nasal and sinus mucosa become inflamed and opacification of the sinuses is common. Symptoms include mucopurulent rhinorrhea and pain and tenderness over the sinuses. Chronic sinusitis may lead to post-nasal drip, adenoidal breathing (with the mouth open), sleep apnea, and halitosis. Chronic mucus impaction and inflammation results in infection that, over time, leads to bronchiectasis. There is usually a history of chronic cough with purulent sputum. Examination reveals clubbing of the fingers and crackles over the involved areas of the lung.

■ MANAGEMENT

The diagnosis should be suspected in children with recurrent sinopulmonary infections particularly if situs inversus is present. The symptoms may start in the newborn period. The diagnosis can be confirmed by biopsy of respiratory epithelium. It is helpful to get tissue from upper and lower airways because ciliary abnormalities may result from chronic infection.

Antibiotics are indicated for infections and the duration of therapy depends upon the recurrence rate. It may be necessary to use continuous antibiotics to keep the infection under control. The most common organisms are *Staphylococcus aureus*, *Haemophilus influenzae* (nontypable), and *Pseudomonas aeruginosa*. The choice of antibiotic will vary with the organism and its sensitivity. Endoscopic sinus surgery may help drainage and surgical treatment may be indicated for lung abscess or localized area of pulmonary infection. The prognosis is usually good with aggressive management of infection.

Pulmonary Hemosiderosis

There are many causes of pulmonary hemorrhage including infection, foreign body, cardiovascular, autoimmune, trauma, and idiopathic. Idiopathic means that no cause is found and that label is applied to idiopathic pulmonary hemosiderosis (IPH). Pulmonary hemosiderosis follows bleeding into the lungs in which iron from red cells collects as hemosiderin in the parenchyma of the lungs. The hemosiderin can be demonstrated by staining macrophages which can be found by bronchoalveolar lavage or lung biopsy. Hemosiderin-laden macrophages may be found in IPH and other disorders associated with chronic pulmonary hemorrhage. Autoimmune disease may be associated with renal involvement.

The classic description of IPH is a young child who presents with respiratory distress, patchy infiltrates on chest X-ray, and iron deficiency anemia. Episodes tend to be recurrent and blood may be coughed up (hemoptysis) or swallowed. The precipitating factor for an episode of bleeding is commonly a viral upper-respiratory infection or exercise. Recurrent episodes of bleeding over many years may lead to chronic lung disease with clubbing of the fingers, persistent oxygen requirement, and pulmonary hypertension.

There are patients who have IPH who demonstrate cow's milk allergy (Heiner's syndrome) and who have less bleeding with exclusion of cow's milk from the diet. Many patients have immunologic findings but there is no consistency among patients.

■ MANAGEMENT

Supportive treatment with oxygen and correction of anemia is indicated. Many patients require corticosteroids to reduce the potential for bleeding and some patients bleed again when the dose is lowered. Immunosuppressants should be considered if bleeding recurs and azathioprine, cyclophosphamide, and chlorambucil have all been reported to be useful. The long-term outcome is variable. Some patients die of an acute bleed or right heart failure, some continue with recurrent bleeding and chronic lung disease, and some appear to resolve.

Sinusitis

Chronic sinusitis is defined as infection of the paranasal sinuses that persists for more than 30 days. Recurrent sinus infections are associated with many chronic illnesses and also in at least 50 percent of cases is accompanied by recurrent ear infections. Sinus infection often is diagnosed when a nasal cold persists for more than 10 days with continued symptoms of nasal discharge and cough. Acute sinusitis may be accompanied by pain and tenderness over the affected area (the cheeks or forehead, for example). Chronic sinus infection also may have discomfort but the dominant symptoms are nasal stuffiness, mucopurulent discharge, and post-nasal drip.

In addition to immune disorders, chronic sinus disease is a feature of asthma, atopy, and cystic fibrosis, all of which are liable to develop nasal polyposis. Sinus X-rays are of little value in children under 1 year as the sinuses are very small. X-rays are taken in at least three views to show maxillary, frontal, ethmoid, and sphenoid cavities. Limited CAT scan of the sinuses is more useful and provides better imaging than regular X-rays. Both show opacification, mucosal thickening, and air-fluid levels.

■ **MANAGEMENT**

Treatment of chronic sinusitis requires antibiotics for 3–4 weeks, and the choice of antibiotics varies with the underlying cause but will often need to be fairly broad spectrum. Decongestants have not been shown to be beneficial but may produce symptomatic improvement. Nasal steroids may improve atopic patients. Surgical drainage of the sinuses may be indicated for recurrent sinusitis that does not respond to medical management.

Obstructive Sleep Apnea Syndrome

The first comprehensive description of obstructive sleep apnea syndrome (OSAS) was as recent as 1976 and it was considered to be rare. Osler had described in 1892 that chronic tonsillar enlargement would disturb a child's sleep with loud and snorting respiration accompanied by prolonged pauses. OSAS is common in adults and the childhood version differs in many ways. While snoring occurs in 7–9 percent of children, OSAS has been reported in 2 percent of 4–5-year-old children. The peak incidence in children corresponds to the period of maximal adenotonsillar hypertrophy which is 3–6 years of age.

Many chronic pediatric disorders are associated with OSAS, especially those that predispose to upper airway obstruction. These include cerebral palsy, achondroplasia, obesity, Down syndrome, Prader–Willi, and more. The prevalence of OSAS is highest in the normal population who have adenotonsillar enlargement and narrowing of the upper airway passage that collapses on inspiration during sleep. It is unclear why some children manifest severe symptoms while others do not.

**TABLE 20-3. FEATURES OF OBSTRUCTIVE
SLEEP APNEA SYNDROME**

Snoring
Difficulty breathing when asleep
Apnea during sleep
Restless sleep
Mouth-breathes when awake
Sweating when sleeping
Excessive daytime sleepiness
Poor appetite
Secondary enuresis
Behavior disorder especially at school
Pulmonary hypertension
Cor pulmonale

There are several clinical manifestations of sleep disordered breathing (Table 20-3). Snoring tends to be loud, restlessness is common, and apnea may be prolonged and associated with arousal. The complications include pulmonary hypertension, which results from hypoxia during sleep, that can lead to cor pulmonale. Sudden death has been reported, especially in relation to general anesthesia. Systemic hypertension and cardiac arrhythmias may occur.

Neurobehavioral complications are the result of disturbed sleep. The most common report is excessive daytime sleepiness which is defined as falling asleep at inappropriate times. Developmental delay, hyperactivity, poor school performance, and other changes in behavior are all common. There may be growth failure and secondary enuresis.

Management involves confirmation of the diagnosis, ideally with polysomnography to quantify the apnea duration and hypoxia. Videotaping is helpful, but audiotaping may only confirm the presence of snoring. Removal of the tonsils and adenoids should be considered if the studies of breathing during sleep reveal hypoxia. Anatomic abnormalities of the airway may need to be corrected if it is feasible to do so. Obesity must be treated if it is a dominant component of OSAS and the complications noted above are present.

21

Chapter Twenty-One

Cardiac Disorders

After birth, the blood circulates successively through the right side of the heart, from the right atrium to the right ventricle, passing through the pulmonary arteries to the lungs. Oxygen is acquired and carbon dioxide excreted and blood returns from the lungs via the pulmonary veins to the left atrium. The left ventricle pumps the blood around the body from the aorta to the regional arteries. Blood passes through the capillary system and collects into the venous system leading to the great veins (venae cavae) which connect to the right atrium. The heart valves include the tricuspid between the right atrium and ventricle and the mitral between the left atrium and ventricle. The valves of the great vessels are pulmonic and aortic from the right and left ventricle, respectively. Between the two sides of the heart there is the atrial septum and the ventricular septum. The normal position for the heart, lungs, and abdominal organs is called *situs solitus* and if they are reversed (mirror image) it is called *situs inversus*. Dextrocardia implies that the heart is mostly in the right chest.

Heart disease in children is either congenital or acquired. Congenital heart disease (CHD) includes structural defects of the heart and great vessels that may lead to heart failure and hypoxia. Acquired heart disease results mostly from infection, autoimmune disorders, and environmental factors.

CHD has been reported to occur in 4–10 per 1,000 live births and, in many cases, other defects are found including renal anomalies, diaphragmatic hernia, or tracheoesophageal fistula. There are multiple etiologies including diabetes, rubella during pregnancy, maternal alcohol or drugs during pregnancy, maternal age more than 40 years, and genetic factors. CHD occurs in many inherited conditions including Down syndrome.

Cardiac output is the amount of blood that is pumped per minute from the heart and is the stroke volume (of each heartbeat) times the number of beats per minute. In adults, the cardiac output is 4–5 liters per minute. Heart rate and blood pressure at different ages are shown in Table 21-1.

The symptoms of heart disease tend to be related to congestive heart failure. Heart failure results when there is strain on the myocardium from excess pressure of overload so that the cardiac output cannot meet the needs of the body. Symptoms and signs include tachypnea, tachycardia, dyspnea (evidenced by retractions), cool extremities, sweating, and tiredness. This leads to difficulty with feeding and failure to thrive. Cough and wheeze may be present. There may be an enlarged liver and edema around the eyes. Unlike the adult, ankle edema is not a feature.

Hypoxia means lack of oxygen and results in cyanosis or a blue hue of the skin which occurs when the oxygen saturation is less than 80–85 percent (desaturation). Central cyanosis implies that the blood leaving the heart through the aorta and going to the body is desaturated. The lips and tongue will be blue as well as the

TABLE 21-1. HEART RATE AND BLOOD PRESSURE AT DIFFERENT AGES

Age	Resting heart rate		Normal blood pressure		Upper limits (95%)	
	Low	High	Systolic	Diastolic	Systolic	Diastolic
			M / F	M / F	M / F	M / F
Newborn	80	160	73/65	55/55	92/84	72/72
1 year	70	120	90/91	56/54	109/110	73/71
6 years	60	90	96/96	57/57	115/115	74/74
12 years	50	90	107/107	64/66	126/107	81/82
18 years	50	90	121/112	70/66	140/112	88/84

body. Peripheral cyanosis occurs if there is increased extraction of oxygen from the blood in the periphery which occurs if the circulation is reduced.

Heart murmurs may be innocent (benign) which means that they are not associated with an organic lesion or structural defect of the heart. They are quite common except in infancy. They are important because there is a stigma to heart disease so that the presence of an innocent murmur should not convey a negative implication. Activity does not have to be restricted and it can be explained to the parents that it is like the noise that water makes going through pipes or hoses.

The electrocardiogram (EKG) is a record of electrical activity of the heart. The sinus (or sinoatrial) node orginates the heart beat and the wave passes in a circular motion around the atria prior to conduction through the atrioventricular (AV) node. The impulse moves rapidly through the conduction system of the ventricles in special pathways starting with the Bundle of His. The P-wave indicates atrial conduction, the QRS indicates ventricular conduction, and repolarization occurs with the T-wave.

The echocardiogram is an ultrasound and provides noninvasive information of structure and function of the heart. The science has expanded so that the procedure has become a standard test and can be performed in the out-patient clinic and even in the operating room (transesophageal echo). Fetal echocardiography is providing prenatal diagnosis of structural heart disease. Doppler color flow mapping allows calculation of the velocity of flow that allows a map of the direction of blood. Septal flow and regurgitation can be evaluated.

Cardiac catheterization is used to calculate flows, shunts, and resistance and provides physiologic information in addition to the anatomic detail and pressures in the heart. Interventional cardiology has become very sophisticated with the ability to enlarge or to create atrial communications, to occlude the patent ductus, and to embolize vascular structures. Embolization of vascular structures might be considered for arteriovenous malformations, bronchial collaterals, or aortopulmonary shunts. Balloon angioplasty, which involves stretching a vessel by inflation of a balloon at the site, has been successful in the treatment of aortic and pulmonic stenosis. Balloon angioplasty in coarctation of the aorta has been associated with complications (especially aneurism) when performed initially but is useful for recoarctation following surgery.

Congenital Heart Defects

Heart defects are classified in many ways. Defects are classified as cyanotic if there is significant hypoxia or acyanotic if oxygenation is normal. They vary in their effect on blood flow so that blood flow to the lungs could be increased or decreased; blood leaving the right or left heart may be reduced; or there may be shunting of blood from one side of the heart to the other. The congenital heart defects in these categories are shown in Table 21-2.

■ ACYANOTIC

Increased Pulmonary Flow

Atrial septal defect is most commonly the secundum (ASD 2) defect which is near the center of the atrial septum. The primum

TABLE 21-2. CLASSIFICATION OF CONGENITAL HEART LESIONS

Acyanotic lesions	
Increased pulmonary blood flow	*Obstructive lesions*
Atrial septal defect (ASD)	Coarctation of the aorta
Ventricular septal defect (VSD)	Pulmonic stenosis (PS)
Patent ductus arteriosus (PDA)	Aortic stenosis (AS)
Atrioventricular (AV) canal	
Cyanotic lesions	
Decreased pulmonary blood flow	*Miscellaneous lesions*
Tetralogy of Fallot (TOF)	Truncus arteriosus
Severe pulmonic stenosis	Total anomalous pulmonary venous
Pulmonary atresia	return (TAPVR)
Tricuspid atresia	Transposition of the great vessels
	Hypoplastic left heart syndrome

(ASD 1), which is close to the A-V junction, may involve the mitral valve. Persistent foramen ovale is also classified as an ASD. The pressure is higher in the left atrium and so blood passes from the left side of the heart to the right, and the amount of flow (shunt) increases the pulmonary blood flow. Many patients are asymptomatic, but heart failure may eventually occur. The murmur is systolic in the pulmonary area with wide fixed splitting of the pulmonary second sound. Cardiac enlargement or atrial arrhythmias may occur. Surgical treatment is performed with patch closure of the defect often before school age.

Ventricular septal defects (VSDs) vary in size from a pinhole to absence of the septum and can be a single defect or multiple. Blood flows from the high-pressure ventricle (left) to the low-pressure (right) ventricle and the amount of flow varies with the pressure difference and the size of the defect. The increased pulmonary blood flow can be excessive, leading to heart failure and pulmonary hypertension. The right side of the heart may hypertrophy. If the right-sided pressures increase over many months, it is possible for the right ventricular pressure to exceed the left (systemic) ventricle. This results in shunt reversal and arterial desaturation (Eisenmenger's syndrome).

There tends to be reduction in size of VSDs in the first few months of life and many small defects close spontaneously (maladie de Roget). Many VSDs are part of other syndromes. VSDs that are symptomatic present with heart failure, which may be severe, in the first few weeks of life. The murmur is holosystolic and usually accompanied by a thrill and is to the left of the lower sternum. Presentation is with respiratory distress and failure to thrive. Medical management is with digoxin and diuretics. Surgical treatment is closure of the VSD which often requires placement of a patch. If there is uncontrolled heart failure, banding of the pulmonary artery to protect the pulmonary vasculature and reduce the chance of pulmonary hypertension may be considered. The results of early repair are excellent and so banding is rarely necessary.

Patent ductus arteriosus (PDA) results when the connection between the left pulmonary artery and the descending aorta, which carries blood in fetal life, fails to close. The high pressure in the aorta allows blood to shunt left-to-right to the pulmonary artery. This commonly occurs in the premature baby and is treated with indomethacin or surgical ligation. Persistence beyond the newborn period is associated with a continuous (systolic and diastolic components) machinery-like murmur under the left clavicle. Pulses tend to be bounding. Patients may be asymptomatic or develop symptoms and signs of heart failure. It is treated by insertion of a coil or ligation and division.

Atrioventricular canal (AV canal) is also called endocardial fusion defect because there is a failure of fusion of this region. There is a low atrial septal defect with high ventricular septal defect with cleft of the mitral and tricuspid valves. It is usually initially acyanotic but cyanosis may occur especially with crying. The flow between the four chambers of the heart depends on the pressure differences between the systemic and pulmonary circuits.

AV canal is the most common cardiac defect in Down syndrome. The clinical symptoms are related to the development of congestive heart failure and there is a risk of pulmonary vascular disease. Pulmonary artery banding may be indicated to reduce pulmonary blood flow. Many centers advocate early repair with closure of the septal defects and reconstruction of the A-V valves.

Obstructive Lesions

Coarctation of the aorta is a narrowing of the aorta in the region of the ductus arteriosus. The narrowing results in upper-body hypertension and congestive heart failure. Females with coarctation may have Turner syndrome. Coarctation is associated with bicuspid aortic valve. Presentation in the infant tends to be because of cardiac failure which can be very acute and life threatening. High upper-limb blood pressure with absent femoral pulses is characteristic. Older children tend to present with symptoms of hypertension including headache and dizziness.

Presentation with acute heart failure may require aggressive ICU management with mechanical ventilation and inotropic support. Stabilization is necessary prior to correction of the defect.

Treatment used to be excision of the narrowed segment but most centers now perform balloon angioplasty.

Pulmonic stenosis (PS) is narrowing of the pulmonary outflow which causes reduced pulmonary blood flow and elevation of right ventricular pressure and eventually hypertrophy of the right ventricle. Valvotomy or balloon angioplasty may be indicated.

Aortic stenosis (AS) is obstruction to the left ventricular outflow because of narrowing or stricture of the aortic valve. Critical aortic stenosis is associated with syncope. Aortic valve stenosis is treated by valvotomy or balloon angioplasty.

■ CYANOTIC LESIONS

Decreased Pulmonary Blood Flow

Tetralogy of Fallot comprises four components: VSD, PS, overriding aorta, and right ventricular hypertrophy. The hemodynamic effects are dependent in the degree of right outflow obstruction which may include valvular stenosis and narrowing of the infundibulum. The VSD may be large with equal pressures of the right and left ventricle. Early correction may be indicated.

Severe pulmonic stenosis results in decreased pulmonary blood flow that may be reduced enough to cause right ventricular hypertrophy and result in flow through the foramen ovale. The combination of reduced pulmonary flow and right-to-left shunt results in cyanosis. If the commisures of the valve are totally fused, the lesion is called pulmonary atresia. Treatment involves dilation of the valve by balloon angioplasty in many cases. If there is atresia, the pulmonary arteries may be under-developed which makes repair difficult.

Tricuspid atresia occurs when the tricuspid valve fails to develop so that there is no flow into the right ventricle. The right atrium is large and the desaturated blood flows through an ASD into the left atrium. Mixing of blood in the left side of the heart results in systemic desaturation. If the only blood supply to the lungs in the newborn period is the patent ductus arteriosus, a continuous infusion of prostaglandin E_1 (PGE_1) is needed until surgical intervention is achieved. Palliative treatment includes a systemic to pulmonary artery shunt to improve blood flow to the lungs. A bidirectional shunt between the vena cava and the pulmonary artery (Glenn) may be helpful at a few months of age. A modified Fontan may be used to direct blood from the right atrium to the pulmonary artery (by-passing the ventricles).

Miscellaneous

Truncus Arteriosus. During the development of the heart, there is one outflow tract and this trunk divides into the aorta and pulmonary artery. If the separation fails to occur there is a single vessel leaving the two ventricles which means that the lungs are perfused at systemic pressures which results in pulmonary hypertension. The truncus receives blood from both ventricles resulting in desaturation and cyanosis. The pulmonary artery may arise from the base of the truncus (type I), right and left pulmonary arteries from the posterior truncus (type II), or from the lateral aspect of the truncus (type III). There is usually heart failure and cyanosis and there is a risk of endocarditis and brain abscess. The repair involves correcting the physiology with closure of the VSD and repositioning of the pulmonary vessels so that they receive blood from the right ventricle. Usually the repair is done when the infant is a few months of age.

Total Anomalous Pulmonary Venous Return (TAPVR). The pulmonary veins are four in number and normally return oxygenated blood from the lungs to the left atrium. Partial anomalous venous drainage means that one or more of the veins return to the right atrium and total anomalous if all the pulmonary veins return to the right side of the heart. The return may be supracardiac to the superior vena cava, cardiac to the right atrium or coronary sinus, or infracardiac with drainage below the diaphragm usually to the inferior vena cava. The infracardiac is associated with venous obstruction and requires immediate correction.

There is usually cyanosis early in life and heart failure may be severe. Correction involves implanting the pulmonary veins into the left atrium.

Transposition of the Great Arteries (or Vessels) (TGA/V). Transposition of the great vessels results when the aorta comes off the right ventricle and the pulmonary arteries arise from the left ventricle. Blood from the body comes back to the right atrium and blood returns from the lungs to the left atrium. TGV without VSD presents with immediate cyanosis and urgently requires cardiac catheterization to create an atrial septal communication which allows mixing of the circulations. PGE_1 is indicated to keep the ductus open. The (Raschkind) procedure involves pulling a balloon inflated with fluid to 15–20 mm back through the atrial septum and creating an interatrial communication. Arterial switch repair is the operation of choice. If this is not possible, then an atrial diversion (Mustard) procedure is performed.

Hypoplastic Left Heart Syndrome. This involves underdevelopment of the left side of the heart and may include severe mitral stenosis, hypoplastic left ventricle, and/or aortic atresia. Most of the left atrial blood goes through the right atrium across a patent foramen ovale. The pulmonary artery then supplies the lungs and then the systemic circulation through a patent ductus arteriosus. As the ductus closes, there is progressive heart failure and cyanosis. Until recently, it was considered to be a fatal lesion. Norwood devised a procedure of anastamosing the main pulmonary artery to the aorta. Additional procedures involve creation of shunts and a modified Fontan are used to improve the heart failure and hypoxemia. Alternatively, heart transplantation is a consideration.

Arrhythmias

Rhythm disturbances occur in CHD both from the defect, its treatment, and as a complication of surgery. Atrial arrhythmias occur more commonly than ventricular arrhythmia in children.

■ PAROXYSMAL SUPRAVENTRICULAR (ATRIAL) TACHYCARDIA

Paroxysmal supraventricular tachycardia is characterized by atrial rates of 200–300 that occur in episodes that cause congestive cardiac failure if they last more than a few minutes. Shorter episodes may not be a problem but infants are particularly at risk for developing shock secondary to the fast rate. There is usually no specific cause found although in older children and adults the episodes may be precipitated by emotion, fatigue, caffeine, or alcohol. Five to 10 percent of individuals with this rhythm show ventricular pre-excitation on the EKG between the episodes (Wolff–Parkinson–White syndrome).

Episodes of tachycardia may be stopped by massaging one carotid (do NOT massage both at the same time) to stimulate the vagus nerve. Alternate methods include stimulation of the diving reflex by placing a towel wrapped in ice on the face for about half a minute. It is not recommended to press on the eyeballs. Injection (intravenous) of adenosine produces a rapid but short-lived correction of the rapid rate. Digoxin is useful for long-term management.

Infants who have supraventricular tachycardia tend to have reduction in episodes after 1 year. Children who start this tachycardia later tend to have recurrences for years.

■ THIRD-DEGREE HEART BLOCK

Third-degree (complete) heart block occurs when the electrical impulse does not travel from the atria to the ventricles. In two-thirds of cases, no specific cause is found. It may be associated with heart disease, the most common lesion being corrected transposition of the great arteries. It is seen with maternal lupus and other connective tissue disorders. In childhood, the lesion may occur following cardiac surgery. The heart rate in complete heart block will be in the 40–60 range.

Most cases are asymptomatic although in childhood there may be fainting episodes (Stokes–Adams attacks) which may be associated with asystole or ventricular tachycardia or fibrillation. The episodes last 5–60 seconds and resolve spontaneously, although there is potential for sudden death. Stokes–Adams attacks require insertion of a pacemaker.

Hypertension

Hypertension is defined as persistent elevation of blood pressure above the levels shown in Table 21-1. There are different numbers that are used to meet the definition but usually the 95th percentile for age is the cutoff. Greater than the 99th percentile is classified as severe hypertension.

The causes of hypertension are multiple and may be primary or secondary. The common causes are shown in Table 21-3 and should be evaluated before treatment is recommended because the underlying cause should be treated first.

It is sensible to measure blood pressure as part of the routine physical examination because the symptoms of hypertension are non-specific. Headaches and dizziness are the most common complaints of older children and younger children and infants may have no obvious symptoms. Most children are discovered during routine exams, such as preschool or for camp.

The work-up of a child who has previously undiagnosed hypertension should include urinalysis, renal function tests, cholesterol and lipid profile, and electrolytes. Chest X-ray and EKG or echocardiogram may be considered.

TABLE 21-3. CAUSES OF SECONDARY HYPERTENSION

Renal
Chronic glomerulonephritis
Chronic pyelonephritis
Renal artery stenosis or thrombosis
Chronic renal failure
Malformations (cystic, etc.)
Obstructive uropathy

Endocrine
Cushing syndrome
Congenital adrenal hyperplasia
Primary hyperaldosteronism
Hyperthyroidism

Cardiovascular
Coarctation of the aorta

Central nervous system
Increased intracranial pressure
Dysautonomia

Respiratory
Bronchopulmonary dysplasia

Tumors
Pheochromocytoma
Neuroblastoma
Wilms tumor

Other
Obesity
Ingestions: contraceptives, steroids, cocaine, amphetamines, phencyclidine
Burns
Lead intoxication

Management of primary or essential hypertension should start with dietary and weight considerations, limitation of salt, increased exercise, and avoidance of stress and smoking.

Many milder cases respond to lifestyle changes and they should be tried first. Pharmacologic treatment is used for more severe hypertension and includes beta blockers (propranolol), ACE inhibitors, and diuretics. Home blood pressure monitoring by one of the caretakers can be useful to follow the effect of therapy.

Infective Endocarditis

Infective endocarditis may be acute or subacute. It most commonly results from tetralogy of Fallot, complex cyanotic disease, VSD, PDA and aortic valve disease. It is rare to occur in the absence of underlying heart disease. Change in heart murmur and splenomegaly are the most common findings with peripheral embolization causing petechiae and splinter hemorrhages of the fingernails.

Streptococci and staphylococci account for 80 percent of the cases. It is increasingly seen in IV drug abusers because of repeated exposure to bacteria, or if there is poor dentition.

Myocardial Disease

There are several glycogen storage diseases that affect the heart. Pompe disease is the most common with onset at about 6 months of age. This results from acid maltase deficiency that causes retardation of growth and development with congestive heart failure. Death usually occurs within a few months.

Anomalous origin of the left coronary artery (arising from the pulmonary artery) results in ischemia when the pulmonary pressures lower. Presentation is with pallor, sweating, and abdominal pain at a few months of age. Cardiac enlargement is seen on X-ray and the EKG is diagnostic, demonstrating findings of myocardial infarction. Medical management is usually ineffective and surgery is indicated.

■ CARDIOMYOPATHY

Chronic myocardial diseases are called cardiomyopathies. Dilated cardiomyopathy is the most common type, hypertrophic is less common, and restrictive is rare in children. Dilated cardiomyopathy is most commonly seen following viral myocarditis.

Primary endocardial fibroelastosis is a disorder of thickening of the endocardium. Symptoms of left ventricular failure develop during the first year of life. Infants have dyspnea and feeding difficulty and the heart is enlarged. Medical treatment can control symptoms in many cases but some fail medical management and require heart transplant.

Rheumatic Fever

Rheumatic fever follows infection with group A streptococci. It occurs about 3 weeks after pharyngitis. During the acute infection, there is an acute migratory polyarthritis. The joints are red, hot, swollen and very tender if touched or moved. Most commonly, it is large joints and when one joint improves another becomes involved. The duration of arthritis lasts less than 1 month. It responds to aspirin so that if aspirin does not cause improvement, another diagnosis is likely. The heart involvement initially is asymptomatic and the endocarditis is manifested by the onset of the heart murmur. The most common murmur is the systolic murmur of mitral regurgitation. Carditis is associated with tachycardia that is more than expected for the degree of fever. Cardiomegaly may be present on chest X-ray. Pericarditis may be evident with friction rub and chest pain. Sydenham's chorea has jerky, purposeless movements of the extremities with weakness. It is associated with clumsiness and the movements may become extreme and produce injury. It is one of the major criteria but can occur in other conditions. Subcutaneous nodules are 0.5–1 cm swellings that occur over bony prominences especially the extendor tendons of the hands, feet, and elbows. The diagnosis is made by the presence of the Jones criteria (Table 21-4), with supporting evidence of post-streptococcal infection.

TABLE 21-4. CRITERIA FOR THE DIAGNOSIS OF RHEUMATIC FEVER

Major manifestations	Minor manifestations
Carditis	Clinical
Polyarthritis	Previous rheumatic fever
Chorea	Fever
Erythema marginatum	Arthralgia
Subcutaneous nodules	Laboratory
	Acute phase reactants:
	ESR
	C-reactive protein
	Leukocytosis
	Prolonged P-R interval

■ MANAGEMENT

After the diagnosis is made, a full course of penicillin is given. In the future, prophylaxis is given. The usual regimen is an IM injection every 3 weeks or oral penicillin daily. Children with severe carditis or heart failure are more likely to develop valvular cardiac disease.

22
Chapter Twenty-Two

Renal Disease

The kidneys regulate the amount of fluid and electrolytes that are excreted so that intake and output are approximately equal. The total body water is the sum of the extracellular fluid (ECF) and intracellular fluid (ICF). Sodium (Na^+) is the dominant cation of the ECF comprising 95 percent of the total body sodium. The volume of the ECF is directly dependent on the quantity of total body sodium. Water loss is from the lungs and skin (insensible loss) and from the kidneys (renal excretion). The pH of the ECF is normally 7.35–7.45 and is regulated by the respiratory system which controls carbon dioxide excretion and by the kidneys, which control bicarbonate excretion. The kidneys are also responsible for regulating the excretion of potassium (K^+) which is in high concentrations in the ICF compared to the ECF. Potassium has a very important role in cellular functions and in the maintenance of volume and pH of the cell. If kidney function is impaired and there is reduced renal excretion of potassium, hyperkalemia results. Metabolic wastes including urea nitrogen, creatinine, phosphorus, and uric acid, are also excreted by the kidney.

The urinalysis is the most useful examination for any patient who has suspected kidney disease. It should be considered when evaluating any child for a health problem and as a screen for unsuspected illness. The specimen should be freshly voided (within 1 hour), and collected into a clean or sterile container after cleaning the external genitalia. The advantage of collecting the first morning specimen is that a more concentrated and acidified urine will be obtained.

Urine color varies with the concentration and presence of pigments, particularly urochrome, carotene, and urobilin. The concentration of the urine is expressed as the specific gravity which ranges from 1.001 (very dilute) to 1.030 (very concentrated). Urine pH varies from 4.5 (acid) to about 8.0 (alkaline). Increased amounts of protein in the urine occur in febrile illnesses, seizures, and as a result of stress or exercise. This is a transient increase that resolves when the condition improves. Orthostatic proteinuria occurs in normal individuals and results from increased protein excretion when standing as opposed to lying down. Persistent proteinuria usually implies glomerular damage but small amounts may be excreted in tubular disease.

Glycosuria implies excess glucose in the urine and is measured by the glucose oxidase method. All reducing sugars, including glucose, are measured by the standard copper-reduction method that is the basis of the Clinitest tablets. If the serum glucose exceeds the renal threshold for glucose, it will appear in the urine. The most common cause for glycosuria is diabetes mellitus. It may also occur with tubular defects and in this situation the serum glucose may be normal.

Hematuria may be microscopic and is detectable with the dipstick method which can detect the equivalent of 3–4 red cells per high-power field of hemoglobin or myoglobin. Macroscopic hematuria implies that the urine is pink or red colored and may appear smokey and clots may be visible. In addition to seeing red cells on microscopy, white cells, bacteria, casts or crystals may be seen. White cells do not always indicate infection because they are commonly increased in inflammatory renal conditions as well as in hypertension and febrile states. Bacteria may indicate urinary-tract infection and a culture of voided urine containing greater than 100,000 colony-forming units per milliliter is abnormal. Casts are formed in the renal tubule; red cell casts imply glomerulonephritis, and white cell casts indicate pyelonephritis. Crystals may be observed in centrifuged urine and phosphate and urate crystals are usually a normal finding. Sulfa crystals may be seen if the patient is taking sulfonamides and cystine crystals suggest cystinuria.

The kidneys produce urine via ultrafiltration of plasma which perfuses through the glomeruli. About 20 percent of the cardiac output passes through the renal arteries. There is selective reabsorption of water and solutes by the renal tubule and 99 percent of fluid, sodium, and bicarbonate is reabsorbed into the blood. The glomerular filtration rate (GFR) reflects the overall excretory function of the kidneys. The best estimation of GFR that is useful in the clinical situation is the creatinine clearance. Creatinine is the metabolic end-product of normal muscle metabolism and the rate of production parallels very closely the rate of excretion.

Chronic Renal Failure

Chronic renal failure (CRF) is the long-term deterioration of renal function resulting in the failure to maintain normal excretory and regulatory balance. There may be four stages including early renal failure when the glomerular filtration rate (GFR) is 50–75 percent of normal. There is decreased renal reserve but fairly normal regulatory and excretory function. The second stage may be chronic renal insufficiency when the GFR is 25–50 percent with impairment of renal function. Chronic renal failure results when the GFR is 10–25 percent. End stage renal disease (ESRD) is defined by a GFR of less than 10 percent so that renal replacement therapy (RRT), including dialysis or transplantation, is necessary to sustain life.

CRF is associated with a variety of congenital and acquired illnesses. The various pathologies include obstructive uropathy, glomerulopathy, collagen vascular disease, metabolic or cystic diseases, and malignancies (see Table 22-1). Children with congenital disorders or whose renal disease begins in infancy are at greatest risk for growth failure and ESRD. It is important to establish the cause of CRF because treatment tends to be

TABLE 22-1. CAUSES OF CHRONIC RENAL FAILURE

Developmental abnormalities of the urinary tract
Hypoplasia, dysplasia or aplasia
Polycystic kidneys
Obstructive uropathy
Hereditary
Alport syndrome
Congenital nephrotic syndrome
Renal parenchymal disorders
Chronic glomerulonephritis
Hemolytic uremic syndrome
Pyelonephritis/Chronic urinary tract infection
Renal vein thrombosis
Hypertensive glomerulosclerosis
Renal tumor
Metabolic
Diabetes mellitus
Cystinosis
Oxalosis

diagnosis-specific and the prognosis varies. Genetic counseling may be important for the family planning other children if there is a metabolic or hereditary disorder.

The kidneys have the potential to adapt to loss of nephrons. Glomerular function as a whole compensates although tubular function does not adapt as well. There may be hypertrophy of remaining renal tissue such that removal of one kidney is followed by an increase in size so that the remaining kidney reaches 80 percent of the mass of the two kidneys. However, if there is loss of 75 percent of renal function, there is gradual sclerosis of the remaining glomeruli resulting in progression to end-stage renal disease. CRF results in various biochemical and systemic manifestations in addition to losing the ability to control fluid, electrolytes, and excretion.

Bone demineralization and impaired growth result from secretion of parathyroid hormone, elevation of plasma phosphate, acidosis, and impaired intestinal calcium absorption. The condition is known as renal osteodystrophy and the effects are varied. The outcomes include osteitis fibrosa cystica from hyper-parathyroidism and osteomalacia or rickets. The condition results from the inability to excrete phosphate with fall in ionized calcium that leads to secretion of parathormone. Eventually, this leads to osteoclastic bone resorption which leads to cystic defects in bones, especially in the hands. Osteomalacia and rickets result from defective mineralization of bone.

Reduction of the effect of renal osteodystrophy is achieved by using a phosphate binder. Characteristically, this has been aluminum, but aluminum may cause osteomalacia and calcium salts may be preferred. Vitamin D analogues may also be pre-scribed.

Anemia results from impaired red cell production and decreased red cell life span. There is a deficiency of erythropoetin (EPO) which appears to be the primary cause. Bleeding results from impaired platelet function contributing to the anemia. Replenishment of iron stores, prescription of EPO, and, on occasions, blood transfusion are all considerations for manage-ment.

Neurologic abnormalities are frequent in CRF with seizures because of hypertension and metabolic abnormalities. Encephalopathy accompanies advanced renal failure. There may be loss of milestones and slowing of head growth in young children.

The incidence of CRF has been estimated at 18 per 1 million children and the incidence of end-stage renal disease is 3–6 per 1 million children.

■ CLINICAL FEATURES

The individual patient may present with different symptoms based on the diagnosis and the severity of involvement:

- Fluid overload with edema, oliguria, hypertension, and congestive heart failure.
- Intravascular volume depletion secondary to polyuria and inadequate fluid intake with dehydration.
- Electrolyte imbalance.

- Hyperkalemia.
- Metabolic acidosis.
- Retention of waste products especially urea and creatinine.
- Calcium and phosphorus abnormalities.
- Anemia or bleeding.
- Growth disturbance.
- Gastrointestinal symptoms including anorexia and vomiting.
- Neurologic changes including seizures, confusion, and encephalopathy.

■ MANAGEMENT

Treatment includes non-specific measures to control the effects of CRF and to reduce the progression toward ESRD. There needs to be aggressive treatment of hypertension. Hypertension may be an effect of CRF but it also can worsen the kidney damage. There may need to be limitation of water and salt intake and pharmacologic methods to correct hypertension. The other clinical features of CRF that can be treated to improve outcome include correction of metablic acidosis with sodium bicarbonate or citrate, control of hyperphosphatemia, correction of anemia, and aggressive management of growth and nutrition.

When conservative management fails to control the metabolic abnormalities, dialysis and transplantation are the options. Peritoneal dialysis involves placement of a silastic catheter which is inserted into the peritoneal cavity through the abdominal wall. A sterile solution of glucose and electrolytes is instilled into the peritoneal space and after equilibration is drained from the abdomen. There is removal of fluid, electrolytes, and waste products dependent on the gradient and diffusion of the substance. Each pass is called an exchange and there may be several passes in a day. Peritoneal dialysis may be a home procedure and most families manage to achieve the skills to perform dialysis. The major complication of peritoneal dialysis is infection.

Hemodialysis involves circulating blood through a dialysis machine that filters fluids, electrolytes, and waste by diffusion across a semipermeable membrane. Vascular access is achieved with an arteriovenous shunt which allows needles or catheters to be attached during dialysis. Hemodialysis is performed in a hospital or clinic setting rather than at home. The usual regimen is 3–4 hours treatment 3 times per week.

Renal transplantation is the definitive treatment for ESRD. The best results have been if the kidney donor is a close relative but cadaveric transplantation is performed if there is no suitable live donor. Most kidney transplant recipients have an immunosuppression regimen that includes prednisone, azathioprine, and cyclosporine. Rejection and infection remain the major problems following transplantation. The 2-year survival rate for related donor is over 80 percent and it is 60–70 percent for cadaveric renal transplantation.

Alport Syndrome

First described by Alport in the early 1900s, Alport syndrome is progressive hereditary nephritis. It is characterized by glomerulonephritis, sensorineural deafness, and ocular abnormalities. The symptoms include hematuria, proteinuria, and progressive renal insufficiency. There is a high-frequency hearing loss in adolescence which may only be detectable on hearing testing. It accounts for 3 percent of children with chronic renal failure.

Inheritance is autosomal male-to-male dominant, autosomal recessive, and X-linked dominant that has been localized to the middle of the long arm of the Y chromosome.

Glomerulonephritis

Chronic glomerulonephritis (CGN) is a group of disorders with injury to the vascular tuft of the renal glomeruli. Most cases are the result of a progression of acute disorders into a chronic

TABLE 22-2. CAUSES OF GLOMERULONEPHRITIS (GN)

Post-infectious glomerulonephritis
  Post-streptococcal GN
Membranoproliferative GN
  Types I and II
IgA nephropathy
Henoch–Schönlein purpura GN
Glomerulonephritis of lupus erythematosis
Hereditary GN
  Alport syndrome
Goodpasture syndrome

condition (Table 22-2). The causes are intrinsic renal diseases and systemic conditions that also involve the kidneys.

■ MEMBRANOPROLIFERATIVE GLOMERULONEPHRITIS (MPGN)

MPGN is also known as mesangiocapillary or hypocomplementemic GN and accounts for 8 percent of children with primary nephrotic syndrome. It also presents as acute nephritic syndrome, rapidly progressive GN, and persistent hematuria or proteinuria. There are various histologic types but there is low plasma complement C3. The presentation also varies from minor urinalysis abnormalities to nephritic–nephrotic syndrome with gross hematuria, edema, hypotension, and azotemia (high blood urea nitrogen). Diagnosis is established by renal biopsy.

Because of the variability of presentation and progression, there is no specific treatment strategy, although alternate day prednisone seems to be the best option.

■ MEMBRANOUS GLOMERULONEPHRITIS (MGN)

There is generalized thickening of the basement membrane of the glomerulus with immune complex deposition. The cause may be idiopathic or it may occur in association with a systemic condition. In children, 50 percent are secondary and the conditions include autoimmune disorders, infections, drugs and toxins, and hemoglobinopathies. The nephrotic syndrome may result and hematuria is common. Although most patients (65–90 percent) do not progress to end-stage renal disease, there are some who have a steady progression of disease. The decision to treat is difficult, and prednisone, cytotoxic agents, or cyclosporine may be indicated.

Nephrotic Syndrome

The nephrotic syndrome (NS) is defined by the presence of massive proteinuria, hypoalbuminemia, edema, and hyperlipidemia. There is glomerular injury that results in increased permeability so that there is a significant loss of protein that is mostly albumin. The amount of protein excreted in the urine in children is greater than 50 mg/kg/day and in adults it is greater than 3.5 g/day. The resultant hypoalbuminemia leads to edema, and there is hyperlipidemia and hypercholesterolemia. The term primary NS replaces the older term idiopathic NS and there are several secondary causes. In children, primary NS is more important than secondary and is classified on the basis of the histological changes. Table 22-3 shows the common primary and secondary causes of the nephrotic syndrome.

The presentation of NS is usually the appearance of edema which is dependent and leads to swollen eyes in the morning and

TABLE 22-3. PRIMARY AND SECONDARY NEPHROTIC SYNDROME

Congenital nephrotic syndrome
  Lipoid nephrosis
  Minimal change disease
Focal glomerular sclerosis
Mesangial nephropathy
Membranous nephropathy
Diabetic nephropathy
Renal vein thrombosis
Lupus nephrotic syndrome
Heavy metal nephrotic syndrome (e.g., gold)

feet in the evening. There may be significant weight gain, abdominal distension with ascites, and pleural effusions leading to respiratory distress.

■ MINIMAL CHANGE NEPHROTIC SYNDROME (MCNS)

The title describes the findings on renal biopsy with normal-appearing glomeruli and some increase in mesangial cellularity. There is no deposition of immunoglobulins except for some cases that show IgM mesangial deposition. MCNS is the commonest (78 percent) cause of the primary nephrotic syndrome in children with a peak occurrence between 2 and 6 years of age. Often there is a mild viral infection, or a history of allergies or immunization, followed by the development of edema. Most patients have normal blood pressure and renal function but some patients may have hypertension and azotemia. Mild hematuria is possible, but if it is gross or there are red cell casts, then the diagnosis is in doubt. Serum complement (C3) levels are normal.

Treatment consists of glucocorticoids and supportive therapies which include dietary restrictions, antihypertensives, and diuretics. Steroids result in a good therapeutic response with reduction of proteinuria and diuresis of fluid. Within 8 weeks, over 90 percent are improved with resolution of proteinuria. Children who relapse may have become either steroid dependent or steroid resistant. Cytotoxic drugs including cyclophosphamide or chlorambucil may be used and remission is often induced. Progression to renal failure does not occur but there may be complications related to treatment or problems of infection.

■ FOCAL SEGMENTAL GLOMERULOSCLEROSIS (FSGS)

The initial presentation of FSGS is similar to MCNS. It tends to be diagnosed when a child who was thought to have MCNS is not responsive to treatment. There is focal and segmental sclerosis of the glomerular tuft with increased mesangial matrix and basement membrane. It is considered that the two conditions are etiologically separate and that FSGS is not a progression of

MCNS. About 7–15 percent of cases of the nephrotic syndrome are FSGS and more than 85 percent are resistant to steroids. Treatment with cyclosporine or cytotoxic agents has not been beneficial. About 25 percent progress to renal failure in 5 years and require dialysis or transplantation. There is a 40 percent risk of recurrence in the transplanted kidney.

Congenital Renal Tract Anomalies

■ POLYCYSTIC DISEASE OF THE KIDNEYS

There are two forms of polycystic kidney: autosomal recessive polycystic kidney disease (AR-PKD), formerly known as infantile PKD, and autosomal dominant polycystic (AD-PKD), formerly known as adult PKD. AD-PKD comprises two forms: PKD1 with a gene locus on 16p and PKD2 possibly on chromosome 2.

AR-PKD has two subgroups, the severe diffuse disease with enlarged kidneys in newborns, and the more limited, sometimes patchy disease that progresses to variable cortical atrophy in older children. Some newborns have innumerable cysts of the collecting ducts and die from the accompanying pulmonary hypoplasia. Both forms are accompanied by hepatic abnormalities that in older children can lead to portal hypertension and have been designated as congenital hepatic fibrosis. AR-PKD may result in hypertension or chronic renal failure requiring dialysis and renal transplantation. AD-PKD usually remains asymptomatic until the fifth or sixth decade but can present at any time.

■ URETEROPELVIC JUNCTION (UPJ) OBSTRUCTION

This is the commonest obstructive lesion of the urinary tract in childhood. The lesion may be disarray of the musculature at this position or extrinsic compression by an aberrant renal artery. UPJ obstruction may be complete with severe renal dysplasia.

Lesser degrees of obstruction lead to hydronephrosis with recurrent urinary-tract infections. It may be detected on fetal ultrasound. Treatment requires surgical removal of the obstructed segment and reanastamosis (pyeloplasty).

■ PRUNE BELLY SYNDROME

The triad of large flaccid abdominal wall with absent musculature, undescended testes, and a hypertrophied, dilated collecting system without obstruction is also called Eagle–Barrett syndrome. In females (without cryptorchidism), the syndrome accounts for 3–5 percent of patients. The incidence is 1 in 29–40,000 and the etiology is unknown. Approximately 20 percent will die in the newborn period as a result of pulmonary hypoplasia secondary to severe renal hypoplasia. There is a group of patients who have reasonable pulmonary function but severe involvement of the urinary tract. Presentation with azotemia, renal failure, and failure to thrive may be static or progressive. The remaining patients have normal pulmonary and renal function.

The abdominal wall defect results in delay in walking and there may be respiratory infections and chronic constipation. Most patients have intra-abdominal testes which have a 30–50 times incidence of malignant degeneration. Orchiopexy is performed before the age of 1 year. GI anomalies, including malrotation, volvulus, and atresia, are common.

■ POSTERIOR URETHRAL VALVES

Posterior urethral valves (PUV) obstruct the urinary outflow from the bladder in boys. Type I valves are folds that radiate anteriorly and are fused as a membrane for most of their course. Type II valves proceed proximally and divide into membranes that are of no clinical significance. Type III are diaphragms that may be proximal or distal. The incidence of PUV is 1 in 5–8,000 males. The cause is unknown and no genetic defect has been found. PUV are part of a dysplastic syndrome that may involve the entire urinary tract. There may be bilateral hydronephrosis. Voiding cystourethrogram (VCUG) will confirm the presence of valves in the urethra. The clinical findings range from severe obstruction to milder obstruction with difficulty urinating and a weak stream. Achievement of adequate urine drainage is the immediate goal. Transurethral surgical ablation can be performed endoscopically. Approximately 26 percent of patients with PUV will eventually develop chronic renal failure.

Hemolytic Uremic Syndrome

There is acute renal failure, microangiopathic hemolytic anemia, and thrombocytopenia. There is an epidemic form which presents with a GI prodrome with abdominal pain, vomiting, and diarrhea. The sporadic form has no prodrome. On occasions (more common in adults) it is secondary to drugs, the post-partum period, collagen vascular disease, malignant disease, and following transplantation. There is thrombotic microangiopathy especially of the kidney and brain. The most common organism has been *Escherichia coli* 0157 : H7 and it has been associated with *Shigella* and *Salmonella*.

Following the prodrome, there is hematuria and protein-uria with anemia and thrombocytopenia. The degree of hemolytic anemia varies from mild to severe and thrombo-cytopenia results from clumping and removal of platelets from the circulation. Central nervous system involvement occurs in 30 percent of cases with seizures, drowsiness, paralysis, or coma.

■ **MANAGEMENT**

Treatment is directed at correcting the anemia and thrombo-cytopenia and electrolyte abnormalities. Some patients develop anuria and may require dialysis. The mortality rate is 5–10 percent so that aggressive treatment is appropriate but the majority of patients improve with time. Prolonged anuria is associated with worse renal prognosis and the potential for chronic renal failure.

Henoch–Schönlein Purpura

Henoch–Schönlein purpura (HSP), also known as anaphylactoid purpura, is a generalized aseptic vasculitis of small blood vessels. The only etiologic agent that has been implicated is beta-hemolytic streptococcus. Seventy-five percent of patients present before 10 years of age. The clinical features include a skin rash which starts as an urticarial-type lesion and progresses to petechial and purpuric over the lower extremities and buttocks. Arthritis affects the majority of patients with joint swelling, mostly of the lower extremities, that is migratory. Abdominal vasculitis results in bowel wall edema and hemorrhage. There is acute abdominal pain, vomiting, and melena. Intussusception or perforation may result. Isolated hematuria or proteinuria or both are the most common. The usual renal pathology is segmental or focal glomerulonephritis.

In most cases, the course is short and symptoms resolve in 6 weeks. In a small number of children, exacerbations recur at intervals for years. Approximately 5–10 percent develop chronic nephritis with eventual renal failure.

IgA Nephropathy

Recurrent hematuria, which usually occurs after a viral infection and is associated with mesangial deposits of IgA, is called Berger disease. The diagnosis is only confirmed by renal biopsy and so the incidence is not known. It is the most frequent diagnosis made on renal biopsy. Progressive glomerular disease occurs in 30–50 percent of patients and 10 percent progress to chronic renal failure.

Renal Tubular Acidosis

Renal tubular acidosis (RTA) is a clinical syndrome in which impaired renal acidification is manifest by a chronic hyperchloremic metabolic acidosis and inappropriately high urine pH.

■ PROXIMAL RTA

There is impaired reabsorbtion of bicarbonate in the proximal renal tubule. There is a metabolic acidosis because of reduced acid excretion. As the plasma bicarbonate decreases, there is no further bicarbonate secretion in the urine and there is enhanced secretion of potassium with resultant hypokalemia. Proximal RTA occurs in a variety of diseases, usually as part of the Fanconi syndrome.

Fanconi syndrome is a generalized dysfunction of proximal tubule transport. The most common cause is cystinosis. The effects of the Fanconi syndrome include hypophosphatemia and often hypocalcemia and hypomagnesemia. There may be retarded bone age with rickets and osteomalacia. Nephrocalcinosis and nephrolithiasis usually do not occur. Primary proximal RTA may be genetically transmitted or idiopathic. Secondary proximal RTA is more common and may be associated with hereditary defects of amino acid or carbohydrate metabolism. The combination of persistent hyperchloremic metabolic acidosis with an acid urine pH is consistent with proximal RTA. The amount of bicarbonate wasting indicates the amount of alkali necessary for replacement. The alkali may lead to a further drop in potassium levels.

■ DISTAL RTA

Hypokalemic distal RTA is an inability to acidify the urine below pH 5.5 with reduced excretion of ammonium, phosphate, and hydrogen ions. Proximal tubular function is normal and, in particular, the Fanconi defect is not present. The effect of the chronic positive acid balance is calcium, magnesium, and phosphate wasting. This results in dissolution of bone.

Primary distal RTA may occur as an inherited defect with metabolic acidosis in the first few months of life. Nephrocalcinosis (renal stones) may result. Many disorders are associated with secondary distal RTA including autoimmune disorders with hyperglobulinemia.

Distal RTA is suggested by hypokalemic–hyperchloremic metabolic acidosis with an alkaline urine pH. The initial management requires correction of the hypokalemia. Oral bicarbonate will usually suffice to correct the acidosis.

23

Chapter Twenty-Three

Gastrointestinal Disorders

The gastrointestinal (GI) tract is a continuous lumen from the mouth to the anus. The primary function is the digestion and absorption of food and the secondary function is the regulation of nutrients and fluids. The esophagus connects the mouth and pharynx to the stomach. The stomach is a reservoir that secretes acid and pepsin which initiates the digestion of protein. The small intestine comprises sequentially the duodenum, the jejunum, and then the ileum. The common bile duct (from the liver) and the pancreatic duct enter the second part of the duodenum at the ampulla of Vater. The jejunum (40 percent) and ileum (60 percent) are 200–250 cm in the neonate and 350–600 cm in the adult. The majority of absorption of amino acids, mono- and disaccharides (sugars), and fats are absorbed in the jejunum. The large intestine reabsorbs fluid and electrolytes and comprises the cecum, the ascending, transverse and descending colon, the rectum, and anus. There is also absorption of short-chain fatty acids in the cecum and proximal colon.

Vomiting is a symptom that is present in a wide variety of disorders, both GI and other illnesses. It must be distinguished from regurgitation which is effortless. Vomiting is associated with nausea which is the feeling that vomiting will occur. Nausea may have other symptoms related to autonomic stimulation including pallor, sweating, salivation, and loss of appetite. Retching is the motor response of the GI tract that does not lead to emesis and emesis is the forceful expulsion of stomach contents. There is a vomiting center in the brainstem which is stimulated by the brain or GI tract as well as by substances (e.g., drugs or ketone) in the blood.

Broad categories of disorders resulting in chronic vomiting are shown in Table 23-1. The causes include both GI and non-GI conditions and the severity varies from mild to severe. The evaluation will be initiated with history and physical examination and the diagnostic work-up will be dependent upon the findings. Vomiting may be the initial symptom of a serious disorder, such as small-

TABLE 23-1. CAUSES OF CHRONIC VOMITING

Esophageal
GE reflux
Hiatus hernia
Congenital vascular ring
Esophageal duplication/diverticulum

Upper GI
Peptic ulcer disease
Superior mesenteric artery syndrome
Intussusception
Malrotation
Small-bowel obstruction
Milk protein intolerance (cow/soy)

Lower GI
Hirschsprung disease
Distal intestinal obstruction syndrome (cystic fibrosis)

Metabolic
Urea cycle defects
Hypercalcemia
Aminoacidopathies
Uremia
Diabetic ketoacidosis

Other
Migraine
Hepatitis
Cyclical vomiting
Anorexia/bulimia nervosa

bowel obstruction, or it may be a symptom of a chronic disorder that will require investigation that might include upper GI series or endoscopy. It is described as bilious if it is yellow. If there is obstruction proximal to the ampulla of Vater (e.g., pyloric stenosis), vomiting will not be bilious.

Diarrhea and constipation can be either acute or chronic. The causes are multiple and the evaluation needs to be methodical. Abdominal pain is a common symptom in children. The diagnostic approach will vary with the age of the patient, the progression of the symptoms, and the additional signs and symptoms that are present. The work-up of GI disorders includes evaluation of growth, including height and weight, relationship of symptoms to eating, presence of discomfort or pain, and implication of associated findings. The presence of bleeding may be indicated by hematemesis (vomiting blood) or blood in the stools. Hematemesis is vomiting blood which varies from streaks to gross bright-red blood or it can be "coffee ground emesis." Bright-red blood in the stool (hematochezia) usually implies bleeding from the lower GI tract whereas upper GI bleeding results in melena which is dark and tar-like. Occult blood implies blood in the stool that is not visible but is positive on Occultest.

Physical examination of the abdomen includes evaluation for abdominal masses. Table 23-2 shows a differential diagnosis of abdominal masses and their location.

TABLE 23-2. LOCATION AND CAUSES OF ABDOMINAL MASSES

Right upper quadrant: Liver, gallbladder, kidney, adrenal
Left upper quadrant: Spleen, stomach, kidney, adrenal
Periumbilical: Pancreas, bowel, mesentery, retroperitoneum
Suprapubic: Bladder, uterus, ovary
Causes

Liver:	Hepatoblastoma
Gallbladder:	Choledochal cyst
Kidney:	Wilms tumor
	Hydronephrosis
	Polycystic kidney
Adrenal:	Neuroblastoma
Bowel:	Mesenteric cyst
Ovary:	Ovarian cyst
	Hydrometrocolpos

GI endoscopy has become a very important component of diagnosis and treatment of GI disorders. Chronic liver disease is becoming more important in pediatrics. There is greater understanding of metabolic and genetic disorders. Liver transplant is being increasingly utilized for childhood conditions.

Inflammatory Bowel Disease

The term inflammatory bowel disease (IBD) encompasses Crohn (or Crohn's) disease and ulcerative colitis. They are similar entities in terms of signs, symptoms, and management (Table 23-3). Both illnesses are chronic GI disorders, but they are not the same pathologically and the associated complications tend to be different. The etiology of either condition is unknown and appears to be a complex inter-relationship between genetic susceptibility and immunology, with psychology altering the course and severity. There are multiple extraintestinal manifestations (Table 23-4).

TABLE 23-3. COMPARISON OF CROHN DISEASE AND ULCERATIVE COLITIS

	Crohn disease	Ulcerative colitis
Diarrhea	Varies	Often severe
Weight loss	Severe	Moderate
Growth retardation	Often marked	Usually mild
Rectal bleeding	Uncommon	Common
Anal & perianal lesions	Common	Rare
Fistulas and structures	Common	Rare
Toxic megacolon	Rare	May occur
Location	Terminal ileum commonest	Colon and rectum
Histology	Transmural involvement	Mucosa and submucosa
Gross appearance	Longitudinal ulcerations	Friable mucosa, pseudopolyps
X-ray findings	String sign: areas of stenosis	Loss of haustral markings

TABLE 23-4. **EXTRAINTESTINAL MANIFESTATIONS OF INFLAMMATORY BOWEL DISEASE**

Fever
Growth failure
Anemia, thrombocytosis
Aphthous mouth ulcers
Arthritis, arthralgias
Ankylosing spondylitis
Clubbing
Erythema nodosum
Pyoderma gangrenosum
Ocular disorders, episcleritis, uveitis
Hepatobiliary disease
Nephrolithiasis
Myocarditis, Pericarditis
Pulmonary fibrosis
Amyloidosis
Thromboembolic disease

■ CROHN DISEASE

The condition was publicized by Drs. Crohn, Ginzberg, and Oppenheimer in 1932, but the original description was probably from an article in a British journal in 1913. Small-bowel Crohn disease is also known as regional ileitis.

Description

Although the major pathology occurs at the terminal ileum and ileocecal junction (50–60 percent), it is isolated to the terminal ileum in 20 percent, or there may be involvement throughout the GI tract from mouth to anus. The inflammation causes non-caseating granulomas with ulceration that produces a cobblestone appearance and normal tissue is interspersed. The characteristic finding is "skip lesions," and there may be bowel thickening with resultant stenosis and stricture. Fistula development is common and is a complication of surgery. The fistulae may be to other loops of bowel, to the skin, or to bladder or vagina. The etiology of Crohn disease is unknown but is considered to be an immune-mediated response because of the extra-intestinal manifestations such as arthritis and the response to immunosuppressive therapies. Genetic influences are suspected because there is a higher incidence in Ashkenazic Jews and there is some familial clustering. Psychological influences appear to play a role in modifying the presentation and course of the disease.

Clinical Features

The incidence of Crohn disease is reported to be from 1–7 cases per 100,000 and appears to be increasing over time. The peak occurrence is between 15 and 35 years of age. Seventy-five percent of pediatric patients present with disease in the terminal ileum and cecum or right colon. The onset is usually slow with diarrhea that is often accompanied by abdominal pain and tenderness and weight loss. It may be a year from the onset of symptoms to the time of diagnosis. Growth retardation is common and may precede clinical symptoms. Blood in the stool may be obvious or occult. Perianal disease is common in children with skin tags, fistulas, fissures, and hemorrhoids. On occasions (10 percent), the onset is acute and sometimes severe and may simulate an acute appendicitis.

The diagnosis is made by radiographic study, usually barium enema, which shows mucosal thickening, cobblestone appearance, scarring, string sign, and areas of stenosis. Endoscopy is used to visualize the lesions and biopsy provides pathologic correlation. Hypoalbuminemia is common.

Management

Medical therapy involves corticosteroids, although there is not good evidence that it alters the long-term course. Remission is induced in about 70 percent of cases. Unfortunately, 70 percent of those treated with steroids will relapse in 1 year. Doses of 2 mg/kg of prednisone (maximum 60 mg) per day are recommended initially for 3–4 weeks and need to be weaned actively although the usual course of therapy will be about 2 months. Growth suppression is a common side effect and alternate-day therapy may lessen this. Recurrence of symptoms is common during the weaning process.

Sulfasalazine does not help in prophylaxis (unlike ulcerative colitis), but it does help with symptomatic treatment in Crohn colitis. Metronidazole has been used when sulfasalazine is ineffective. It is useful if there is *Clostridium difficile* colitis and if there is perianal disease. Immunosuppression with azathioprine or 6-mercaptopurine may be tried to maintain remission and to reduce the need for prednisone. Close monitoring of blood counts and liver function is necessary during the immunosuppressive treatment.

Nutritional management is important both for overall health and to improve growth and aid sexual maturation. Growth failure is common from steroids as well as being a feature of Crohn disease. The goals of nutritional management include adequate caloric intake, especially protein, as well as to correct vitamin and mineral deficiencies. Ideally, the needs can be met by mouth and there should be supplementation with multivitamins, iron, and folic acid. Tube feedings may be necessary if oral feeding is inadequate and, on occasions, parenteral (IV) nutrition will be required.

Elemental formulas may be beneficial to improve the overall status and help in inducing remission and have the advantage of being fully absorbed in the small bowel. There is no evidence that nutritional avoidance or elimination makes a difference.

Surgical management is indicated only in the management of the complications of the disease. These include intestinal perforation, obstruction, significant bleeding, abscess, or fistula. The hesitation to perform surgery is important because of the complications that tend to be more problematic each time the abdomen is entered surgically.

Although the risk of carcinoma of the colon is much less than with ulcerative colitis, it is still 20 times more common than in the general public. Carcinoma of the distal ileum has been reported in cases that are more than 10 years. Appropriate surveillance, including colonoscopy, is necessary in long-standing cases.

■ ULCERATIVE COLITIS

Ulcerative colitis occurs in all pediatric age groups with an incidence of 2–4 per 100,000 with equal sex distribution. It is an inflammatory bowel disease that involves the colon and rectum. In half of the cases, pan-colitis occurs. Disease involving only the descending colon occurs in 20–35 percent of cases and 15 percent have rectal involvement only.

Clinical Features

Ulcerative colitis presents with diarrhea that is usually bloody. The diarrhea may be chronic and mild or it may be acute and similar to infectious diarrhea. Tenesmus (painful desire to defecate) and urgency with incontinence may occur in 25 percent of cases. The symptoms relate to the degree of bowel involvement. If disease is confined to the rectum, there may be painless blood-streaked stools, whereas pan-colitis will be associated with bloody, mucoid diarrhea, and severe abdominal pain. Anorexia and nausea are common, contributing to the weight loss. Hypoalbuminemia and iron deficiency anemia are characteristic. Hepatobiliary complications are seen in 5–10 percent of cases and extraintestinal manifestations are common (Table 23-4).

Management

Contrast studies should not be performed during an acute episode of colitis because of the risk of perforation or precipitating toxic megacolon. Colonoscopy with biopsy can confirm the diagnosis and define the extent of involvement. Care should be taken when the procedure is performed during an acute episode of severe inflammation.

Medical management is with sulfasalazine which acts as a prophylaxis as well as a treatment. It is a combination of 5-amino-salicylic acid (5-ASA) and sulfapyridine. The combination is poorly absorbed until it reaches the colon where it is split by bacteria and 5-ASA exerts local anti-inflammatory effects. It can be used to treat minor flare-ups often obviating the need for steroids. There are side effects in 15–30 percent of patients with anorexia, headache, and nausea and less commonly neutropenia, hemolytic anemia, and oligospermia. These effects are related to the sulfapyridine component of sulfasalazine so that alternative agents are being evaluated. Sulfasalazine is given once daily and the dose is increased slowly. Blood tests need to be taken every few weeks to identify side effects.

Corticosteroids may be necessary in severe cases but the complications of long-term oral usage are considerable and the relapse rate is significant. Local treatment with Budesonide or similar enemas has been encouraging. Immunosuppressive agents, such as azathioprine or 6-mercaptopurine, are useful for steroid-dependent cases. Surgical treatment by total colectomy is curative. Alternative strategies include subtotal colectomy with either an ileostomy or a pull-through. The long-term risk of colon cancer is significant. After 10 years of active ulcerative colitis, the risk of developing colon cancer is 0.5–1 percent per year. Strategies for anticipatory management include serial biopsies after 7–10 years or, alternatively, colon cancer is preventable by total colectomy prior to 10 years of active disease.

Celiac Disease

Children with celiac disease have an intolerance to gluten which is a protein found in wheat and rye but not in corn or rice. The incidence varies widely and is highest in western Ireland (1 in 300) and most common in countries where wheat is an important staple in the diet. This includes Europe, North America, and Australia. Genetic factors are important but the cause is unknown. The small intestinal mucosa is flat with resultant reduction in absorptive surface.

The age of onset tends to be 1–2 years of age following introduction of gluten into the diet. The presenting symptom is diarrhea which is usually bulky and offensive. Failure to thrive is common and growth failure may result. The diagnosis is made by intestinal biopsy and the clinical response to removal of gluten from the diet. The biopsy should precede the removal of gluten from the diet. Clinical response includes weight gain and resolution of symptoms.

Treatment requires removal of wheat, rye, barley, and oats for life. If the diet is not strict, there is increased risk of cancer of the mouth, pharynx, and esophagus as well as lymphoma. With complete removal of these items, the risks are the same as the general population.

Chronic Abdominal Pain

The definition is three or more episodes of abdominal pain during a 3 month or longer period. It may initially appear to be acute but with time the chronic nature of the problem becomes clearer. The challenge is to distinguish organic causes from functional. The principal causes comprise both GI and other causes (Table 23-5). Pre-school children tend not to have abdominal pain as the sole complaint. Children from 5–14 years of age have a reported prevalence of chronic abdominal pain of 10–15 percent.

TABLE 23-5. CAUSES OF CHRONIC ABDOMINAL PAIN

Functional (non-organic) 95%
Organic 5%
Hiatus hernia
Esophagitis
Peptic ulcer disease
Choledochal cyst
Chronic appendicitis
Constipation
Pinworms
Mesenteric lymphadenitis
Abdominal migraine
Lactose intolerance
Sickle cell disease
Diabetes mellitus
Abdominal tumor (Wilms, neuroblastoma)
Pelvic inflammatory disease
Ovarian cyst
Endometriosis

Functional abdominal pain is considered to be a complex relationship between physical or psychological stressors and autonomic control of GI function. The history is most important and there are clues that the diagnosis may be functional and there are signs and symptoms that suggest organic causes. The child and parents should be interviewed separately. Stress factors should be sought which may include a change in the family situation or problems at school. The pain tends to be periumbilical, paroxysmal, and unrelated to eating. The work-up will depend on the index of suspicion of other disorders.

The treatment of recurrent abdominal pain that is functional is reassurance. The pain is "real" and the treatment plan should include normalization of routine activities, including returning to school (if it has been missed).

Chronic Diarrhea

The definition of chronic diarrhea is persistence of diarrheal stools for more than 2 weeks. Chronic diarrhea may result from the same organisms that cause acute diarrhea. There are many conditions that have persistent diarrhea as an accompanying symptom (Table 23-6). The seriousness of the problem often relates to the degree of failure to thrive.

The history relates to the duration, type, and frequency of diarrheal stool. Small-volume frequent stools with tenesmus suggest distal colon inflammation, whereas large-volume and less frequent stools suggest small bowel or proximal colon disease. The presence of blood suggests inflammatory or infectious conditions of the colon, and mucus tends to be seen with irritable bowel syndrome or allergy. Failure to thrive supports consideration of Hirschsprung disease, cystic fibrosis, or celiac disease.

Stool examination helps to differentiate malabsorption, infection, bleeding, or protein loss and to narrow the diagnostic considerations. Stool culture and examination for ova and parasites may be indicated.

TABLE 23-6. CLASSIFICATION OF CAUSES OF CHRONIC DIARRHEA

Infection in immunocompromised host
  Bacterial
    Salmonella, Campylobacter
  Viral
    CMV, rotavirus
  Parasitic infections
    Entamoeba, Giardia, Cryptosporidium
Metabolic disorders
    Lactose intolerance
    Congenital lactase deficiency
Pancreatic malabsorption
    Cystic fibrosis
    Shwachman syndrome
    Chronic pancreatitis
Celiac disease
Intestinal lymphangiectasia
Immunodeficiency syndromes
    SCID
    HIV infection
Short bowel
    Surgical resection
Inflammatory bowel disease
    Ulcerative colitis
    Crohn disease

Chronic Intestinal Pseudoobstruction Syndrome

There are signs and symptoms of intestinal obstruction without physical obstruction. It is common for children to undergo laparotomy to try and define an abdominal cause and no reason for the obstruction is found. There is a group of disorders of GI smooth muscle that result in ineffective GI motility, some of which are familial and some are not. Children have cramping abdominal pain that may be accompanied by vomiting or diarrhea. Many have symptoms from birth and on occasions there is progression of symptoms to severely disrupt their daily lives.

The radiographic signs demonstrate intestinal obstruction with dilated loops of small intestine and in neonates there may be microcolon. Failure to thrive is common and tube feedings may be necessary to gain weight. Pharmacologic treatment is usually not beneficial. It may be years between the onset of symptoms and the making of the correct diagnosis.

Gastroesophageal Reflux

When gastroesophageal reflux (GER) becomes problematic, it is often referred to as GER disease (GERD). Regurgitation of stomach contents varies from spitting up a small amount after feeding to a constellation of symptoms that are associated with significant morbidity. There may be failure to thrive, esophagitis with hematemesis, or esophageal stricture. Pulmonary symptoms are common with apnea, cough, wheeze, and aspiration pneumonia. Reflux and pulmonary aspiration are more common in neurologically impaired infants.

Esophogram and barium swallow (upper GI) are performed to evaluate other disorders that produce similar symptoms, such as vascular ring. The upper GI is not a sensitive test to confirm reflux and the 24-hour pH probe measuring esophageal acidity is more useful.

The majority of infants have improvement in reflux in the second 6 months of life. Simple measures such as positioning, smaller feeds, and thickening with rice cereal may reduce regurgitation. Esophageal symptoms may be improved with H_2 receptor antagonists or proton pump inhibitors. The prokinetic agent cisapride can no longer be prescribed in the United States. Metoclopramide can be tried to improve esophageal motility and aid in stomach emptying.

Persistence of symptoms despite aggressive medical management may lead to consideration of surgery. The procedure is fundal plication (wrapping the fundus of the stomach around the lower end of the esophagus) and should be performed only if there is significant failure to thrive, severe esophagitis, or major pulmonary disease.

Hirschsprung Disease

Hirschsprung disease occurs in 1 in 5,000 live births and is the commonest cause of lower intestinal obstruction in the neonate. There is absence of enteric ganglionic neurons beginning at the anus and extending proximally for a variable distance. Aganglionosis is limited to the rectum and sigmoid in 75 percent of cases, involves the total colon in 8 percent of cases, and very rarely affects the whole intestine. The more common rectosigmoid disease shows a male predominance of 4 : 1 with a sex-modified multifactorial or recessive pattern of inheritance. Associated anomalies include congenital heart disease or Down syndrome in 5–10 percent of patients.

Because of the loss of intrinsic innervation of the rectum, there is overexpression of extrinsic sympathetic and parasympathetic nerves. The net result is that the aganglionic segment, internal sphincter, and anal canal are in a constant state of contraction with resultant obstruction, and there is proximal dilatation of the bowel before the site of obstruction. Hirschsprung disease may present as complete intestinal obstruction with bilious vomiting and abdominal distension. There may be delayed passage of meconium or there may be enterocolitis. In 1976, a survey showed 15 percent of cases were diagnosed within the first month of life, 64 percent of cases by 3 months of age, and 80 percent by 1 year. It is thought that the diagnosis is now made more commonly in the newborn period. Ninety percent of normal-term infants pass meconium within 24 hours of birth and 99 percent within 48 hours. Ninety-four percent of newborns with Hirschsprung disease fail to stool within the first 24 hours after birth. Enterocolitis occurs most commonly at 2–4 weeks in those cases where the diagnosis has been delayed. It presents as fever, and explosive, foul smelling, often bloody stools. It is associated with a significant mortality.

The diagnosis of Hirschsprung disease is suspected by barium contrast enema and confirmed by suction rectal biopsy and acetyl-cholinesterase staining. Occasionally, it is necessary to do a full-thickness rectal biopsy to demonstrate aganglionosis. If the diagnosis is made in the newborn period, it is necessary to create a stoma proximal to the site of obstruction. It is usual to delay removal of the involved segment followed by a pull-through procedure to restore the continuity of the bowel until 6–12 months of age. In older children, it may be possible to perform primary removal of the affected segment.

Irritable Bowel Syndrome

Irritable bowel syndrome (IBS) is also known as spastic colon and is a common cause of abdominal pain in children and adults. The pain tends to be episodic and cramping and is most common in the lower abdomen but may be mid- or upper-abdominal. Eating may bring on the pain, which leads to a desire to defecate, often with a diarrheal stool. After evacuation, the pain may resolve. There is a relationship with stress, which may direct treatment strategies. The only other measure that improves the condition is addition of fiber to the diet.

Liver Disease

■ α_1-ANTITRYPSIN DEFICIENCY

α_1-Antitrypsin deficiency is a deficiency of a protease inhibitor, synthesized in the liver, which acts to inhibit potentially destructive enzymes including trypsin. The presentation is with jaundice, acholic stools, and enlargement of the liver. Phenotyping of the various forms are designated as Pi (protease inhibitor) with MM being normal and the ZZ most commonly (10–20 percent) associated with liver disease. Some of these patients progress to cirrhosis.

■ BILIARY ATRESIA

This is the most common indication for liver transplantation. It is an inflammatory process that scleroses the intra- and extra-hepatic bile ducts. Jaundice is present from birth, stools are acholic, and liver enzymes are elevated. In 25 percent of cases, there is a delay in presentation for up to 4 weeks. Splenomegaly is present in half the patients.

Surgical treatment success often depends on finding some patent bile ducts and establishing connection to the duodenum. A hepatic portoenterostomy (Kasai procedure) is performed in the absence of bile-containing ducts. Successful improvement of bile flow occurs in 60–90 percent of infants under 2 months of age. After 90 days of age, long-term survival is unusual. Less than 50 percent of the survivors are alive at 5 years of age. Liver transplantation has an 80 percent, 5-year success rate.

■ CHOLEDOCHAL CYST

This is an extrahepatic bile duct cyst that presents after 1 year of age with abdominal pain, jaundice, and abdominal mass. The cyst occurs on the free portion of the common bile duct and produces prestenotic dilatation with distal obstruction. Half are detected after 10 years of age. Ultrasound demonstrates the cyst and treatment is excision. Five to 10 percent of infants develop cholangitis, which may lead to biliary cirrhosis.

■ CHRONIC HEPATITIS

Chronic viral hepatitis may result from hepatitis B or hepatitis C in 10 and 40 percent of acute infection, respectively. A small percentage progress to cirrhosis. Autoimmune hepatitis type I, which used to be called lupoid hepatitis, presents with lethargy, jaundice, and chronic liver disease and usually responds to steroids.

■ CIRRHOSIS

Cirrhosis of the liver is the replacement of normal hepatic tissue by nodules that are separated by fibrous tissue. The causes of cirrhosis are varied and include abnormalities of the hepatobiliary tree, chronic hepatitis due to infection and inflammation, toxins or accumulation of abnormal metabolites. The liver damage is irreversible. The result is elevation of portal venous pressure to more than 10 mm Hg and is called portal (venous) hypertension. Elevation of portal pressure may result from cirrhosis or obstruction in the portal venous system. The effects of portal hypertension result from the development of collaterals between the portal and systemic circulations and from splenomegaly. The most clinically important collaterals are to the stomach and esophagus which lead to the development of varices. Bleeding varices lead to hematemesis and melena. The splenic enlargement results in hypersplenism which is associated with excessive removal of red and white blood cells and platelets from the circulation. Ascites (fluid in the abdomen) may develop from the increased portal pressure as well as from hypoalbuminemia. End-stage liver disease is commonly associated with coagulopathy not only from the low platelet count but also because of prolonged prothrombin time (PT).

If the cause of portal hypertension is cirrhosis, there may also be signs of liver disease. The liver itself tends to be smaller and firmer than normal. There may be jaundice, spider nevi, and palmar erythema. Esophageal varices may be evident on radiographic study (upper GI) but are best visualized by endoscopy. Portal hypertension can be assessed with abdominal ultrasound, which shows enlargement of the portal vein.

Management

Children with significant enlargement of the spleen should not participate in contact sports. If there is acute bleeding from esophageal varices, blood transfusion may be necessary. Varices may be sclerosed endoscopically which usually temporarily stops the bleeding. Portal hypertension causes collateral circulations to decompress the high venous pressure. If bleeding from varices continues, it may be necessary to provide a shunt between the portal and systemic circuits with or without removal of the spleen. Portocaval (to the inferior vena cava) shunt and splenorenal shunts may be considered. A temporizing procedure that is sometimes used is the TIPS which is trans-hepatic to inferior vena cava, portal shunt which is performed transvenously and may be useful if the child is too sick for an operative shunt.

■ CRIGLER–NAJJAR SYNDROME (CONGENITAL NON-HEMOLYTIC UNCONJUGATED HYPERBILIRUBINEMIA)

Type I Crigler–Najjar syndrome is due to the absence of hepatic glucuronyl transferase and type II is due to deficiency of the enzyme. In the neonatal period, type I produces rapidly rising indirect (unconjugated) bilirubin without evidence of hemolysis. Kernicterus develops unless treatment is aggressive. Kernicterus is bilirubin encephalopathy with staining of the basal ganglia, hippocampal cortex, and subthalamic nuclei of the brain with bilirubin. There is a triad of choreoathetosis, loss of upward gaze, and deafness that characterize kernicterus but the most important component is severe mental retardation.

Type I defect is autosomal recessive and the absence of the enzyme means that exchange transfusions will be needed during the initial 10 days and then nightly phototherapy is necessary to keep the bilirubin less than 15 mg/dL. Type II defect is autosomal dominant and presents at any time from newborn to adulthood, commonly with an intercurrent illness and sudden rise in bilirubin. Phenobarbital has no effect in type I but can help lower bilirubin levels in type II. Liver transplantation is a consideration.

Recurrent Cyclical Vomiting

This is a poorly understood condition of vomiting that occurs in cycles with periods of time of normal health between the cycles.

Most often a girl of 6 or 7 years of age presents with vomiting that lasts 6–48 hours that repeats every 2–3 weeks. Because many chronic conditions are associated with vomiting, these must be ruled out. Renal, metabolic, or endocrine conditions as well as GI disorders need to be considered. When no cause is found, there is thought to be a relationship to abdominal migraine and appropriate medications can be tried. On occasions, the vomiting may be severe enough to merit intravenous fluids to treat dehydration.

Short-Bowel Syndrome

This is a severe malabsorption syndrome resulting from resection of large amounts of the small intestine. The reasons for the resection include necrotizing enterocolitis, volvulus, multiple atresias, and gastroschisis. Loss of surface for absorption is the major cause of malabsorption but loss of bile acids and bacterial overgrowth contribute. Resection of the duodenum results in poor absorption of iron, folate, and calcium which leads to anemia and osteopenia. Loss of the duodenum is rare. Isolated jejunal resection is well tolerated, whereas loss of the ileum has profound effects on the loss of fluids and electrolytes. In addition, there is malabsorption of bile acids, fat, and vitamin B_{12}.

Shwachman–Diamond Syndrome

After cystic fibrosis, Shwachman–Diamond syndrome is the second most common cause of pancreatic insufficiency. It is an autosomal recessive disorder and involves all ethnic groups. The presentation is with diarrhea (or rather steatorrhea) and failure to thrive, and the key to the diagnosis lies in the neutropenia and other signs of bone marrow suppression. This includes anemia, thrombocytopenia, and elevated levels of fetal hemoglobin.

Steatorrhea implies fatty stools, because of pancreatic insufficiency, which are bulky, smelly, and float. The stool frequency increases and growth failure results, despite good appetite.

The characteristic age of onset is 2–12 months although symptoms in the neonatal period are common. Other findings include pulmonary and skin infections. Also there may be dysmorphic features, neurologic findings, and psychomotor retardation as well as liver and kidney dysfunction. Delayed puberty occurs and another late complication that has been reported is diabetes mellitus. The work-up will include the sweat test to rule out cystic fibrosis. The pancreatic enzymes, duodenal trypsin, amylase, and lipase are all reduced.

■ MANAGEMENT

The management of Shwachman syndrome is replacement pancreatic enzymes and nutritional interventions to reduce growth retardation. The tendency to infection and neutropenia place the infant at risk for overwhelming sepsis and aggressive management may be necessary. The malabsorption improves with time and the long-term prognosis depends on the hematologic abnormalities.

Wilson Disease

This is hepato-lenticular degeneration which is an autosomal recessive disorder of inadequate biliary secretion of copper. The metabolic defect has not been defined but involves impaired synthesis of ceruloplasmin which is a protein that binds to copper. The result is the accumulation of copper in the hepatocytes with resultant cellular necrosis of the liver. Copper is released into the circulation and is deposited in the iris of the eye producing the Kayser–Fleischer rings at the junction of the iris and the conjuctiva and readily seen with a slit-lamp. In addition, copper is deposited in the central nervous system and kidneys. Decreased serum ceruloplasmin levels are found. Bilirubin may be elevated but serum transaminases tend not to be elevated.

The clinical features relate to the enlarged liver and abnormal liver function, with, in more advanced cases, the development of portal hypertension. Minor neurologic dysfunction and abnormal behaviors, especially at school, may be discernible.

■ MANAGEMENT

Treatment of Wilson disease involves increasing urinary copper excretion by means of the copper-chelating agent D-penicillamine. The copper levels fall slowly and the symptoms improve with time. If the disease is advanced, plasmapheresis and even liver transplant should be considered. Without treatment, Wilson disease is fatal.

24

Chapter Twenty-Four

Hematology and Oncology Disorders

Hematopoiesis is the production of red blood cells, white blood cells, and platelets. During the last trimester of pregnancy, fetal blood cells are produced mainly in the bone marrow which fills the bony cavities of most of the skeleton. During childhood, hematopoietic tissue is mostly in the vertebrae, pelvis, proximal femur, and humerus. Extramedullary hematopoiesis is increased production of blood cells that occurs outside the bone marrow, and the liver and spleen are the main sites.

The red cell contains hemoglobin that comprises four subunits (chains) each with one iron atom linked to a porphyrin ring which is the heme component. The four globin chains are designated with a Greek letter. Fetal hemoglobin (hemoglobin F) has either 4 epsilon or 2 epsilon and 2 alpha chains (Gower 1 and 2, respectively). Fetal hemoglobin averages 75 percent of hemoglobin at birth, 20 percent at 4 months and less than 2 percent by 1 year of age. Adult hemoglobin (hemoglobin A) comprises 2 alpha and 2 beta chains.

Hemoglobin acts to transport oxygen from the lungs to the tissues and carbon dioxide from the tissues to the lungs. In the fetus, the oxygen tension is about 25 mm Hg and in children about 90 mm Hg and adults 97 mm Hg. The oxygen dissociation curve of fetal hemoglobin favors extraction of oxygen from maternal blood but not its release at the tissues compared to adult hemoglobin which facilitates release of oxygen to the tissues.

Anemia

Anemia implies that the hemoglobin and hematocrit are below the lower limit of normal for age and that there is not enough oxygen-carrying capacity for normal activity. Hemoglobin is the major compound in the red blood cell and it carries oxygen from the lungs to the tissues. Normal values of red cell indices for age are shown in Table 24-1. Anemia is classified by cause (Table 24-2). There may be impaired production of red cells and hemoglobin, accelerated destruction of red cells, or blood loss.

The most common causes in children are iron deficiency and the anemia associated with an acute infection. Anemia is found in many chronic conditions. History is important to include diet, evidence of chronic disease, or acute infection. Cows milk fed to infants less than 9 months is associated with GI hemorrhage and iron deficiency anemia.

Anemia presents to the clinician in many ways. The diagnosis may be made during a check of the hemoglobin either during a routine well-child visit or as part of the work-up for a medical condition. The child may present with pallor and tiredness and anemia may be suspected by the parent. On occasions, the child may be seriously ill with pallor and jaundice.

Anemia may present with rapid onset accompanied by tachycardia or shock whereas gradual onset leads to pallor. Many

TABLE 24-1. NORMAL RED CELL INDICES FOR AGE

Age	Hemoglobin (g/dL)	Hematocrit (%)	RBC Count (10^6/ml)	MCV (fL)	MCH (pg)	MCHC (g/dL)
Birth	16.5	51	4.7	108	34	33
1 month	14.0	43	4.2	104	34	33
0.5–2 years	12.0	36	4.5	78	27	33
2–6 years	12.5	37	4.6	81	27	34
6–12 years	13.5	40	4.6	86	29	34
12–18—female	14.0	41	4.6	90	30	34
12–18—male	14.5	43	4.9	88	30	34

TABLE 24-2. CAUSES OF ANEMIA

Pure red cell aplasia
    Congenital hypoplastic anemia (Blackfan-Diamond)
    Transient erythroblastopenia of childhood

Nutritional anemias
    Iron deficiency
    Megaloblastic anemia
        Folic acid deficiency
        B_{12} deficiency

Anemias of chronic disorders
    Chronic renal failure
    Hypothyroidism
    Chronic inflammatory disorders (e.g., GI)

Congenital hemolytic anemias
    Red cell membrane defects
        Hereditary spherocytosis
        Hereditary elliptocytosis
    Hemoglobinopathies
        Alpha thalassemia
        Beta thalassemia
        Sickle cell anemia
        Sickle cell trait
        Hemoglobin C and E disorders
    Disorders of red cell metabolism
        G-6PD deficiency
        Pyruvate kinase deficiency

Acquired hemolytic anemia
    Autoimmune hemolytic anemia
    Non-immune hemolytic anemia

anemias have a hereditary basis. A dominant inheritance suggests a defect of the red cell or of hemoglobin whereas recessive or sex-linked inheritance is characteristic of enzymopathies. The diagnosis of an inherited anemia such as spherocytosis is suggested by a family history of anemia, jaundice, gallstones, or splenomegaly. Bruising may suggest a clotting disorder and petechiae suggests a low platelet count. Jaundice with or without splenomegaly is characteristic of hemolytic anemia.

Analysis of hemoglobin by spectrophotometry is the standard and the hematocrit is measured as packed cell volume following centrifugation. Hemoglobin is roughly one-third of the hematocrit so that hemoglobin of 10 g/dL is equivalent to hematocrit of 30 percent. In most clinical settings, values less than the third percentile are considered abnormal.

The approach to the laboratory diagnosis of anemia involves MCV, blood smear, and reticulocyte count. Iron deficiency anemia is the commonest cause of anemia in the United States. It is less common now than previously. It is important to treat iron deficiency anemia in infants because it is associated with developmental delay if untreated. The symptoms of iron deficiency anemia are non-specific and when mild there may be no symptoms. Severe iron deficiency anemia has similar symptoms to other anemias which include fatigue, shortness of breath on exertion, loss of appetite, and pallor.

Low hematocrit and low MCH and MCV support the diagnosis of iron deficiency anemia but it does not rule out thalassemia minor. Serum ferritin concentration less than 10 µg/L indicates depletion of iron stores. Serum ferritin <15 mcg/L in the presence of anemia indicates iron deficiency. Erythrocyte protoporphyrin (EP) accumulates in red blood cells when insufficient iron is available to combine with protoporphyrin to produce heme. The EP is elevated in both iron deficiency anemia and lead poisoning and is therefore used to screen infants and young children in urban low-income areas that have high incidences of both conditions.

■ MANAGEMENT

The usual treatment is ferrous sulfate by mouth on an empty stomach. GI symptoms are less in children than adults. Response is best monitored by checking the hemoglobin or hematocrit after 1 month of treatment at which time there should be one-half to two-thirds correction. Treatment for 2–3 months more helps to rebuild iron stores. If the anemia is associated with infection, the infection may need to be treated before the anemia is corrected.

It is reasonable to give a therapeutic trial of iron for 1 month for mild anemia with the goal of avoiding an expensive work-up. Intramuscular or intravenous iron should be avoided because of the potential of a rare but severe anaphylactic reaction.

Iron deficiency anemia is becoming less with better dietary habits. Megaloblastic anemia is uncommon in children. The causes include cancer therapy, folate deficiency, and even more rarely vitamin B_{12}. Aplastic anemia implies pancytopenia which is anemia, plus white cell and platelet reduction because of suppression of the bone marrow function. Presentation is usually pallor and tiredness from low hemoglobin, bruising, epistaxis, and bleeding from the gums because of thrombocytopenia. Infections from low white count are a late complication.

Hematologic Disorders

■ SICKLE CELL DISEASE

Sickle (HbS) and normal adult hemoglobin (HbA2) differ in the substitution of valine, a neutral amino acid, for glutamic, an acidic amino acid, in the sixth position from the N-terminal end of the beta-globin chain. This substitution of a hydrophilic for a hydrophobic amino acid changes the physical properties so that the hemoglobin becomes susceptible to oxidation and predisposed to polymerization upon deoxygenation. The abnormal properties of HbS result in the sickle shape that produces the clinical effects.

The incidence of sickle cell anemia in newborn African-Americans is estimated to be 1 : 600; sickle-hemoglobin C (HbC) disease 1 : 800; and sickle beta-thalassemia 1 : 1,700. The frequency of the sickle cell gene is 8 percent, the HbC gene is 4 percent, and the beta-thalassemia gene is 1 percent. The sickle cell is easily damaged by mechanical stresses during passage through the vasculature. This results in hemolytic anemia with the rate of red cell destruction being 2–8 times normal. Normal red cells last

120 days versus about 16 days for sickle cells. Sickling occurs during periods of reduced oxygen that result in polymerization which is in part reversible when oxygenation improves, but, characteristically, a significant percentage (10 percent) remain distorted.

Clinical Features

There are two types of crises, anemic, and vaso-occlusive, that result in the clinical features of sickle cell disease. Anemic crises occur when the bone marrow reduces the production of red cells, most usually with viral infections. The parvovirus is most common and the reticulocyte count declines. There may be sudden sequestration of red cells in the spleen with acute life-threatening drop in hemoglobin. This occurs within a few hours either spontaneously or following a viral infection. The spleen acutely enlarges and this scenario is a major cause of death under 5 years of age.

Vaso-occlusive crises are the dominant cause of symptoms in sickle cell disease. Often the initial presentation is the hand-foot syndrome with painful swelling of the hands and feet that lasts a few days to 2 weeks. X-rays may show aseptic necrosis of bone. Abdominal pain in infants may be similar to colic and in any child an acute abdomen may be suspected. There may be long bone pain or back pain.

The newborn appears normal and pallor and jaundice may be evident at 4 months of age. By 1 year of age, the spleen may be enlarged and there may be functional asplenia. Older children who have continued infarction may no longer have an enlarged spleen. Growth is usually normal for the first few years but height and weight usually fall below normal in later childhood. At 1 year of age, it is usual for the hematocrit to be in the 20s with the reticulocyte count also in the 20s (reflecting hemolysis). The peripheral blood smear shows sickled cells and Howell–Jolly bodies.

The clinical severity is very variable and visceral organ involvement may result in damage to kidney, liver, lung, and central nervous system. Pain crises can occur regularly, more often than once a month, or may be spaced out by years. Many pain crises can be managed at home with oral hydration, rest, and pain medications.

TABLE 24-3. CAUSES OF SPLENOMEGALY

Congestive splenomegaly
  Portal hypertension
Chronic infections
  Tuberculosis
  Histoplasmosis
  Coccidioidomycosis
  Subacute bacterial endocarditis
Infectious mononucleosis
Hematologic
  Leukemia
  Lymphoma, Hodgkins disease
Hemolytic anemia
Reticuloendotheliosis
  Histiocytosis X
Storage diseases
  Gaucher, etc.
Splenic cyst or hemangioma

Additional problems include cerebrovascular accidents, myocardial infarction, delayed sexual maturation, and priapism (painful penile erection).

Management

Newborn screening of cord blood of the populations at risk (African American and Hispanic) is the best way to define the infants with sickle cell anemia. If the diagnosis has not been made, hemoglobin electrophoresis is used to identify the predominance of hemoglobin S. Penicillin must be given to prevent pneumococcal sepsis. Surveillance is necessary for emergence of penicillin-resistant pneumococci. Treatment must be directed at general and preventive care in addition to the management of the crises. A multidisciplinary comprehensive plan can reduce the complications. Regular transfusions are used to suppress hemoglobin S levels.

Adequate hydration and avoidance of hypoxia are crucial in the management of crises. Pain management needs to be aggressive and narcotics may be indicated. It is important to avoid using inadequate analgesia because of the risk of addiction.

Hydroxyurea for stimulation of hemoglobin production may be beneficial.

■ SPLENOMEGALY

There are many causes of chronic splenomegaly as shown in Table 24-3. This often results in hypersplenism which is associated with increased destruction of circulating red and white cells and platelets. In many cases there is life-threatening thrombocytopenia. This is particularly seen with splenomegaly secondary to portal hypertension.

Thalassemia

Thalassemia syndromes result from reduced synthesis of one or more globin chains of hemoglobin.

■ ALPHA-THALASSEMIA

Deletion of one or more of the alpha-globin genes on chromosome 16 results in alpha-thalassemia. Persons with one alpha-globin gene deletion are asymptomatic silent carriers. If 2 genes are deleted, it is alpha-thalassemia trait which results in a mild anemia with microcytosis. Hemoglobin H disease results if 3 alpha-globin genes are deleted and there is moderately severe anemia. If all 4 alpha-globin genes are deleted, the result is fetal demise due to hydrops fetalis.

Alpha-thalassemia occurs in individuals of African, Mediterranean, Middle Eastern, Chinese, or Southeast Asian ancestry. The clinical findings are dependent upon how many alpha-globin chains are deleted. If alpha chains are deleted, there is increasing amounts of hemoglobin Barts. Hemoglobin Barts comprises four gamma-globin chains. Normally there is no hemoglobin Barts, with 1 deletion there is 0–5 percent, 2 deletions there is 2–10 percent, 3 deletions there is 20–27 percent, and if there are no alpha genes, there is more than 75 percent hemoglobin Barts.

Alpha-thalassemia results in microcytic anemia which must be distinguished from iron-deficiency anemia. There will be increased amounts of ferritin and serum iron and free erythrocyte protoporphyrin is not elevated. The principal complication of alpha-thalassemia is the needless administration of iron. Treatment is with folic acid.

■ BETA-THALASSEMIA

Beta-thalassemia occurs in African, Mediterranean, Middle Eastern and Asian ancestries. Heterozygotes for beta-thalassemia genes result in beta-thalassemia minor and homozygotes have beta-thalassemia major (Cooley's anemia).

Beta-thalassemia minor causes a mild microcytic, hypochromic anemia which does not respond to iron therapy. There are usually no symptoms. No treatment is necessary. Beta-thalassemia major is a major cause of transfusion-dependent anemia. There may be significant hepatosplenomegaly. The requirement for repeated transfusion means that chelation therapy is necessary to avoid hemosiderosis (iron deposition). Failure to thrive is not uncommon and viral hepatitis may occur. Splenectomy may be necessary. Bone marrow transplant may be indicated.

Coagulation Disorders

■ HEMOPHILIA

Hemophilia A is Factor VIII deficiency and is the most common hereditary deficiency of clotting factors. Hemophilia A accounts for 80 percent of cases and hemophilia B accounts for 20 percent of cases. Hemophilia B is deficiency of factor IX and is also known as Christmas disease and tends to be milder than hemophilia A.

They are both X-linked recessive disorders so that female carriers are not affected and all patients are male. The initial presentation occurs after cutting the umbilical cord or circumcision in many cases. Mild hemophilia may go unsuspected for years until a surgical procedure or trauma is associated with prolonged bleeding which is the first indication of any problem. Hemorrhage can be internal or external and may result from minor injury. The effect of large hematomas can be problematic and can occur into muscle or joints. The leading cause of death is intracranial bleeding.

Hemophilia should be suspected in any male who presents with prolonged bleeding. A family history of bleeding diathesis is not unusual. The major laboratory finding is prolonged PTT (partial thromboplastin time) which should lead to specific factor assay. The clinical severity of hemophilia A depends on the factor VIII level so that a level of 10–30 percent corresponds to mild disease, moderate disease 2–10 percent, and severe 0–2 percent. Spontaneous hemorrhage is a feature of severe disease and minor trauma results in major hemorrhage.

Hemophilia occurs in all racial and ethnic groups with an incidence of 1 : 7,500 males. The diagnosis is usually made before 18 months of age either by a bleeding episode or family history in severe cases of hemophilia. It is not unusual for child abuse to have been suspected because of the bruising that may result from minor trauma. Intracranial hemorrhage occurs in the neonatal period in 1–5 percent of patients with severe hemophilia. If family history is positive, it is reasonable to suspect that the deficiency is likely to be similar and therefore the severity.

Management

Treatment of patients with hemophilia involves replacement of concentrated factor VIII. Many preparations are available including recombinant forms. Comprehensive medical care programs are necessary to optimize treatment. Multidisciplinary care is indicated, usually at a hemophilia treatment center. In addition to keeping the factor VIII levels in a reasonable range, it is necessary to immunize against hepatitis B as soon after diagnosis as possible. Other areas of concern include dental work, especially extraction.

Unfortunately 10 percent of patients with severe hemophilia develop antibody to factors in the concentrate. This may require exchange transfusion or the use of immunosuppression. Additional concentrate may need to be given to saturate the blocking antibody and provide sufficient coagulation ability.

■ VON WILLEBRAND DISEASE

Von Willebrand disease is a defect in platelet aggregation resulting from deficiency of platelet glycoprotein. This results in bleeding because the lack of von Willebrand factor reduces adherence of platelets to damaged endothelium and there is reduced transport of factor VIII. There are various forms with most being an autosomal dominant, but rarely there are autosomal and sex-linked recessive cases. The common form is type I and desmopressin (DDAVP) is the treatment of choice. It is important to evaluate cases because there are different defects that should be treated differently. The incidence of von Willebrand disease is not known and it is thought that there are many mild cases that are not even diagnosed.

Von Willebrand disease commonly results in bleeding from mucous membranes and epistaxis. The PTT will be abnormal and may be discovered in pre-operative testing when the history of mouth bleeding or epistaxis is obtained. Because the condition also occurs in females, increased menstrual bleeding may be the first indication of the problem.

There is increased information available concerning the genetics of bleeding disorders. Carrier detection using the factor VIII coagulant–antigen ratio is accurate to about 90 percent. DNA testing is even more accurate but multiple relatives may need to be checked. Hemophilia A is associated with an inversion wherein the distal end of the X chromosome containing part of the factor VIII gene flips and this has been shown to be present in 50 percent of cases. The inversion occurs also in the female carriers who are relatives. Prenatal diagnosis may be performed by chorionic villus sampling at 8–12 weeks or by fetal blood sampling at 18–20 weeks.

Leukemia

Cancer is the leading cause of death from disease in children age 3–15 years of age. In the United States, the occurrence in this age group is about 13 cases per 100,000 Caucasian children and 10 per 100,000 African American children. Leukemia is the most common disorder (30 percent of all cancers), followed by brain tumors and lymphomas. There are 6–7,000 children diagnosed with cancer each year. More than 60 percent of children with cancer are surviving.

The different types of leukemia are based on the morphology of the cells and the course of the disease. Ninety-seven percent of leukemia in children is acute with proliferation of immature white cells which are called blasts. The commonest leukemia in children is acute lymphoblastic leukemia (ALL), which accounts for 80–90 percent of childhood leukemia. Non-lymphoid leukemia refers to myelogenous leukemia which originates from bone marrow cells other than the lymphoid series.

Cell surface immunologic markers (antigens) have allowed differentiation of ALL into 3 types: non-T, non-B which is also known as pre-B cell; B-cell ALL; and T-cell ALL. Children with non-T, non-B have the best prognosis especially if they have the acute lymphocytic leukemia antigen known as CALLA positive on their cell surfaces.

Cancer involves tumor cells which have rapid growth rates. The cells often function differently with loss of differentiation and organization and this process is called anaplasia. Cancer means "crab" and the features that make it dangerous are invasion and destruction of adjacent tissue by cancer cells and distant spread, or metastasis, by cells that travel by blood stream or lymphatics to other sites to form secondary tumors.

Many cancers will present with generalized as well as local findings. Fever and night sweats, persistent or localized pain, easy bruisability, and decreased appetite with weight loss are typical. There may be changes in behavior, balance or vision, or finding of a palpable mass. Pallor and tiredness are common.

■ ACUTE LYMPHOBLASTIC LEUKEMIA (ALL)

ALL occurs in 4 per 100,000 Caucasian children, 2.4 per 100,000 African American under 15 years of age, and the peak incidence is at the age of 4 years.

The main consequences of leukemia result from infiltration of the bone marrow which results in anemia, thrombocytopenia, and neutropenia. Anemia results in tiredness, thrombocytopenia (low platelet count) leads to bleeding, and neutropenia results in infection. The bone involvement may lead to pathological fractures. The spleen, liver, and lymph nodes are infiltrated which leads to enlargement. Involvement of the central nervous system may cause increased intracranial pressure.

Involvement of other organs systems is seen more commonly because of the longer survival. Leukemia cells may invade the testes, kidneys, lungs, gastrointestinal, and genitourinary tracts which may result in symptoms referable to these organs.

Leukemia is suspected from the history and physical examination and the presence of immature cells in the blood. Bone marrow is performed to confirm the diagnosis and lumbar puncture is done to establish the presence of CNS involvement.

Management

Treatment of leukemia involves induction therapy to cause a remission and removal of leukemic cells. Central nervous system (CNS) prophylaxis reduces the chance of CNS invasion. Then, when remission is induced, there will be maintenance therapy.

The combination of drugs and radiation that is used in an individual patient varies according to the risk characteristics of the leukemia as well as the protocol followed by the oncologist. The following comments provide an approach that is similar to that used for many patients.

Induction therapy is begun immediately after diagnosis and the principal agents are corticosteroids, vincristine, and L-asparaginase. Doxorubicin is added to the regimen in high-risk patients. Approximately 95 percent achieve remission within the first month. The maintenance protocol includes methotrexate and 6-mercaptopurine with pulses of prednisone and vincristine. Additional agents that have been beneficial in various protocols include cyclophosphamide, anthracyclines, 6-thioguanine and cytosine arabinoside in a reinduction phase.

Prophylactic therapy for the CNS is very important and involves intrathecal chemotherapy with methotrexate and usually cytosine arabinoside and hydrocortisone. Cranial irradiation is employed in many cases and definitely those with CNS involvement. The testes are the next most common site of metastasis and irradiation may be indicated. Surveillance of the need for replacement androgen therapy is necessary.

Complications of therapy are, unfortunately, common. There is a high risk for infection and bleeding because of bone marrow suppression and many of the agents used in treatment are toxic, especially to the CNS. Hyperleukocytosis and tumor lysis syndrome is a metabolic derangement caused by rapid lysis (disintegration) of tumor cells with release of phosphate, uric acid, and potassium producing a load that the kidneys are unable to excrete rapidly enough. Uric acid, calcium, and phosphate may precipitate in the kidneys causing obstruction. Aggressive, anticipatory treatment is necessary including maximizing urine output, alkalinizing the urine (with sodium bicarbonate), and closely monitoring electrolyte status and cardiac function. Occasionally, dialysis may be indicated. The major long-term effect of treatment relates to neurologic damage from chemotherapy and radiation. Most children have a mild reduction in IQ or subtle learning problems but some have a more severe leukoencephalopathy with ataxia, seizures, and intellectual impairment.

The reappearance of leukemic cells indicates a poor prognosis and the prognosis becomes worse with each relapse. Chemotherapeutic agents or bone marrow transplant (BMT) are then indicated. BMT, when it is successful, replaces the bone marrow with normal cells after destroying the leukemic cells. Selection of the donor is dependent upon finding a match related to human leukocyte antigen (HLA) typing.

ACUTE NON-LYMPHOBLASTIC LEUKEMIA

This includes various disorders that affect the non-lymphoblastic precursors which develop in the bone marrow and inhibit the normal functioning of hematopoiesis. The conditions occur throughout childhood and have a worse prognosis than lymphoblastic leukemias. The cause is unknown but there is an increased incidence with Down, Fanconi, Diamond-Blackfan and other syndromes. Fever is the most common presenting symptom which may accompany anorexia, pallor or bleeding.

LYMPHOMA

Lymphomas are usually divided into Hodgkin disease and non-Hodgkin lymphoma.

Hodgkin Disease (HD)

This is common in adolescents with the same frequency as leukemia in 15–19 year olds. It is very rare in young children. There are 4 types of HD that vary with the type of cells that dominate: Nodular sclerosis is the commonest type with bands of scar-like tissue in the lymph nodes. There are multiple Reed–Stromberg cells which are abnormally large cells characteristic of HD; some are lymphocyte predominant, some mixed cellularity, and some are lymphocyte depleted. Identification of the tumor type allows staging of the tumor which is the basis for treatment protocols.

HD causes lymphocytes to proliferate in the lymph nodes in the neck, axilla, or groin with painless swelling. Unexplained fevers are common and there may be tiredness, night sweats, and weight loss. Metastasis may occur to the spleen, liver, and bone marrow. Lymph node biopsy is essential for diagnosis and staging. Laparotomy may be necessary for staging if there is suspicion of disease below the diaphragm.

- Stage I is involvement of a single lymph node or single organ (stage 1E)
- Stage II is involvement of 2 or more lymph nodes on the same side of the diaphragm
- Stage III is involvement of lymph nodes on both sides of the diaphragm, an extralymphatic site (IIIE), the spleen (IIIS), or both (IIIES)
- Stage IV is widespread involvement of one or more sites other than lymph nodes, with or without lymph node involvement

Each of these stages is also subclassified as A for asymptomatic or B for symptoms present including fever, sweats, and weight loss. HD was one of the first cancers that was cured with chemotherapy. The approach to therapy includes radiotherapy for early stages and in combination with chemotherapy for the later stages. Radiation therapy usually lasts for 3–6 months. Chemotherapy is given in monthly courses lasting for 9–12 months. The combinations include MOPP [mechlorethamine (nitrogen mustard) + vincristine (Oncovin) + procarbazine + prednisone] and ABVD [doxorubicin (Adriamycin) + bleomycin + vincristine + dacarbazine].

The 5-year prognosis for the stages varies from 90 percent for the early stages to 60–80 percent for stage IV. Long-term follow-up is important because radiation therapy may induce other cancers and patients who have splenectomies are more susceptible to infection.

■ NON-HODGKIN LYMPHOMA (NHL)

The implication is that any lymphoma that does not have Reed–Sternberg cells is NHL. It is more common in inherited immune deficiencies, autoimmune diseases, HIV, and following transplantation. NHL tends to be more diffuse than HD and spread throughout the lymphatic system. Thirty to 60 percent develop into a more aggressive form (conversion).

Presentation is with painless lymph node enlargement and systemic symptoms are unusual. There are many different forms of NHL involving different organs and staging and classification are difficult. Radiation and/or single or combination chemotherapy are all considerations for treatment. Overall, the survival for NHL is about 50 percent for 5 years.

Childhood Cancer

The presentation of cancer in children is often suggested by the onset of one of the manifestations shown in Table 24-4. Many of these symptoms and signs are non-specific and so a high index of suspicion is necessary. It is not unusual for the diagnosis of cancer to be suspected during a routine visit to the doctor's office. This produces a devastating change in the life of a family who is told that their child has a potentially life-threatening illness. There may be some delay until the diagnosis is confirmed which leads to great anxiety. Early referral for consultation is important and if the diagnosis of cancer is made then prompt staging will allow the development of a treatment protocol. Cancer centers participate in multicenter treatment studies that have markedly improved the prognosis in childhood cancer. The care has to be coordinated by an oncologist and the non-specialist should not treat cancer because the field is expanding so rapidly and the community physician does not have the resources. Managed care plans may be reluctant to refer to cancer centers that are outside their network.

TABLE 24-4. PRESENTATIONS OF CHILDHOOD CANCERS

Mass lesion
Lymph node enlargement that persists
Unexplained bruising or bleeding
Petechiae
Hematuria
Pallor
Bone pain
Morning headache and vomiting
Fever—persistent or unexplained
Tiredness
Weight loss
Diarrhea

There are general approaches to all cancer treatments. The treatment options include surgery, chemotherapy, radiation, biologic response modifiers, and bone marrow transplantation. The National Cancer Institute sponsors the Children's Cancer Group (CCG) and the Pediatric Oncology Group (POG) and the majority of children (2/3) with cancer are cared for by protocols from these two groups.

Surgical approaches include biopsy of the tumor or organ to provide a specimen for pathology or to determine the extent of the lesion. On occasions, it will be indicated to remove all or part of the primary or secondary tumor and sometimes surgery will be necessary if the tumor is causing symptoms that need to be relieved.

Chemotherapy has the potential to alter the cell cycle of pro-liferating tumor cells, hopefully without affecting normal cells. Drugs may be cell-cycle specific which means that they kill cells only during a specific phase of cell development and are most useful if the cell is growing rapidly. These drugs also cause damage to cells in the bone marrow which increases susceptibility to infection; to hair follicles, resulting in hair loss; and to the intestine. The non-specific drugs kill cells regardless of their state of development. Radiation inhibits cell division by affecting DNA. Accurate staging is performed with molecular genetics and immunohistochemistry so that the appropriate specimen must be acquired for study. The prognosis for malignant disease is improving all the time. For an individual child, the outlook depends on age, the site of the primary, the extent of spread, and the cell type.

■ BRAIN TUMORS

Brain tumors are the second most common cancer found in children after leukemia, and the most common solid tumor. The majority (60 percent) are infratentorial which is below the tentorium cerebelli and are related to the cerebellum and brainstem. The remainder (40 percent) are supratentorial, accounting for two-thirds of the brain mass comprising principally the cerebral hemispheres. The majority of infratentorial tumors are medulloblastomas, cerebellar astrocytomas, brainstem gliomas, and ependymomas (Table 24-5).

Headache is the commonest presentation in school age children, whereas ataxia and vomiting are the commonest presentations in pre-school children. Headache tends to be recurrent and progressive, frontal or occipital, and is worse on rising and improves through the day. The headache is exacerbated by coughing or straining. The vomiting tends to be without nausea and is more severe in the morning. It tends to be progressively more projectile.

TABLE 24-5. CLASSIFICATION OF PRIMARY BRAIN TUMORS

Glial cell (50–60%)
   Astrocytoma
   Optic nerve glioma
   Brain stem glioma
   Ependymoma
Neuroectodermal (25–35%)
   Medulloblastoma
   Pinealoblastoma
Craniopharyngioma (5–10%)
Germ cell tumors (< 10%)
   Teratoma
   Dermoid
Meningeal tumors (< 5%)
   Meningioma
   Meningeal sarcoma
Lymphoma (< 1%)

The neuromuscular changes tend to be incoordination or clumsiness with loss of balance and poor fine motor control. The behavior changes include irritability, mood changes, fatigue, and lethargy which may progress to coma. Cranial nerve disorders and visual defects are common. Signs of raised intracranial pressure include decreased pulse and respiration with increased blood pressure. Temperature instability may occur with high and low temperatures.

The diagnosis requires a high index of suspicion. Fundal examination is important to look for papilledema. Imaging studies, including CAT scan and MRI, should be considered in any child that has persistence of the symptoms described.

Cerebellar astrocytomas comprise 12 percent of brain tumors in children. They grow slowly in the cerebellar hemisphere and consist of a large cyst with a mural nodule. The peak incidence is from 5–9 years of age. The presenting symptoms tend to persist which leads to the consideration of the diagnosis. Because of its position, it is associated with raised intracranial pressure.

If there is life-threatening hydrocephalus, immediate treatment is to perform a procedure to relieve the pressure. Steroids may be helpful in relieving the pressure. The 5-year survival after surgical removal approaches 95 percent. The mural nodule needs to be removed or the tumor may recur.

Medulloblastoma is a primitive neuroectodermal tumor with the capacity to differentiate into neuronal and glial tissue. Most tumors are in the vermis or fourth ventricle and may extend into the cerebellar hemisphere. The tumor grows rapidly and the interval between onset of symptoms and medical consultation is often only a few weeks. Vomiting is the commonest presenting symptom, followed by headache and unsteady gait. Two-thirds have papilledema when first evaluated.

■ NEUROBLASTOMA

Neuroblastoma is derived from the neural crest which is the origin of the adrenal medulla, sympathetic ganglia, and thymus. Neuroblastoma may develop anywhere along the sympathetic nervous system chain. Forty percent of the tumors are in the adrenal medulla and they are also seen in the paraspinal ganglia, the neck, chest, and pelvis. They are the most common malignancy of infancy and second only to brain tumor of solid tumors in the first 10 years of age.

The tumor tends to be silent and so 50 percent of infants and 70 percent of children have metastases at the time of diagnosis. On occasion, the presentation is with an abdominal mass or sometimes a mass on chest X-ray. Older children tend to have non-specific symptoms including fever and weight loss. A bruising pattern around the eyes is a well-recognized presentation. Urinary catecholamines are increased. The location of tumor requires CT scan or MRI. Calcification may be seen on abdominal studies.

Neuroblastoma is staged and various combinations of surgery, chemotherapy, and radiation will be used for treatment. Attempts to remove the tumor surgically will be tried, but the most important component is often chemotherapy. The outlook for infants is considerably better than for older children. Bone marrow transplantation is a consideration for advanced disease.

■ WILMS TUMOR

This is cancer of the kidney that is seen mostly in children 3–4 years of age. The incidence is about 10 per 1 million children. The diagnosis usually results from the discovery of an abdominal mass by the parent and sometimes because of hematuria or hypertension. Tumors may be unilateral or bilateral. Surgery is performed in the hope of removing the tumor. Chemotherapy and radiation may be beneficial. Relapse is quite common during the first 2 years of treatment and close follow-up is indicated. A cure rate of 80 percent can be anticipated.

■ OTHER CANCERS

Rhabdomyosarcoma is a cancer of muscle tissue that tends to occur in the head and neck. It occurs in about 8 per 1 million children.

Osteogenic sarcoma affects the long bones with an incidence of 2.5–3.4 million children. Presentation tends to be because of pain at the site of the tumor.

Ewing's sarcoma occurs in the bones of the pelvis, humerus, and femur. Presentation tends to be from metastatic disease with symptoms of fever, malaise, or weight loss.

Chapter Twenty-Five

Neuromuscular Disorders

The nervous system is divided into central, including brain and spinal cord, and peripheral which comprises the nerves that connect to the end organs. The autonomic nervous system comprises sympathetic and parasympathetic systems. A careful history and physical examination is vital to the diagnosis of neurological disorders. The history is taken with the objective of establishing the nature of the problem and how long it has been present. Many disorders are present from birth or soon after and the details of family history and pregnancy and delivery may be important. The evolution of the disorder is important because the progression of neurologic symptoms may be episodic, static, or progressive.

The physical examination includes a general evaluation with vital signs and anthropometric data. Neurologic disorders may be primary, or secondary to systemic disorders. Head circumference should be recorded, especially under 2 years of age, and other family members should be measured when it might be relevant. The head shape should be noted. Vision and hearing can initially be tested simply by observing the response to the surroundings, including lights and sounds. The examination encompasses mental state, cranial nerves, motor and sensory system, autonomic system, and the muscles. Observation of communication and movement continues throughout the evaluation.

Assessment of cerebral dysfunction has become much more sophisticated in the last two decades. The variety of tests has increased and it is tempting to order a scan (CT or MRI) but they should not replace clinical skills of evaluation and rather should be used to localize and confirm the findings.

Diagnostic evaluation includes the lumbar puncture (LP, and also called spinal tap), to collect cerebrospinal fluid (CSF). The LP must be carefully performed. It is a safe procedure and the parents (and child) should be reassured before the procedure. If there is potential for raised intracranial pressure, it is usual to perform a CT or MRI scan prior to performance of the LP. Very raised intracranial pressure may cause brainstem herniation when CSF is removed.

The information provided by the LP can be vital in the evaluation of neurologic disease. The pressure is measured before much of the CSF has been removed and then checked for oscillation (with abdominal pressure) to imply free flow of CSF. Normal CSF is clear with very few cells (usually less than 5 white blood cells/mm^3) and the glucose and protein are measured. Low glucose is associated with infection and high protein is abnormal. Bacterial and viral cultures of CSF provide information of central nervous system (CNS) infection. The presence of blood in the CSF may be from a traumatic tap when the needle hits a blood vessel. Usually, this clears so that if blood is uniformly present in all three tubes that are collected, it is implied that the blood is distributed throughout the CSF and probably originates from the brain or surrounding membranes. If the bleeding occurred more than a few hours prior to the LP, the fluid may be xanthochromic (yellow tint).

Electroencephalography (EEG) is most useful in the evaluation of convulsive disorders but it also provides information of brain function globally and locally. The EEG is recorded when awake and asleep and activation procedures, such as flashing lights, used to bring on seizure activity. The absence of EEG abnormality does not exclude a seizure disorder. Simultaneous video recording of the child allows correlation between the EEG findings and the movement of the child.

Evoked potentials are helpful in defining response to a sensory stimulus. These include visual evoked response (VER), brainstem auditory evoked response (BAER), and somatosensory evoked response (SER). These potentials are abnormal in demyelinating disorders and brain stem abnormalities (including tumors). BAER is most useful in evaluating hearing under 2 years of age because the test does not require cooperation. Electromyography (EMG) is useful in the assessment of nerve and muscle disorders. Nerve conduction velocities are abnormal in various peripheral neuropathies and degenerative neurologic diseases.

Plain X-rays of the skull and spine can be useful in the evaluation of CNS pathology. Newer neuroradiology techniques have advanced the science of diagnosis and the CT scan and MRI are the most widely used. CT is computerized axial tomography (also called CAT) and the images of the brain and surroundings are useful in hemorrhage and trauma as well as assessing ventricular size. Intravenous injection of contrast enhances the brain substance resulting in better definition of pathology. MRI is magnetic resonance imaging and produces images of brain tissue that are much clearer than the CT scan and are able to identify lesions in the brain stem and spinal cord.

Abnormal head size correlates with an abnormal brain. Microcephaly results from craniosynostosis (premature closure of sutures) or from a small brain. There are many causes of microcephaly including genetic, metabolic, infectious, drugs, and malnutrition. Insults during delivery and the newborn period, including hemorrhage and asphyxia, may also cause failure of normal development of the brain. Macrocephaly may be caused by a large brain (megalencephaly) but more commonly there is distension of the ventricles called hydrocephaly.

Cerebral Palsy

Cerebral palsy (CP) was first described in 1862 by Dr. George Little, who reported that difficult births resulted in mental and physical abnormalities in the child. It can be defined as a disorder of physical and mental development resulting from injury to the brain, usually in the perinatal period. The incidence of 2–3 per 1,000 live births has not changed in 30 years which is remarkable considering the changes in obstetric and neonatal care. What has changed is the type of defects that are seen because the survival of extremely immature and sick neonates results in different problems than are seen with the more mature baby. It is difficult to diagnose cerebral palsy because there is not a strict definition. CP is recognized by pediatricians, neurologists, and developmentalists as a specific entity.

■ PATHOPHYSIOLOGY

Several factors seem to interact to produce the outcome of CP. Birth asphyxia is an important factor as evidenced by the fact that a very low Apgar score is associated with a greatly increased incidence of CP. In many cases, it is thought that the brain abnormality arises prenatally from events occurring before the delivery. In 24 percent of cases, no specific cause is found. The neurologic injury is classified as a static lesion which means that the brain injury is not progressive. The cause of CP is still unclear. In many cases, significant potential brain injury is not associated with abnormal neurologic development whereas, in other cases, a mild insult results in a devastating outcome. Certainly, asphyxial changes with hypoxia and reduced cerebral perfusion are most implicated as well as significant intracranial hemorrhage.

■ CLINICAL FEATURES

The diagnosis of CP tends not to be made until after 1 year of age. Suspicion that an infant may have CP results when there is a delay in the developmental milestones. Many of the milestones are a function of motor development (gross and fine) and delay in sitting, standing, or walking, in association with physical findings such as abnormal muscle tone or neurologic signs, may suggest the diagnosis.

It is useful to classify cerebral palsy on the basis of the movement disorder that predominates as well as the involved parts of

TABLE 25-1. CLASSIFICATION OF CEREBRAL PALSY

Spastic forms (75%)
Quadriplegia (4 extremities)
Diplegia (legs more than arms)
Hemiplegia (one side more than the other)
Paraplegia (legs only)
Mono- or triplegia (1 or 3 limbs)
Ataxic (15%)
Dyskinetic (choreoathetosis) (5%)
Hypotonic ($< 1\%$)
Mixed

the body. The defects are classified as spastic, dyskinetic (abnormal voluntary movement), ataxic (abnormal balance and coordination), or mixed which is a combination of the above (Table 25-1).

Spasticity occurs with increased tone of muscles which results in tightness of the extremities with movement. Deep tendon reflexes tend to be increased and ankle clonus is common. Over time, the increased tone leads to contractures. Limb deformities and scoliosis develop. Spastic diplegia affects all extremities but lower tends to be more affected than upper. Examination reveals positive Babinski, tight heel cords, and scissoring. Scissoring results from increased adductor muscle tone. This form of CP accounts for 10–30 percent of cases and is seen following birth asphyxia and especially in the premature infant.

Spastic quadriplegia implies 4-limb involvement and sometimes the face is also involved and called pentaplegia. Hemiplegia implies that the arm and leg on one side are involved and double hemiplegia means that four limbs are involved with one side more involved than the other. All of these classifications are arbitrary, but they can be useful as descriptive terms.

Abnormal movements are called dyskinesias which are involuntary movements that occur after voluntary movement. The common form is choreoathetosis which results from basal ganglia involvement in kernicterus and is rare now compared to 30 years ago. Ataxia involves disorders of the cerebellum which leads to

TABLE 25-2. PROBLEMS OF CEREBRAL PALSY

Impaired motor functioning
Static (non-progressive) muscular weakness
Failure to reach developmental milestones

Symptoms
   Poor head control after 3 months of age
   Moro or atonic neck reflexes persist beyond 6 months of age
   Irritability
   Weak cry, poor suck
   Excessive sleep

problems of balance and coordination. Some of the children with ataxic CP inherit this as an autosomal recessive disorder.

Table 25-2 provides a listing of the various problems that are associated with CP. The key to the diagnosis is the failure to achieve the milestones that are associated with normal development. Neonatal follow-up of the high-risk infant is important to identify infants at risk.

Diagnostic radiologic and laboratory studies should be performed to assist in the diagnosis and to rule out other disorders. Structural abnormalities are evaluated with CT scan and MRI as well as head ultrasound. Evidence of cerebral hemorrhage in the newborn period, especially the preterm infant, and its resolution and brain atrophy may accompany CP. EEG may be useful, metabolic work-up should be performed, and genetic studies may be indicated.

The features of the diagnosis are that there is no progression of the neurologic injury; that there is failure to meet the normal motor milestones; and that the neurologic evaluation is abnormal. Examples of early signs include poor head control, increased tone in the hamstrings or achilles tendon, abnormal moro, and atonic neck reflexes. Later signs of CP include abnormal gait and weakness.

■ **MANAGEMENT**

The disorder is permanent and relatively static. The therapy is directed at prevention, reducing the effect of complications and allowing the child to achieve full potential. The major problems are secondary to the neurological damage and orthopedic complications. The treatment plan must be devised in light of the symptoms that are present. Some patients have dominantly physical limitations, while others have mental retardation and some have both. There are multiple secondary effects as listed in Table 25-3 and prevention and treatment of these are important.

During the early years, treatment is primarily physical and occupational therapy. One treatment program that has been tried is the Bobath method to improve motor development and to reduce contractures. During childhood, the goal is to allow the child to achieve functional capacity in the real world. This has to be planned within the framework of the current medical and educational systems.

Orthotic devices are used to supplement the therapies. They include braces and splints which serve to provide stability to joints and to reduce the contractures. Various equipment from crutches to wheelchairs may be needed to assist in care.

Orthopedic surgery is used to correct deformities and contractures. Heel-cord lengthening, release of spastic wrist flexor muscles, and correction of hip and adductor muscle spasticity are used to improve mobility. It is important to be selective about surgical intervention.

Selective dorsal rhizotomy is a procedure that has been tried with some success. It involves cutting the nerves along the spinal

TABLE 25-3. SECONDARY EFFECTS OF CEREBRAL PALSY

Seizures
Mental retardation
Sensory and speech deficits
Learning disability
Visual defects (strabismus, retinopathy of prematurity, cortical blindness)
Hearing deficit
Hip dislocation
Scoliosis
Contractures
GE reflux
Bowel and bladder deficits
Pulmonary infections

cord but not in the spinal cord to reduce the spasticity. The abnormal nerves are identified by electrical stimulation and are divided. The result is reduction of the spasticity but the resulting flaccidity requires considerable retraining. Many practitioners consider the procedure to be experimental and the results are unpredictable. There does not appear to be improvement in patients more than 8 years of age. Consent should only be sought and accepted when there is full understanding of the risks.

The treatment of associated problems is important. Mental retardation and seizures are commonly associated and may be severe. Sensory disorders, including speech disorders and visual and auditory impairment, need to be evaluated and treated. Most systems can be involved: feeding and GI problems, lung infections and aspiration, skin and dental problems, and psychological and behavior problems. Learning disabilities and attention-deficit hyperactivity disorder are all commonly seen. Neuropsychological testing is necessary to evaluate these and include the interventions in the treatment plan. About half of the children with CP suffer from seizures which run the gamut of generalized tonic-clonic and partial complex to absence spells. Blindness may be associated because of retinopathy of prematurity. Deafness may be a complication of medications received in the neonatal period resulting in auditory nerve damage and also commonly from recurrent otitis media.

Coma/Persistent Vegetative State/Brain Death

Coma is a deep state of unconsciousness from which the patient cannot be aroused. *Stupor* is a lighter state and the patient can be aroused by vigorous or painful stimuli. Persistent vegetative state occurs following coma and there is a lack of awareness of surroundings or self, although arousal may occur.

The causes of coma are multiple and most are acute disorders. Recovery from coma after a prolonged period may be possible if there has not been irreversible extensive brain injury.

Brain death implies that there is no electrical function of the brain as measured by EEG or absence of perfusion as shown on radionuclear scan or angiogram.

Epilepsy

A seizure is the result of an aberrant electrical charge which results in overexcitation of neurones that discharge abnormally. The result is variable and may have no clinical effect or there may be seizure activity which will manifest in different ways depending on which part or parts of the brain are involved. Epilepsy is the constellation of repeated seizures that originate in the brain. In many cases no specific cause is found. Childhood absence epilepsy is a genetic disorder with autosomal dominant inheritance.

■ ETIOLOGY

The causes of repetitive seizures are multiple and categorized in Table 25-4. Seizures accompany many other disorders. Four percent of all children have a febrile seizure which is defined as occurring between the age of 6 months and 3 years. The seizure is brief, lasting less than 5 minutes, and it is generalized. The fever usually exceeds 38.8°C (101°F) and tends to accompany respiratory or GI illness. Less than 5 percent of children who have febrile seizures go on to develop epilepsy.

Epilepsy can occur because of a defect of the CNS or alternatively a disorder that affects the CNS. They are commonly noted first in the newborn period. Childhood absence epilepsy tends to start between 4 and 8 years and juvenile absence epilepsy tends to occur during puberty and may be associated with generalized tonic-clonic seizures.

TABLE 25-4. CAUSES OF REPETITIVE SEIZURES (EPILEPSY)

Localized—focal or partial
  Idiopathic
    Benign childhood partial seizure
    Benign centrotemporal (Rolandic) epilepsy
    Benign occipital epilepsy
  Secondary
    Tumor
    Trauma
    Infection
    Ischemia
Generalized
  Idiopathic
    Benign neonatal convulsion
    West syndrome
    Lennox–Gastaut syndrome
    Childhood absence "petit mal"
    Tonic-clonic "grand mal"
Local and general
  Progressive myoclonus epilepsy
Special syndromes
  Febrile convulsion
  Seizure caused by metabolic, toxic or drug-induced event

■ CLINICAL FEATURES

Generalized seizures imply that the electrical discharge is widespread. They used to be called "grand mal" and the new terminology is "tonic-clonic." Generalized tonic-clonic seizures may be preceded by a prodrome of anxiety or apprehension. The seizure commences with an immediate loss of consciousness with widespread contraction of muscles. There may be forcible expiration of air (epileptic cry) and the eyes are deviated up. This tonic phase usually lasts 10–20 seconds and is followed by the clonic phase that lasts about 30 seconds. The clonic phase is alternate contraction and relaxation leading to shaking (that cannot be stopped by holding the limbs in place). There are marked autonomic changes that accompany this phase including salivation, sweating, and elevation of heart rate and blood pressure. Incontinence of urine is usual and there may also be fecal incontinence. After the seizure, there is a slow return to consciousness with post-ictal confusion and somnolence often lasting a few hours. There is amnesia for the event.

Partial or focal seizures are less common in children than in adults. In most cases, no etiology is found, although they may be a feature of metabolic disorders including low glucose, low calcium, and water intoxication. In children, they may be related to lesions acquired early in life, for example atrophy, and may be the presenting sign of subdural hematoma in infants. Complex partial seizures arise in the cortex, most often the temporal lobe, but can also start in the frontal or parietal lobes. A non-specific aura precedes the seizure in 30 percent of cases and the seizure tends to last 1–2 minutes. The seizure may start with staring, automatic behavior, tonic extension of one or both arms, or loss of body tone. Staring is associated with a change in facial expression and is followed by automatic behavior which may be fumbling movements of the fingers, facial grimaces, walking, or resisting restraint. The behavior tends to be similar for an individual from seizure to seizure and is followed by confusion or lethargy. Generalized seizures may follow if the child is not treated.

Complex partial seizures have EEG abnormalities that may be a spike or slow wave focus in the area of origin. The study may be normal and may need to be repeated to demonstrate the abnormality because hyperventilation or photic stimulation tends not to provoke the seizure. MRI should be considered in all cases as low-grade gliomas may be the cause of the seizure.

Absence seizures (petit mal) are often not recognized initially. The child stops what he is doing and stares vacantly, sometimes with rhythmic eyelid movements, and then resumes the previous activity. There is no aura or post-ictal confusion. The absence tends to occur for 5–10 seconds but may last as long as a minute. There may be up to 100 episodes a day. About 50 percent of children with absence seizures have at least one generalized tonic-clonic seizure and this may be the event that brings the disorder to medical attention. In addition, there are forms of absence epilepsy that are associated with myoclonic movements.

Myoclonic seizures are characterized by brief jerking movements that tend to be symmetrical and can be vigorous enough to cause a patient to fall. They are usually not associated with loss of consciousness—rather the patient tends to be aware of the event. They may be the only symptom of epilepsy or be part of another form such as absence. There is a juvenile myoclonic epilepsy that is inherited and features myoclonic movements (sometimes with tonic-clonic seizures) shortly after waking up.

The diagnosis of absence seizure is confirmed with the EEG which shows a bilaterally synchronous and symmetric paroxysms of 3-cps spike-wave complexes that coincide with the seizure. Hyperventilation can usually be used to activate the EEG pattern.

Infantile Spasms (West Syndrome)

This disorder starts before 2 years of age, with two-thirds of cases occurring first before 6 months of age. The feature of this disorder is the salaam attack (Blitzkrampf) with sudden flexion of the head and trunk at the same time with flexion and adduction of the arms and legs. The spasms may only be partial movements in the beginning but they increase and may occur several times a day. The EEG is grossly abnormal and shows high-voltage irregular slow waves with spikes over wide areas of the brain. This pattern has been named hypsarrhythmia. The infantile spasms and hypsarrhythmia tend to reduce over time so that by 2 years of age 50 percent have stopped and almost all by 5 years of age. Unfortunately the prognosis is bad and treatment unsatisfactory. The mortality is about 15–20 percent and two-thirds of the survivors will have severe mental retardation and seizures. Some children do respond to steroids and ACTH or prednisone should be tried. Clonazepam or valproate may help with the spasms.

Pseudoseizures (Psychogenic Seizures)

These are behavioral manifestations that result in seizure movements without any changes on the EEG. They may be present in a child or adolescent who has a seizure disorder. The episodes will tend to be different from true seizures although some patients learn to be very realistic. The spells are emotionally triggered and require a psychological approach to manage.

Status Epilepticus

This is defined as continued or recurring seizure activity, often despite treatment, with duration that may be as long as 30 minutes or more. It constitutes a medical emergency and immediate treatment is necessary.

Management

Management of epilepsy involves treatment of the individual seizure, suppression of seizure activity, as well as addressing the cause of epilepsy, which may be amenable to treatment. Tonic-clonic seizures are managed with phenobarbitone, valproate, carbamazepine, and phenytoin.

Complex partial seizures can be treated with carbamazepine, phenytoin, primidone, or valproate. Temporal lobectomy has been recommended if the seizures do not respond to medications.

Absence seizures can be managed with either ethosuximide or valproate and the seizures are controlled in 80 percent of children. The former has fewer side effects and should be the first consideration. When the treatment is successful the EEG becomes normal.

Myoclonic seizures respond best to valproate or diazepines. A ketogenic diet may be effective in children with myoclonic seizures related to brain damage. The ketogenic diet involves fat to carbohydrate in a ratio of 4 : 1.

If seizures are persistent and difficult to control surgical treatment has been successful, particularly if a specific focus can be identified.

The management of seizures requires support and education for the patient and the family. Seizures are frightening and it is important to stress safety. Intervention at the time of the seizure involves maintaining an airway and avoiding injury. Supervision of children with seizures is essential, particularly in relation to heights and water.

Compliance with medications is a major issue. Older children and adolescents do not like to be different from their peers. Alcohol and other drugs can alter the seizure threshold. Drug levels should be checked if there is an alteration in mental status or if there is increased seizure activity.

Fetal Alcohol Syndrome

Alcohol is the leading abused drug worldwide and prenatal alcohol exposure results in many fetal abnormalities. Lemoine in France in 1868 and Jones in the United States in 1973 reported the multiple effects of alcohol on the developing fetus. The spectrum of effects is broad and even with 2 drinks a day smaller birth size may result and 4–6 drinks a day is associated with evident clinical features. Infants born to alcoholic mothers result in the fetal alcohol syndrome (FAS). The incidence is not known, but Olegaard in Sweden showed that 1 in 300 babies had effects of alcohol. They estimated that 10–20 percent of children with IQs in the 50–80 range and 1 in 6 cases of cerebral palsy were the result of heavy alcohol exposure in utero.

FAS is characterized by distinctive facial features and with microcephaly. There is a flat midface with narrow palpebral fissures, a low nasal bridge with short upturned nose, and a rather long convex filtrum with a thin long upper lip. There is usually pre- and post-natal growth deficiency with failure to thrive. The newborn is often tremulous. Mental retardation and developmental delay results in an average IQ of 63.

It is estimated that as many as 1 in 200 children born to women in the United States may have developmental problems related to prenatal alcohol drinking. It is recommended that no alcohol be taken during pregnancy.

Hydrocephalus

When there is an excessive amount of cerebrospinal fluid (CSF) with dilatation of the ventricular system, the condition is called hydrocephalus. CSF is produced continuously by the choroid plexus within the cerebral hemispheres and circulates through the ventricular system. The lateral ventricles are within the cerebral hemispheres and connect at the foramen of Monro to the single third ventricle in the midline. The third ventricle connects via the aqueduct of Sylvius to the fourth ventricle in the brainstem. CSF drains out of the brain through the foramen of Magendie and Lushke which are in the posterior fossa. Hydrocephalus is caused by obstruction to the passage of CSF as it circulates. It may be congenital or acquired. Communicating hydrocephalus occurs when the obstruction is outside the ventricular system and fluid circulates from the ventricular system to the subarachnoid space and cisternal system. Non-communicating hydrocephalus implies that the blockage is within the ventricular system.

The congenital form can be isolated or in association with many neurologic disorders. The incidence is estimated to be 1–4 per 1,000 live births. The cause may be infectious or from congenital malformation of the CNS. The Dandy–Walker malformation consists of a posterior fossa cyst continuous with the fourth ventricle, partial or complete absence of the cerebellar vermis, and hydrocephalus. Acquired hydrocephalus may also be infectious and is associated with cerebral tumors and intracranial hemorrhage.

The symptoms directly related to hydrocephalus (rather than the underlying condition) include full fontanelle, enlarging head, vomiting, lethargy, and posturing. In children there will be headache, vomiting, lethargy, and visual changes. Depending on the cause of the raised pressure, the progression may be acute or chronic.

■ MANAGEMENT

Surgical treatment will attempt to remove the obstruction and if necessary divert the flow of CSF so that drainage can occur. Shunting procedures involve placement of a catheter from the ventricle to another site for absorption. The most common site is the peritoneum, and the atria and pleural cavity are alternate sites. The ventricular catheter is placed via a burr hole and the catheter tunneled under the skin. There is a one-way valve with a reservoir to test shunt function. Shunt malfunction may be associated with infection and bleeding. Most children need shunt revision at intervals during childhood.

Muscle Disease

The major group of muscle diseases of children is muscular dystrophy (MD). These are genetic disorders associated with degeneration of muscle fibers that result in weakness with slow progression throughout childhood. There are no specific therapies for the conditions but supportive therapies, especially physical therapy, can make a real difference. Contractures and deformities are common and the area of disability varies with the involved muscle groups.

Facioscapulohumeral (Landouzy-Déjerine) MD is an autosomal disorder that affects adolescents. There is slow progression with difficulty raising the arms over the head, forward slope of the shoulders, and facial weakness. Limb-girdle MD is an autosomal recessive disorder with weakness of the shoulder and pelvic girdles. It manifests in late childhood and adolescence and is slow to progress.

■ DUCHENNE MUSCULAR DYSTROPHY

The most well-known muscular dystrophy is Duchenne, also known as pseudohypertrophic, muscular dystrophy (DMD). It is an X-linked recessive disorder with an incidence of 1 per 3,500 live male births. The child appears normal until he starts to walk and play at which time he begins to suffer trips and falls, and to walk on tiptoe, and he may have difficulty with coordination. The progression of symptoms is variable but tends to be obvious by 3–5 years of age. The physical finding that suggests the diagnosis is enlarged calf muscles. The clinical problems are listed in

TABLE 25-5. CLINICAL FEATURES OF DUCHENNE MUSCULAR DYSTROPHY

X-linked recessive disorder
Males aged 2–6 years
Early clumsiness, walking on toes
Pelvic girdle weakness
Hypertrophy of gastrocnemius
Eventual cardiomyopathy
CK 4,000–5,000
Chromosome deletion Xp21

Table 25-5. Gower's sign is the turning onto the side or abdomen and then kneeling. In order to get to an upright position, the torso is raised by walking the hands up the legs.

Contractures of the lower limbs develop, particularly the Achilles tendon, and lumbar lordosis becomes prominent. The child gradually becomes unable to walk and most boys are in a wheelchair by the age of 13 years. Death tends to occur in the late teens or early 20s because of respiratory failure.

The serum creatine kinase (also known as creatine phospho-kinase—CK or CPK) level becomes elevated to 10 times the normal value. If an infant older than 3 months is found to have a creatine kinase greater than 2,000 U/L, the diagnosis is made and muscle biopsy confirms the diagnosis. The pathologic changes are degeneration of muscle fibers, phagocytosis, and fiber changes including variable size and shape.

The genetic defect has been located to the chromosome Xp21. The gene protein product that is lacking is called dystrophin. About 25–30 percent of cases are spontaneous mutations; the remainder receive the gene from their mother.

There is a mild form of pseudohypertrophic MD, which is known as Becker's. Weakness tends to start later in life and to progress gradually and intelligence tends to be normal. CPK is elevated and muscle biopsy is abnormal.

■ MANAGEMENT

There is no specific treatment for childhood MD. Activity is beneficial in improving muscle strength and delaying the need for the wheelchair. Physical therapy is used for range-of-motion exercises and braces to improve their potential for activities of daily living. Orthopedic procedures may be indicated for relief of contractures. As there is progress in disability, there needs to be a plan for care for the child and the family. While the child will hope to remain independent, there reaches a point when the activities become very restricted. Respite care for the family, and even institutional care in a skilled nursing facility, may be indicated. Support for the family is beneficial and the Muscular Dystrophy Association can be most helpful.

Neural Tube Defect

Myelodysplasia is the term used to describe defective formation and development of the spinal cord. The defect can occur at any level and results in altered function below that level. The incidence of neural tube defects is approximately 0.7–5 per 1,000 live births and varies with geographic location. The cause is unknown but there is some familial tendency and an increased risk if there is poor maternal nutrition and lack of prenatal care. Spina bifida occulta occurs when there is a defect in the vertebra because of failed fusion of the arch. It is associated with cutaneous lesions, including tufts of hair, hemangioma, or a dermoid cyst over the defect. If the neural tube fails to close, there is a cystic dilatation of meninges through the vertebral defect, known as meningocele. If the spinal cord protrudes through the vertebral defect the lesion is meningomyelocele.

The recurrence risk is 5 percent if one sibling is affected and 10–15 percent if two siblings are affected. Affected mothers have a 3 percent chance of having a child with a similar defect.

Antenatal diagnosis may be made if the neural tube is open because there will be elevation of maternal serum alpha-feto-protein. The best time to detect the elevation is at the 3rd to 4th months of the pregnancy.

■ CLINICAL FEATURES

Spina bifida occulta is usually asymptomatic although in time bladder and/or bowel dysfunction or other neurologic abnormality may ensue. The protruding sac of the meningocele is evident at birth and may be covered with thin layers of skin or muscle. There may not be any neurologic deficits initially.

Meningomyelocele has a much more severe outlook with virtually all cases demonstrating hydrocephalus and 85 percent of these requiring an internal shunt. One of the associated defects is the Arnold Chiari II malformation. There is downward displacement of the cerebellum, brainstem, and fourth ventricle. There may be compression of the brainstem and cerebellar tonsils if they are displaced below the foramen magnum.

The site of the defect dictates in part the neurologic deficit. Most lesions are lumbar or sacral and Table 25-6 lists the potential

TABLE 25-6. MYELODYSPLASIA AT DIFFERENT LEVELS

Thoracic
  Flaccid paralysis of lower extremities
  Abdominal wall weakness
  Respiratory compromise (high thoracic)
  Absent bowel and bladder control

High lumbar
  Flaccid paralysis of knees, ankles, and feet
  May walk with devices/braces
  Absent bowel and bladder control

Midlumbar
  Flaccid paralysis of ankles and feet
  Absent bowel and bladder control

Low lumbar
  Weakness of ankles
  Limited bowel or bladder control

Sacral
  Essentially normal lower limb function
  Essentially normal bowel and bladder control

problems at the different levels. It is usual for the spinal cord to be dysplastic and motor and sensory deficit below the level of the lesion to be significant with complete paralysis and absence of sensation. There may be some central connections so that some sensation or movement is possible. There is almost always incontinence of bladder and bowel.

■ MANAGEMENT

If there is a significant defect, it is recommended to deliver the baby by cesarean section. The meningocele is evident at birth. The defect is corrected surgically and manipulation of the sac may result in neurologic deficits. Meningomyelocele requires multidisciplinary team management. Table 25-7 lists some of the associated problems that need to be addressed. Until the defect has healed, skin problems, especially infection, are possible. Sensory defects below the lesion increases the risk of skin breakdown. CT scan or MRI is necessary to evaluate ventricular size. MRI scan provides a better look at the brainstem and may be more useful to delineate the Chiari malformation. Hydrocephalus may be more prominent after the spinal defect is closed if CSF was draining at the site. Hydrocephalus will be managed with a shunt, usually a ventriculoperitoneal shunt.

Cranial nerve defects may occur with visual problems. Overall the children with myelodysplasia have normal intelligence. The impact of the hydrocephalus and seizures may result in intellectual impairment. Motor defects require physical therapy

TABLE 25-7. MENINGOMYELOCELE-ASSOCIATED PROBLEMS

Hydrocephalus
Seizures
Visual and perception problems
Cognitive deficit
Skin breakdown at back and below level of lesion
Urinary-tract infection
Latex allergy

and assistance with wheelchairs. Scoliosis is a common problem. Restrictive pulmonary disease may develop.

Maternal treatment with folic acid appears to reduce the chance of myelodysplasia and should be started a few months before the pregnancy for optimal results.

Neurofibromatosis Type I

Also known as von Recklinghausen disease, this is one of the most common autosomal dominant defects with an incidence of 1 per 3,000 live births with many cases being new mutations (30–50 percent). The gene has been localized to 17q11.2. The features include pigmented skin lesions called café-au-lait spots which slowly grow during childhood. To be diagnostic there should be 6 or more spots over 5 mm in diameter prepuberty and over 15 mm postpuberty. The spots tend to be smooth and darken with age. If they are irregularly shaped, the diagnosis of McCune–Albright syndrome should be considered. There may be freckling in the axilla and groin region or pigmented nevi. Ninety-five percent of patients more than 6 years of age have Lisch nodules which are small pigmented hamartomas of the iris.

The neurofibromas may be few or multiple and may develop on any nerve. They tend to be soft and can enlarge to produce significant deformity. Plexiform neurofibromas are large, occurring along nerve bundles and may be present at birth. Most of the tumors are benign but there is a 5 percent malignancy rate. The majority of patients have normal intelligence but there are learning disorders in 50 percent and mental deficiency in 5 percent of cases. Seizures occur in 20 percent of cases. Bone lesions are fairly common and may produce deformities. Involvement of the spine may cause scoliosis. The diagnostic features are shown in Table 25-8.

Neurofibromatosis type 2 is also called central or acoustic neurofibromatosis. It is a dominant disorder (gene 22q11.2) with an incidence of 1 per 50,000 live births. The main features are

TABLE 25-8. CLINICAL FEATURES OF NEUROFIBROMATOSIS

Two or more of the following:

More than 6 café-au-lait spots (5 mm pre-puberty, 15 mm post-puberty)
Two or more neurofibromas of any type or one plexiform neurofibroma
Freckles of axilla or inguinal areas
Optic glioma
Two or more Lisch nodules (hamartomas of the iris)
Osseous lesions
First-degree relative with neurofibromatosis using these criteria

bilateral acoustic neuromas with spinal cord and brain tumors. Skin lesions are sparse in this condition. The lesions appear late in childhood and tend to be more severe than neurofibromatosis type 1.

■ MANAGEMENT

The majority of affected individuals have a benign course but still require regular (1–2 times a year) follow-up to screen for complications. Surgical removal of lesions is indicated only if complications arise. Complications may result from local pressure from the enlarging tumor or the development of malignant change. Suspicion of malignant change includes pain, increasing size, and neurologic deficits. Optic gliomas are suggested by visual field changes.

Spinal Muscular Atrophy

■ PROGRESSIVE (INFANTILE): WERDNIG–HOFFMANN

This is progressive spinal muscular atrophy and is characterized by weakness of skeletal muscles. There is degeneration of the anterior horn cells in the spinal cord and the motor neurone cells in the brainstem. These cells innervate the skeletal muscles. It is an autosomal recessive disorder with an incidence of 1 per 10,000 births. The disorder has been subdivided into three groups.

Group 1 has the onset at birth or before two months of age and has severe generalized weakness and is the classic "floppy infant syndrome." The baby lies in the frog position and cannot lift against gravity. The breathing is diaphragmatic and secretions tend to pool in the pharynx. Death tends to occur within months. Group 2 starts between 2 and 12 months of age with initial limb weakness followed by generalized weakness. The progression is slower with death occurring before age 8 years. The third group has onset of symptoms in the second year of life with weakness of the thigh and hip muscles that makes walking difficult so that they tend to become wheelchair-bound by adolescence. The gene has been localized to 5-q12–q13 and prenatal diagnosis is possible.

■ MANAGEMENT

Group 1 is the floppy baby with progressive severe weakness leading to respiratory failure within a few months so that most infants die in the first 2 years. With intensive nursing and medical care, the rate of progression can be reduced. The condition causes severe floppiness and with weakness there is impaired swallowing and cough with the result that aspiration and pneumonia are common. Frequent changes of position and nasopharyngeal suctioning and careful attention to feeding can reduce the complications. Chest physiotherapy may be helpful.

If the condition is rapidly progressive with the potential for early death, it is probably inappropriate to be too aggressive. The decision to perform gastrostomy, usually with fundal plication, as well as tracheostomy should be made if the quality of life can be improved. The difficulty with assigning an accurate prognosis is that there is a wide spectrum of severity and rate of deterioration. The family needs to be encouraged but it is necessary to be aware that many patients become progressively worse despite exemplary care.

■ JUVENILE: KUGELBERG–WELANDER

This is juvenile proximal hereditary spinal muscular atrophy. There is anterior horn cell and motor neurone degeneration. The genetics that have been reported are autosomal dominant and recessive as well as X- linked recessive. The onset starts any time from one year to adulthood and is similar to group 3 infantile muscular atrophy. There is lower limb girdle weakness that is slowly progressive such that the inability to walk may result 10–30 years after onset.

Tuberous Sclerosis ....

Tuberous sclerosis (TS), also known as Bourneville disease, epiloia, is an autosomal dominant disorder with a 60–70 percent new mutation rate. The incidence is 1 per 25,000 live births. The genetic disorder is on chromosome 9 or 16. The features include adenoma sebaceum, seizures, and mental retardation. The skin lesion starts as an ash-leaf shaped depigmented macule in infancy and is strongly suggestive of the condition. It is best seen with a Wood's lamp (ultraviolet light source). Adenoma sebaceum lesions are fibroangiomatous nevi that are usually not seen until 4–7 years of age. They are on the bridge of the nose, the cheeks, and along the nasolabial folds in a butterfly distribution. They may also occur on the forehead, neck, and trunk. They change in color from red to brown but they do not enlarge in size, ulcerate, or suppurate.

The brain lesions are cortical and subependymal firm nodules which are benign tumors called hamartomas. The lesions are calcified and CT scan or MRI will demonstrate them. In 5 percent of patients, they cause obstruction to the flow of CSF leading to hydrocephalus which usually requires a shunt procedure. Seizures in infancy present as infantile spasms and 25 percent of children with infantile spasms have TS. In older children, the seizures tend to be generalized but partial complex and myoclonic seizures may occur.

Additional findings include retinal hamartomas, cardiac rhabdomyomas, and angiofibromas of the kidney. Subungual fibromas at the base of the fingernails are characteristic.

■ **MANAGEMENT**

Although mental retardation is listed as a cardinal feature, about 40 percent of patients have normal intelligence. The patients at risk for retardation are those with early onset seizures, particularly infantile spasms. Aggressive management of seizures may reduce long-term complications. If there are learning problems, special schooling should be considered.

Parents of children with tuberous sclerosis should be carefully evaluated before deciding that the mutation was sporadic. There is a great deal of variation and there may only be occasional skin lesions or a single internal hamartoma. It is recommended to perform fundoscopic evaluation and Wood's lamp evaluation of the skin. Negative examination does not completely rule out the condition and it is recommended to perform CT scan and renal sonography to check for internal hamartomas. If a parent has tuberous sclerosis, then each pregnancy is accompanied by a 50 percent chance of the offspring being affected.

26

Chapter Twenty-Six

Psychological Disorders

Mental health treatment has changed markedly in the last few years because of the impact of managed care. Long-term institutional care, month-long hospital stays, and ongoing out-patient care are no longer the norm if the patient is under managed care. The mental health practitioner is prevented from spending the time that may be necessary to make a diagnosis, to try different treatment strategies, and to follow-up to ensure that the patient is responding.

The psychiatrist may be put in the position of prescribing medication and the therapy services will be provided by non-physician professionals and therapists. Child psychiatry is even worse off than adult psychiatry. Certainly the amount of research that is performed with children is limited, partly in view of the fact that the drug companies do not want to fund studies in the smaller market.

Chronic mental health disorders in children are also evolving in terms of our understanding and treatment. Affective or mood disorders can be unipolar (depression) or bipolar (manic depression). They may be primary or as a result of another psychiatric or medical disorder and they commonly accompany chronic illnesses.

Anxiety disorders comprise a group of illnesses that include:

- general anxiety disorder (GAD)
- separation anxiety disorder (SAD)
- panic disorder

- phobias
- obsessive-compulsive disorder
- post-traumatic stress disorder

The features that characterize anxiety disorders are the physiologic changes that accompany them. Depression and anxiety disorders are characterized as internalizing disorders. The externalizing disorders are attention-deficit hyperactivity disorder, oppositional defiant disorder, and conduct disorders. There is constant referral to the Diagnostic and Statistical Manual of Mental Disorders (DSM). The present version is DSM-IV, 1994, which is published by the American Psychiatric Association. This is the source for the diagnostic nomenclature for mental health disorders. The recent edition has improved the classification of childhood psychological disorders and they are now much more consistent with the adult classification.

Attention-Deficit Hyperactivity Disorder

Attention-deficit hyperactivity disorder (ADHD) is one of the most common psychiatric disorders in childhood and may comprise 50 percent of the evaluations performed by child psychiatrists. ADHD was referred to in a Shakespeare play and George Still, an English physician, in 1902 reported 20 children who had aggressive, passionate, lawless, inattentive, impulsive, and over-active behavior. In this study, he noted male more than female and increased alcoholism, criminal conduct, and depression in the family history. The DSM-II described the hyperkinetic reaction of childhood. In the DSM-IV, the disorder is defined as including inattention and hyperactivity/impulsivity with an onset prior to 7 years of age.

One description from Weiss indicates the important diagnostic features including: inappropriate or excessive activity, unrelated to the task at hand, which generally has an intrusive or annoying quality; poor sustained attention; difficulties in inhibiting impulses in social behavior and cognitive tasks; difficulties getting along with others; school underachievement; poor self-esteem; and other behavior disorders, learning disabilities, anxiety disorders, and depression.

Children with ADHD generally spend more of their life in motion. This behavior provides problems at school because of the disruption to other children as well as at home because it places everybody in the family on edge. The behavior also varies at different times so that on occasions the child may respond in a more usual fashion to a teacher that he likes, or to please a parent, or to avoid a problem at the doctor's office. More usually the behavior is manifest in many areas.

Some children are able to concentrate on video games for hours on end and yet when they have to accomplish a small amount of homework their behavior is impossible to control with tantrums and screaming. Impulsive behavior may be associated with disruptive actions that often are without regard for the feelings of others and done because the child wants instant gratification. The behavior often results in difficulty making friends and alienating peers as well as family. Learning disorders are common and there is generally underachievement that is not related to intelligence.

It is estimated that 3–5 percent of children display characteristics of ADHD. More boys are diagnosed than girls at a ratio of 4 : 1 for the impulsive type and 2 : 1 for the inattentive type. The etiology is unknown with some genetic factors based on the fact that the disorder tends to run in families. ADHD may be associated with various conditions as a manifestation of their symptoms, for example seizure disorder, fragile X, and many chronic illnesses. In addition, there is high co-morbidity with other mental health disorders including anxiety or depression which may be present in more than half the cases diagnosed ADHD.

■ MANAGEMENT

The diagnosis is made based on the presence of a constellation of symptoms (Table 26-1) that are listed in the DSM-IV in the

TABLE 26-1. SYMPTOMS OF ATTENTION-DEFICIT HYPERACTIVITY DISORDER

A. Either 1 or 2:

1. Six (or more) of the following symptoms of *inattention* have persisted for at least 6 months to a degree that is maladaptive and with developmental level:

   Inattention
   (a) Often fails to give close attention to details or makes careless mistakes in schoolwork, work, or other activities
   (b) Often has difficulty sustaining attention in task or play activities
   (c) Often does not seem to listen when spoken to directly
   (d) Often does not follow through on instructions and fails to finish schoolwork, chores, or duties in the workplace (not due to oppositional behavior or failure to understand instructions)
   (e) . Often has difficulty organizing tasks and activities
   (f) Often avoids, dislikes, or is reluctant to engage in tasks that require sustained mental effort (such as schoolwork or homework)
   (g) Often loses things necessary for tasks or activities (e.g., toys, school assignments, pencils, books, or tools)
   (h) Is often easily distracted by extraneous stimuli
   (i) Is often forgetful in daily activities

2. Six (or more) of the following symptoms of *hyperactivity-impulsivity* have persisted for at least 6 months to a degree that is maladaptive and inconsistent with developmental level:

   Hyperactivity
   (a) Often fidgets with hands or feet or squirms in seat
   (b) Often leaves seat in classroom or in other situations in which remaining seated is expected
   (c) Often runs about or climbs excessively in situations in which it is inappropriate (in adolescents or adults, may be limited to subjective feelings of restlessness)
   (d) Often has difficulty playing or engaging in leisure activities quietly
   (e) Is often "on the go" or often acts as if "driven by a motor"
   (f) Often talks excessively

   Impulsivity
   (g) Often blurts out answers before questions have been completed
   (h) Often has difficulty awaiting turn
   (i) Often interrupts or intrudes on others (e.g., butts into conversations or games)

B. Some hyperactive/impulsive or inattentive symptoms that caused impairment were present before age 7 years.
C. Some impairment from the symptoms is present in two or more settings (e.g., at school [or work] and at home).
D. There must be clear evidence of clinically significant impairment in social, academic, or occupational functioning.
E. The symptoms do not occur exclusively during the course of a pervasive developmental disorder, schizophrenia, or other psychotic disorder and are not better accounted for by another mental disorder (e.g., mood disorder, anxiety disorder, dissociative disorder, or a personality disorder).

absence of another diagnosis to explain the symptoms. This requires a careful history from the parents and child and possibly input from school teachers. Physical examination is important to rule out other medical conditions. There are no laboratory tests to rule in the diagnosis but they may be necessary for confirmation of other disorders.

Treatment planning requires an individualized plan with the clinician as the coordinator of care. The plan should include consideration for medication as well as behavioral and psychosocial interventions that are dependent on the symptoms displayed by the patient. The initial report of therapy involved the use of benzedrine which caused benefit in a group of disturbed hospitalized patients. The most widely prescribed medicine is methylphenidate (Ritalin) and it has been extensively studied. The onset of action is rapid and dose can be titrated to response. Despite being stimulant medications, methylphenidate and dextroamphetamine have a response rate of about 70–80 percent. There are longer lasting preparations but in many cases they are not as beneficial as the shorter acting preparations. The commonest side effect is appetite suppression and so it is recommended to give the dose after meals. There may be autonomic effects, especially with heart rate and blood pressure increases, but these are usually mild. If there is inadequate response to stimulant medications, it is usual to consider tricyclic antidepressants and they may be particularly useful if depression is the co-morbid condition.

It is reported that 30–80 percent of children with ADHD continue to have features into adolescence. There appears to be an increase in risky behaviors and continued antisocial behavior in some adolescents. These vary from drinking alcohol and smoking to an increase in motor vehicle accidents. Persistence of symptoms into adult life has not been well studied and so it is difficult to give a prognosis beyond adolescence.

Mental Retardation

The definition of mental retardation is reduction of intellectual functioning that is usually stratified on the basis of IQ (Table 26-2). The IQ less than 70, or equivalent low level functioning, is the basis for the definition. The onset will be before 18 years of age. This is the definition in the DSM-IV. The American Association on Mental Retardation implies substantial limitations in functioning without defining an IQ number (Table 26-3).

Formal testing of intellectual performance includes the Stanford–Binet and the Wechsler Intelligence Scales for Children. The results are expressed as a ratio of measured performance to chronologic age. The scores are normally distributed in the population so that an IQ of 70 is approximately 2 standard deviations below the mean and each standard deviation is approximately 15 points. Adaptive functioning is measured by various tests including the Vineland Adaptive Behavior Scales and the Adaptive Behavior Checklist.

■ ETIOLOGY

Mental retardation affects approximately 1–2 percent of the population. It is not a disease but the developmental consequence of impaired mental function caused by a pathogenic process. The identification of genetic abnormalities has allowed a greater understanding of the etiology of many patients but there are still many in whom the cause is not yet defined. Many of the genetic and metabolic causes of mental retardation are discussed elsewhere in the book.

TABLE 26-2. FORMER CLASSIFICATION OF MENTAL RETARDATION BY IQ

IQ 68–83 borderline
    52–67 mild
    36–51 moderate
    20–35 severe
   < 20 profound

TABLE 26-3. PRESENT CLASSIFICATION OF MENTAL RETARDATION BY DIMENSION

1992 Definition by American Association on Mental Retardation
Dimension I—Intellectual functioning and adaptive skills
Dimension II—Psychological and emotional considerations
Dimension III—Health, physical, and etiological considerations
Dimension IV—Environmental considerations

Intensity of supports
Intermittent
Limited
Extensive
Pervasive

■ CLINICAL FEATURES

The clinical manifestations include cognitive impairment with delayed expressive and receptive language skills. Developmental milestones are not achieved. Neuromuscular developmental delay, both motor and sensory, are possible. Associations with other conditions are common, including cerebral palsy, seizure disorder, and ADHD. Microcephaly is often present and the important causes of microcephaly are shown in Table 26-4.

■ MANAGEMENT

Increasingly it is encouraged to manage adults and children with mental retardation in the home setting, either with a family or in a group home with community-based education and training. Referral to programs that can provide family support and inter-disciplinary treatment is indicated. Behavioral techniques can be tried to enhance good behaviors and to reduce behavioral excesses. Caring for a child that is retarded is a major commitment. It can be very rewarding but it requires considerable work and patience.

A developmentally delayed child has the potential to learn skills and some make considerable improvement compared to those who do not receive training. Behavioral techniques have been shown to be effective in managing mental retardation.

TABLE 26-4. CAUSES OF MICROCEPHALY

Chromosomal
  Trisomy 13, 18, 21
Brain malformation
  Lissencephaly
Syndrome
  Cornelia de Lange
Toxins
  Alcohol
  PKU
Intrauterine infection
  STORCH
Perinatal
  Placental insufficiency
  Birth asphyxia, trauma
  Infections
    Group B streptococcus
    Viral encephalitis
Metabolic
  Hypoglycemia
  Kernicterus
  Maple syrup urine disease
Degenerative
  Tay–Sachs
  Krabbe's

Various approaches need to be tried to find the most useful. Rewards may be given for behavior that reduces the frequency of unwanted behaviors or for achieving tasks that are difficult for the child. Psychotrophic medications may be useful in the management of the child with destructive behavior.

Autism

Pervasive developmental disorders (PDDs) are a group of syndromes with autism as the most recognized condition. Other variants defined in the DSM-IV include Asperger's syndrome, pervasive developmental disorder—not otherwise specified (PDD-NOS), Rett's syndrome, and childhood disintegrative disorder.

Autism has an estimated prevalence of 4–5 per 10,000, but if all PDDs are included, an estimate of 20 per 10,000 is accounted for by the incidence of Asperger's which is significantly more common than autism. Asperger's disorder and autism occur more commonly in males than females (4 : 1) and Rett's syndrome occurs only in females.

Autism is characterized by impaired socialization, abnormal language and communication development, and a restricted, repetitive, stereotype of behaviors. There is a wide variation in behavior and intellectual development. Approximately 25–30 percent of autistic children have an IQ less than 50, and 20–30 percent have an IQ greater than 70. All children with childhood integrative disorder have mental retardation. IQs tend to be stable over time and are the most important predictors of outcome.

The etiology and pathogenesis of PDDs are very unclear. Present theory suggests a genetic or early developmental disruption in brain functioning with overt clinical manifestation potentially modified by environmental experiences. Neurotransmitter abnormalities have been suspected after Freedman's observation of hyperserotoninemia in many individuals with autism and confirmed by others. Most children with fragile X have a PDD, but fragile X only accounts for a small number of cases of PDD. Misconceptions are common about autism. There are many differences between autism and schizophrenia so that it would be wrong to classify autism as childhood schizophrenia.

In most children with autism, there is an initial period of normal development and abnormal symptoms tend to start before the age of 3 years. Either a lack of, or an unusual, interaction with the parents is often the first sign of concern. Eye contact (avoidance or staring) is usually inappropriate and social interactions tend to be different than other children the same age. As they get older, the behavior tends to be more obviously different; symptoms that may be observed are shown in Table 26-5. An estimated half of autistic children develop functional speech. Children with autism display unusual behaviors with stereotyped movements such as hand clapping or flapping and may engage in

TABLE 26-5. DIAGNOSIS OF AUTISM

6 criteria including at least 2 from (1) and one each from (2) and (3):

(1) Qualitative impairment in social interaction
- Marked impairment in the use of multiple nonverbal behaviors (eye-to-eye gaze, facial expression, body postures and gestures)
- Failure to develop peer relationships appropriate to developmental level
- A lack of spontaneous seeking to share enjoyment, interests, or achievements with other people
- Lack of social or emotional reciprocity

(2) Qualitative impairments in communication
- Delay in, or total lack of, the development of spoken language
- In individuals with adequate speech, marked impairment in the ability to initiate or sustain a conversation with others
- Stereotyped and repetitive use of language or idiosyncratic language
- Lack of varied, spontaneous make-believe play or social imitative play appropriate to developmental level

(3) Restricted repetitive and stereotyped patterns of behavior, interests, and activities
- Preoccupation by stereotype and restricted patterns of interest (abnormal intensity or focus)
- Apparently inflexible adherence to specific, nonfunctional routines or rituals
- Stereotyped and repetitive motor mannerisms (finger, hand, or whole body)
- Persistent preoccupation with parts of objects

self-injurious habits such as biting themselves or banging their heads. Traditional play with toys tends not to occur.

Asperger's syndrome differs from autism and also shares many characteristics. The major difference is that Asperger noted that the children he studied started to talk at the same time as other children and achieved normal language and syntax. There was a repetition of certain words or phrases and focus on particular topics. Cognitive development is not delayed in Asperger's syndrome. The social interaction and restrictive and repetitive interests are the same as in autism.

Rett syndrome is a developmental disorder that occurs only in females and differs from autism after the toddler stage. At some point between 6 months and 4 years of age, there is a slowing of head growth with impaired language and social development. There is a loss of acquired language and serious psychomotor retardation develops. Hyperventilation and sleep-disordered breathing are common.

■ MANAGEMENT

Because there are no specific markers for the diagnosis of PDDs including autism, it is often difficult to make an accurate diagnosis. There is also considerable overlap with other disorders causing language or speech delay and difficulty and disorders associated with mental retardation. The natural history of the disorder is also very variable; some do improve in adolescence but others have persistent symptoms into adulthood. Studies have shown that as many as two-thirds of autistic children remain seriously impaired and incapable of supporting themselves independently.

There is no medication that has potential to cure the disorder. The goals of treatment are to promote the development of social, communication and adaptive living skills, to reduce aberrant behavior, and to help the family to cope. Psychosocial interventions are geared to structure the environment and build self-esteem and improve social behaviors. The programs need to be individualized to strengthen each patient's deficient areas. Medication including haloperidol, clomipramine, or naltrexone may be tried to improve behavior. Selective serotonin reuptake inhibitors, such as fluoxetine, sertraline, paroxetine, and fluvoxamine, may be effective for ritualistic behaviors. Seizures accompany autism in 25–33 percent of cases and carbamazepine or valproate may be useful. Barbiturates, including phenobarbitone, should be avoided.

Affective Disorders

Perhaps 20–30 percent of people will have a depressive episode in their lifetime. For some people it affects them once and for others it is a chronic problem. A significant proportion of the population, including young people, commit suicide during a depressive episode. Symptoms of a mood disorder occur in many mental and physical conditions. It was not until 1975 that childhood depression was officially accepted as a diagnosis. The DSM-IV defines major depressive disorder as the presence of a single episode of depression with 5 or more of the following symptoms in a 2-week period and it has to include either number 1 or 2 or both.

1. Depressed mood for most of the day and nearly every day.
2. Markedly diminished interest or pleasure in almost all activities nearly every day.
3. Significant weight loss or gain due to a decrease or increase in appetite resulting in 5 percent change in body weight in a month.
4. Insomnia or hypersomnia nearly every day.
5. Psychomotor agitation or retardation nearly every day.
6. Fatigue or loss of energy nearly every day.
7. Feelings of excessive worthlessness or guilt.
8. Diminished ability to think or concentrate.
9. Recurrent thoughts of death and/or suicidal ideation that may include a plan or an actual suicide attempt.

There are additional features to the diagnosis which are discussed in the DSM-IV and review of this is appropriate. Melancholia is a more severe form of depression and uncommon in children.

Depression appears in many forms and affects people differently. The ability to continue daily life also varies from mild impairment to a complete inability to do anything. Dysthymia is the diagnosis that is made when the depressive episodes occur over a long time such that the symptoms occur most days and are milder than the major depressive episode and do not cause much impairment of daily living. The symptoms last for 2 years in adults and 1 year in children and a period of greater than 2 months without symptoms excludes the diagnosis.

Bipolar disorder has only recently been regularly diagnosed in children. It is characterized by manic periods where there is greatly elevated mood as well as periods of depression, hence the term manic-depression.

■ SIGNS AND SYMPTOMS OF DEPRESSION

Women tend to suffer from depression more than men and this is noted also during adolescence. Children who have one depressed parent are 2–3 times more likely to suffer from depression before age 18 than if neither parent has a history of depression and the risk is doubled if both parents have depression.

Depressed, sad, despondent mood is the most important feature of depression although it is not always obvious to the sufferer. The spectrum of feelings can vary from "I don't feel great" to "I don't care if I live or die." Crying and feelings of hopelessness are common. Because of these symptoms, people with depression lose interest in activities that used to be pleasurable, for example in toys or dolls or wanting to participate in games or sports with others. The negative feelings lead to a loss of self-esteem and the apathy that results may lead to an inability to make decisions that might help to improve the situation.

Because of their feelings, depressed children tend to withdraw from contact with others. Their response to communication with others may appear angry or irritable which discourages others from wanting to help. In addition to the emotional problems, there may be physical problems that may be the reason that medical help is sought. These complaints may be vegetative or somatic. Examples of vegetative problems include sleep disorders, which are characteristically early morning waking; appetite problems which may be anorexia or excess appetite, leading to weight increase or decrease. The energy loss and tiredness may be severe enough for the child or parent to think that there is a serious medical problem causing the symptoms. The somatic complaints cover a variety of symptoms which include headaches, constipation, various aches and pains, especially back and chest, and shortness of breath not related to the amount of exercise.

There is a high risk of missing the diagnosis and certainly the child or parent may not have the insight into the problem that will accept the diagnosis. It is also important to remember that chronic illness carries with it the potential for depressive symptoms and the two conditions may co-exist.

■ MANAGEMENT

The assessment will indicate the direction of treatment and will include important components of life of the child including family, friends, and school. Therapy will include personal therapy and family therapy and the addition of medications will be dependent upon the potential for improving the psychological state of mind. Pharmacotherapy for depression is an extension of therapy used in adults. There are no officially approved (by the FDA) drugs for treatment of depression in adolescents and children. Tricyclic antidepressants in research studies have not been as beneficial in children as they are in adults. Despite this, they do seem to be useful in some children and the reason that they were not shown to be better than placebo in many studies was because the placebo effect was as high as 70 percent. If tricyclics are used, it is recommended to check the electrocardiogram because of the problems with arrhythmias. It is often 4–6 weeks before there is a treatment effect and it is important not to stop the treatment too early if it is initially not immediately beneficial.

The introduction of selective serotonin reuptake inhibitors (SSRIs) has resulted in their use in children although there is still not a great deal of experience. There are fewer side effects than with TCAs and overdosage is less likely to be lethal.

The diagnosis of bipolar disorder in children is not easily made. If the manic component is sufficiently disruptive, it may be necessary to stabilize the child in hospital. The mood stabilizers that are used include lithium, valproate, and carbamazepine (Tegretol). There is an interaction that needs to be considered when prescribing SSRIs.

Anxiety Disorders

Anxiety disorders, together with mood disturbances, are classified as internalizing disorders and are among the most common psychiatric disorders. They are reported to occur in 7–15 percent of children and adolescents. There are various disorders that are considered separately.

■ GENERAL ANXIETY DISORDER (GAD)

The previous term for GAD was overanxious disorder. The definition includes excessive anxiety and worry that is difficult to control. It implies that the anxiety occurs more days than not during a 6-month period. Only one item in the following list is required in children versus the adult definition which requires 3 or more symptoms.

- restlessness or on edge
- easily fatigued
- difficulty concentrating or mind going blank
- irritability
- muscle tension
- sleep disturbance which may be difficulty falling or staying asleep or unsatisfactory sleep.

The diagnosis is not necessarily so simple and may overlap another anxiety disorder. Medical conditions, especially hyper-thyroidism and diabetes mellitus, may present with similar symptoms. GAD tends to occur more in girls than boys and in higher socioeconomic status.

Management is with cognitive-behavioral approaches. Children need to be aware that anxiety is often an exaggerated normal response. Relaxation, visual imagery, and replacement with adaptive thoughts will often be beneficial. If the symptoms interrupt daily life and are not controlled with behavior therapy, medications can be considered. Benzodiazepines or anti-depressants may be helpful.

■ SEPARATION ANXIETY DISORDER (SAD)

SAD is excessive anxiety brought on by separation from major attachment figures or the home environment that lasts at least 4 weeks. The DSM-IV definition requires three or more of the following categories.

- recurrent excessive distress when separation from home or major attachment figures occurs or is anticipated
- persistent or excessive worry about losing or harm occurring to major attachment figures
- persistent or excessive worry that something will happen (getting lost or kidnapped) resulting in separation from a major attachment figure
- refusal to go to school or elsewhere because of fear or separation
- fear of being alone without adult presence
- persistent reluctance to go to sleep without major attachment figure or to sleep away from home
- repeated nightmares about separation
- physical symptoms (e.g., headache, stomach ache, nausea, or vomiting) when separation occurs or in anticipation.

The most common age for SAD is 7–9 years but it may occur during adolescence. It is more frequent in girls and in lower socioeconomic status. It tends to come to the clinician's attention when there are problems with school attendance. Many children have a co-morbid condition—either another anxiety disorder or another medical or psychological condition. The symptoms of SAD vary from reluctance to refusal and may be expressed with agitation or temper tantrums.

Behavior and cognitive therapies can be successful with positive reinforcement of non-fearful behavior and withdrawing rewards for anxious behavior. Exposure-based treatment is beneficial for school refusal with gradual reintroduction to the school setting. If the school refusal has been present for several weeks it may take considerable time and coaxing to overcome the problem. Rewarding successful accomplishments is appropriate. Pharmacologic approaches may be needed and imipramine may be useful.

■ PANIC DISORDER

This is uncommon in childhood but occurs in adolescence. It is characterized by sudden, unexpected periods of intense fear and anxiety that lasts a few minutes to a few hours. They may be unexpected or tend to occur in a specific context or situation. They can occur with SAD or with phobic anxiety disorder. The peak age of onset is 15–26 years of age and it is more common in females. The symptoms tend to be trembling, palpitations, shortness of breath, sweating, dizziness, and chest discomfort. Many medical conditions need to be considered in the differential diagnosis. Hyperthyroidism, diabetes, asthma, mitral valve prolapse, and seizures may present with similar symptoms.

■ PHOBIAS

Specific phobia has replaced the term simple phobia and is defined as an unreasonable, excessive, and persistent fear in response to actual or anticipated exposure to a specific object or situation. The object could be an animal or a needle, for example, and the situation could be fear of flying or elevators (Table 26-6). Exposure to the stimulus results in an immediate anxiety response which in children tends to be expressed as crying, tantrums, freezing (staying still), or clinging.

It is important to differentiate phobias from normal childhood fears. A list of developmentally appropriate fears is shown in Table 26-7. The appropriate management is usually a graded exposure with systemic desensitization. If direct exposure is not possible, then visual imagery can be employed. Systemic desensitization combines exposure with relaxation techniques. Psychosocial treatments are clearly more beneficial than medications.

TABLE 26-6. CATEGORIES OF PHOBIAS

Animals (e.g., snakes, rats, dogs)
Natural environmental (e.g., thunder and lightning, heights, water)
Medical—blood (e.g., blood, injections, needles)
Situational (e.g., flying, enclosed or confined spaces)
Other (e.g., loud noises)

TABLE 26-7. FEARS THAT ARE AGE-APPROPRIATE

Birth to 6 months	Loud noises, loss of physical support, rapid change of position
7–12 months	Strangers, unexpected confrontations with objects or people
1–5 years	Storms, animals, the dark, separation from parents, loud noises, monsters, the toilet
6–12 years	Being alone, punishment, injury or disease
12–18 years	School or athletic performance, social embarrassment

■ OBSESSIVE-COMPULSIVE DISORDER (OCD)

OCD comprises either obsessions or compulsions. Obsessions are recurrent or persistent thoughts, impulses, or images that are experienced as intrusive and inappropriate and cause distress. They are not simply excessive responses to real-life problems. The person will attempt to suppress the thoughts, impulses or images and recognizes that they are the products of their own mind. Compulsions are repetitive behaviors or mental acts that the person feels driven to perform in response to an obsession. Examples of behaviors are hand washing or checking and rechecking and, of mental acts, are praying or counting.

The behaviors become intrusive and inappropriate and cause impairment or significant distress. They are aimed at preventing some dreaded event or situation or needing to get something exactly right. Adults are aware that the behavior is unreasonable or excessive but children may not be aware. The disorder affects males and females equally and prevalence estimates range from 0.3–1.9 percent in children and adolescents.

Exposure and response prevention is the preferred treatment in which the behaviors are identified and a planned response to avoid the aberrant behavior is derived. The serotonin agonists (SSRIs) have been noted to be effective in treating OCD which has led to the acceptance of the role of serotonin in the cause of OCD. The serotonergic agents clomipramine and fluoxetine have been shown to be beneficial in children and adolescents. It is likely that the newer SSRIs may also be useful.

■ POST-TRAUMATIC STRESS DISORDER

There are two syndromes induced by trauma named acute stress disorder (ASD) and post-traumatic stress disorder (PTSD) which are important to recognize because early intervention can reduce morbidity. The experiences of soldiers during World Wars I and II led to the term shell shock and combat fatigue. The term PTSD was introduced in the 1970s after the Vietnam War. Extension of the diagnosis to the general population, women and children, has occurred more recently. PTSD results from an overwhelming circumstance or disaster that is experienced by the child. Children of all ages are susceptible to the effects of trauma. The most studied psychological sequelae have related to physical and sexual abuse and the children can be victims or witnesses. Children who are exposed to violent crime or who are involved in accident situations (e.g., a motor vehicle accident) are at risk for psychological problems. Natural disasters such as earthquakes, floods, or hurricanes are all potential for psychological sequelae. Children who suffer life-threatening illness are also at risk.

Gathering the information from the child or family may be difficult. Children may internalize feelings so that they may not remember or connect the traumatic events to the emotional symptoms. Young children fantasize, and it is important to try and separate truth from fiction.

There is an initial response at the time of the initial trauma which may last a few minutes or hours and is characterized by intense arousal. It is the immediate hormonal response to stress and is the "fight-or-flight" reaction. There may be a second phase which tends to last about 2 weeks and is the numbness phase so that it is as if nothing had happened and is associated with absence of emotion. Denial that anything is wrong is often observed. The third phase is one of coping which extends over a period of months. Psychological reactions such as depression, repetitive phenomenon, phobic and anxiety symptoms may ensue.

Management

There is very little data in children that would support a particular strategy for the treatment of PTSD. Various interventions including psychoanalysis, hypnosis, cognitive therapy, and medications have been tried in adults with varying success. Individual psychotherapy has the most potential to be beneficial. Education of the parents in coping skills is important as they may well be confused by the behavior of the child. Group therapy may be useful in many situations. Family therapy may be beneficial because often the whole family suffers when the child experiences trauma. Group therapy, for example at school, may be helpful for incidents that have the potential to affect a number of children. If a school-child dies or is killed or if a major disaster occurs (e.g., gunshots being fired), counseling of the pupils may reduce psychological sequelae.

Somatization Disorder

According to the DSM-IV, this is a pattern of recurring multiple clinically significant complaints that are not explained by a medical condition. Each of 4 criteria need to be met before the age of 30 and sustained over a number of years: (1) there must be pain symptoms related to 4 sites or functions; (2) a history of 2 GI symptoms other than pain; (3) 1 sexual or reproductive symptom; and (4) 1 symptom. The criteria are a modification of what was previously called Briquet syndrome.

Somatization is the process wherein a child and family seek help for symptoms misattributed to physical disease. Recurrent physical complaints in children and adolescents fall into the categories of pain and/or weakness, referable to the heart or GI tract and neurologic problems. Headache, chest pain, abdominal pain, dizziness, and tiredness are among the common complaints.

Tics

Tics are stereotyped, rapid, recurring movement, or vocalizations that are non-rhythmic and tend to be sudden and difficult to control. Transient tics are common in children and occur in up to 15 percent. Tics involve 1 muscle (simple) or muscle groups (complex). Simple tics include eye blinking, facial grimace, shoulder shrugging, or head nodding. Complex tics could be jumping or some purposeful movement. Vocal tics include throat clearing, coughing, or echolalia (echoing someone's words). Tics need to be differentiated from myoclonus, focal seizures, tremors, and drug effects.

The parents need to be aware that tics are not voluntary. Treatment is reasonably effective with the dopamine receptor antagonists haloperidol or pimozide. Clonidine or SRIs (serotonergic agents) such as fluoxetine have assisted in the management of some patients.

Tourette Syndrome

Gilles de la Tourette syndrome is multiple tic disease and is thought to be a disorder of dopamine metabolism affecting the basal ganglia. The disorder usually starts before the age of 12 and by definition before the age of 18 years. Tics usually begin in the shoulders and face and later involve all parts of the body. The movements are blinking, twitching, grimacing, and jerking. They are repetitive, semi-purposeful, and can be suppressed momentarily. Multiple tics with a respiratory component are typical. The respiratory involvement may be coughing, snorting, hiccups, or swallowing. The condition is chronic and fluctuating and tends to persist into adult life. There is no relationship to seizure disorder or psychosis but learning disability is not unusual.

Tourette syndrome is more common in males. It can be precipitated by methylphenidate and dextroamphetamine and made worse by L-dopa. Treatment of the condition is most effective with dopamine receptor antagonists (haloperidol or pimozide). As in the management of simple tics, clonidine or SRIs (serotonergic agents) such as fluoxetine (Prozac) have assisted in the management of some patients.

27

Chapter Twenty-Seven

Rheumatology Disorders

Rheumatic diseases are also known as connective tissue diseases. They are a group of conditions with inflammation, as opposed to infection or neoplasia, as the cause, and the treatments are strategies to reduce inflammation. The dominant symptom is arthritis which results from inflammation of the joints. Most of the conditions are chronic and although they are uncommon they are associated with considerable morbidity because of the effect that they have on the daily life of the patient. Many of the conditions are more common in adults but the onset may start in childhood and juvenile rheumatoid arthritis is different from rheumatoid arthritis that affects adults.

Juvenile Rheumatoid Arthritis

George Still (1897, London) reported the first detailed description of "a chronic joint disease in children." He described 12 children with polyarthritis that was different from rheumatoid arthritis and 6 children who had a disease that was clinically the same as the adult form. He noted the lymphadenopathy, splenomegaly, pericarditis, and the involvement of the cervical spine.

■ DESCRIPTION

Specific criteria for the diagnosis of juvenile rheumatoid arthritis (JRA) have been developed and are shown in Table 27-1. There are 3 principal forms of JRA, systemic JRA, which is Still's disease, and pauciarticular with asymmetric large joint involvement, and polyarticular with multiple symmetric joint involvement. The major distinguishing features are shown in Table 27-2. The disease begins before the child is 16 years of age. The terms juvenile arthritis and juvenile chronic arthritis continue to be used but they have slightly looser criteria. The etiology is unclear although it is considered to be an immune disorder that results in inflammation and fibrosis although the mechanism is unknown. Infectious, psychological and genetic factors, and trauma are all thought to impact the onset and course of the disease.

JRA is one of the commonest chronic diseases and the most common rheumatic disorder of children. The reported incidence is from 9–25 per 100,000 and there are approximately 70,000–100,000 children with JRA in the US. It is twice as common in girls than boys.

■ PATHOPHYSIOLOGY

There is chronic inflammation of the synovium of the joints which is the lining membrane. There is effusion of fluid into the joint space. The inflammation extends to the articular cartilage which erodes and is destroyed. There is soft tissue edema around the joint and hypertrophy of the synovial membrane. The rate of progression is variable so that changes may be present for months or years before

TABLE 27-1. DIAGNOSTIC CRITERIA OF JUVENILE RHEUMATOID ARTHRITIS

Onset before age 16 years
Arthritis (swelling or effusion, tenderness or pain on motion) in one or more joints
Lasting for 6 weeks or more
Polyarthritis is 5 or more inflamed joints
Oligoarthritis is 4 or less inflamed joints
Systemic is arthritis with fever
Other diagnoses excluded

TABLE 27-2. CHARACTERISTICS OF JUVENILE RHEUMATOID ARTHRITIS

	Systemic	Polyarticular	Pauciarticular
Frequency of cases (%)	10	40	50
Number of joints with arthritis at onset	Variable	≥ 5	≤ 4
Sex ratio (F : M)	1 : 1	3 : 1	5 : 1
Frequency of uveitis (%)	1	5	20
Frequency of rheumatoid factor positivity (%)	< 2	5–10	< 2
Frequency of ANA positivity (%)	5–10	40–50	75–85
Frequency of ≥ 5 joints involved any time during course of JRA (%)	50–60	100	40
Frequency of active disease > 10 years follow-up (%)	42	45	41
Frequency of erosions or joint space narrowing on radiographs (%)	45	54	28
Median time to develop erosions or joint space narrowing on radiographs (years after disease onset)	2.2	2.4	5.4
Frequency of adult height < 5th percentile (%)	50	16	11

there is clinical evidence of arthritis or there may be rapid destruction of the joints.

■ CLINICAL FEATURES

The presentation of the different types of JRA varies. The three subtypes are systemic (10 percent), polyarticular (25–40 percent), and pauciarticular (40–65 percent). There is inflammation of joints with swelling, warmth, and limited range of movement. The signs include heat, redness, tenderness, and reduced movement. To make the diagnosis, there has to be more than pain and tenderness. The arthritis is chronic, persisting for more than 6 weeks in a given joint. It is usual to have morning stiffness as well as generalized symptoms including malaise, fatigue, anorexia, and weight loss.

■ SYSTEMIC JRA

Although this is the least common type of JRA, it is the most troublesome. It affects both sexes and all age groups so that in adults it is referred to as "adult-onset Still disease." The peak age of onset is 1–6 years of age. Systemic JRA has constitutional symptoms that commonly predate the arthritis by several weeks or months. Fever is high (>39°C) and spikes daily to 40 or 41°C in the afternoon. There is a discrete salmon-colored macular rash on the trunk and extremities. There may be a Koebner phenomenon wherein the rash appears at the site that the skin is rubbed. Anorexia and irritability are common and there may be intense arthralgia and myalgia. Growth delay is common and there are many extra-articular features which are listed in Table 27-3. The extra-articular features tend to be self-limited and mild-to-moderate in severity. Serious complications include pericardial tamponade (sometimes accompanied by myocarditis) and secondary consumptive co-agulopathy.

Anemia may be profound, particularly if there is associated iron deficiency, and there may be marked leukocytosis and thrombocytosis. Rheumatoid factor (RF) and antinuclear antibodies (ANA) are absent but the erythrocyte sedimentation rate (ESR) is very high.

■ PAUCIARTICULAR JRA

The definition of pauciarticular JRA requires involvement of 4 or less joints. The knee is most commonly involved followed by the ankle, wrist, and elbow. There is an early (1–5 years old) onset group, predominantly girls (4:1), who are ANA positive with a high incidence of chronic uveitis. This group comprises more than 90 percent of pauciarticular JRA and has an excellent

TABLE 27-3. EXTRA-ARTICULAR FEATURES OF JRA

Uveitis
Anemia
Hepatosplenomegaly
Pericarditis
Pleural effusion
Growth retardation
Osteopenia
Thrombocytosis

articular outcome. The inflammatory process (uveitis) involves the anterior chamber of the eye and 80 percent have mild changes but there is a potential for cataracts, visual loss, or glaucoma. The late onset group (usually more than 9 years) tends to involve boys and the arthritis affects the shoulder, hips, knees, or spine. Fifty percent are HLA B-27 positive and there is often a positive family history of associated conditions including inflammatory bowel disease, psoriasis, or Reiter's syndrome (see below).

■ POLYARTICULAR JRA

Polyarticular JRA requires arthritis in 5 or more joints in the first 6 months of illness. There are 2 distinct forms depending on whether they are seropositive or seronegative for RF. Children who are seropositive are almost all girls with the onset after 8 years of age and they have HLA-DR4 positive. There is symmetric small-joint arthritis of the hands and feet and various large joints. There is a risk for erosions, nodules, and poor functional outcome compared to RF-negative patients. This subgroup of RF-positive polyarticular JRA most closely resembles adult-onset RA. There are variable clinical manifestations that include growth retardation, anemia, delayed sexual maturation, and osteopenia.

Laboratory Studies

Rheumatoid factor is only positive in 15 percent of cases, principally those with polyarticular disease. Positive ANA (antinuclear antibody) is present in 40 percent of cases especially pauciarticular disease. Disease activity and response to treatment is followed with the ESR and C-reactive protein, although they tend to be normal with pauciarticular disease.

Management

Treatment is directed to reducing the inflammatory process, to preserve and improve joint function, and reduce pain. Because of the chronic nature and the morbidity associated with JRA, supportive services are needed to improve the quality of life for individuals with the advanced forms of the disease. The progression of arthritis is difficult to predict although exacerbations do appear to coincide with periods of stress and illness. Remission can occur although reduction of therapy may be associated with worsening. A remission is defined as 6 months symptom free on medications followed by 6 months free of medication.

The approach to treatment is to start with milder medications and to escalate to stronger preparations. The goal is to improve growth and to reduce the complications that perpetuate the disability. This involves early aggressive management. The algorithm that follows indicates a progression of treatments. Non-steroidal anti-inflammatory drugs (NSAIDs) are the starting point. They have replaced aspirin as the treatment of choice both from easier dosing as well as the lack of association with Reyes syndrome. The complication of GI irritation is reduced by taking NSAIDs with meals.

There is a group of medications that have been called slow acting, or disease modifying, antirheumatic drugs (SAARD or DMARD). They include D-penicillamine, gold, hydroxy-chloroquine, methotrexate, and sulfasalazine. They are used if NSAIDs are not controlling the symptoms. Next in line are corticosteroids which are given orally or intravenously either by pulse or bolus. It is necessary to be very discriminatory with steroid therapy because there are significant side effects with long-term therapy. If steroids are required for more than six months, alternate day therapy should be tried. Immuno-suppressive and cytotoxic agents are used for severe illness that do not respond to the previously described treatments.

There are several treatments that some patients are convinced are helpful but that have not stood up to strictly controlled clinical trials.

Physical and occupational therapy play an important part of the long-term management. It is important to balance exercise to help with mobility and reduce contractures and rest particularly when a joint is acutely inflamed. Swimming and bicycling are good low-impact exercises that can be graded to ability.

Nutritional strategies can be beneficial particularly when there are significant problems with systemic effects, anorexia, and malnutrition.

Systemic Lupus Erythematosis

Systemic lupus erythematosis (SLE) is a chronic inflammatory condition that principally affects collagen and other connective tissues. There are two basic types that affect children, one being the neonatal form, that result from transmission of maternal autoantibodies from the mother and SLE which is essentially the same condition as the adult form. It is an autoimmune disorder that results from production of antibodies to nuclear constituents and immune-mediated vasculitis. The organs that are affected are throughout the body. In the first decade, the female-to-male ratio is 3 : 1 and after it is 7 : 1. It is more common in African American, Asian, and Hispanic children. The prevalence is estimated to be 5–10 per 100,000.

■ CLINICAL FEATURES

The neonatal form is of interest because the mother has SLE. Transplacental passage of maternal autoantibodies leads to complete heart block in the fetus. The heart block arises from maternal anti-Ro antibody which binds to the fetal conduction system and is permanent. Thrombocytopenia, photosensitivity, and hepatitis may occur and tend to last for a few months as the maternal antibodies decrease.

The diagnosis of SLE should be based on the criteria developed by the American College of Rheumatology in 1982. This is shown in Table 27-4. The presence of four criteria is 96 percent sensitive and specific. The most common symptoms include arthralgia and arthritis with fatigue, headache, and weight loss which are similar to those of JRA. However, the varied organ systems that are involved should provide clues to the diagnosis. The

TABLE 27-4. DIAGNOSTIC CRITERIA OF LUPUS

Presence of 4 of 11 criteria:
  Malar rash
  Discoid rash
  Photosensitivity
  Oral ulcers (usually painless)
  Arthritis (2 or more peripheral joints)
  Serositis (pleuritis or pericarditis)
  Renal disorder (proteinuria or urinary cellular casts)
  Neurologic disorder (seizure or psychosis)
  Hematologic disorder (hemolytic anemia or leukopenia or lymphopenia or thrombocytopenia)
  Immunologic disorder (positive LE cell or abnormal titer anti-DNA or presence of antibody to Sm)
  nuclear antigen or false positive TPI following positive test)
  Antinuclear antibody abnormal titer (in absence of drug-induced)

---

malar butterfly rash, Raynaud phenomenon, and photosensitivity are suggestive. Renal involvement occurs in 50–70 percent of cases and may be mild but some children develop diffuse proliferative glomerulonephritis or membranous nephritis that may progress to renal failure.

The onset of SLE in children tends to be gradual and the malar rash may not be present. Fatigue and malaise with multisystem disease including pleural effusions, hemolytic anemia, proteinuria, and synovitis of the small joints of the hands or feet are characteristic. The onset may be dramatic with a combination of many of the symptoms listed in Table 27-4.

■ MANAGEMENT

Treatment is predicated on which organ system is involved. Corticosteroids are very effective in reducing the inflammatory symptoms of SLE but there are significant side effects because of the dosage and duration of treatment required. If patients are unable to be weaned from steroids, azathioprine or cyclophosphamide may be tried. Hydroxychloroquine has been successful in those with primarily skin involvement (discoid lupus).

Estrogen containing oral contraceptives should be avoided. Sunscreens are indicated if photosensitivity is a problem and avoidance of direct sun exposure by clothing may be necessary.

■ **PROGNOSIS**

Ten-year survival rates for children with SLE are greater than 90 percent

Juvenile Dermatomyositis

Juvenile dermatomyositis (JDM) is a multisystem disease with vascular inflammation of the skin and muscles. It differs from the adult form in that both skin and muscles are involved (adults may have no skin involvement), there is a low rate of malignancy, and the prognosis is better. In addition, there may be vasculitis of the GI tract. The condition is thought to be an autoimmune phenomenon with increased frequency of HLA-B8 and DR3. ANA is positive in 30 percent of cases and immune complexes have been identified in many patients. The peak incidence is 10 years of age.

Presentation may be acute or gradual. Acute JDM has fever, violaceous discoloration of the eyelids, Gottren's papules (inflammatory vasculitic lesions overlying the interphalangeal joints), with generalized muscle pain and weakness. The insidious form has muscle weakness and it may be weeks or months before medical attention is sought. There may be a periorbital rash or facial telangiectasia.

Respiratory symptoms may result from involvement of the diaphragm. Vasculitis of the small bowel may lead to abdominal pain. There is usually elevation of creatine kinase and aldolase, AST, ALT, or LDH may be abnormal. The diagnosis is established with muscle biopsy or electromyography.

Treatment with corticosteroids produces significant improvement and the mortality of the condition is now less than 5 percent. Exacerbations of disease are common and additional treatments may be tried including methotrexate, cyclophosphamide, IVIG, or cyclosporine.

Kawasaki Disease/Syndrome ....

■ CLINICAL FEATURES

Kawasaki syndrome (KS) was described by Dr. Tomasaku Kawasaki in 1967. It was originally called mucocutaneous lymph node syndrome. There is vasculitis of small and medium vessels with distinctive clinical features which constitute the diagnostic criteria: fever lasting for more than 5 days with 4 of the 5 criteria or only 3 of the criteria if there are coronary artery aneurisms (Table 27-5). First reported in Japan, 80 percent of cases involve children less than 4 years of age. The cause is unknown and 3 associations have been reported: antecedent respiratory illness, carpet cleaning, and proximity to water.

The fever is remittent and high and lasts usually 1–2 weeks. The rash is often the clue to the diagnosis and is erythematous, macular, scarlatiniform, or maculopapular. The perineal region is involved in 60 percent of cases and 10–14 days after onset of fever there is distinctive superficial peeling of the skin of the perineum and the fingertips. There may be conjunctival injection that is bulbar and bilateral and there are oral mucosal changes. Associated manifestations are shown in Table 27-6.

Without treatment, 50 percent of children have coronary artery abnormalities and 15–25 percent have aneurisms. Myocardial infarctions occur most often in the first year with a mortality of 32 percent. There are no laboratory studies that confirm the diagnosis. There may be marked thrombocytosis in the second week.

TABLE 27-5. KAWASAKI SYNDROME DIAGNOSTIC CRITERIA

Febrile illness ≥ 5 days' duration, with at least four of the five:
1. Bilateral conjunctival injection
2. Oral changes (erythema of lips or oropharynx, strawberry tongue, or fissuring of the lips)
3. Peripheral extremity changes (edema, erythema, or generalized or periungual desquamation)
4. Rash
5. Cervical lymphadenopathy (at least one lymph node ≥ 1.5 cm diameter)

TABLE 27-6. ASSOCIATED MANIFESTATIONS OF KAWASAKI SYNDROME

Aseptic meningitis
Seizures
Transient paralysis
Transient hearing loss
Pneumonia
Hydrops of the gallbladder
Pancreatitis
Arthritis

■ MANAGEMENT

High-dose aspirin suppresses the inflammation but does not alter the development of aneurisms. Aspirin is often continued for several months until the sedimentation rate and platelet count are more normal. There is a beneficial effect of intravenous immunoglobulin (IVIG) to reduce the development of coronary artery aneurisms. The prognosis is quite good but there are cases of sudden death from myocardial infarction that often occur during sleep.

Polyarteritis Nodosa

Polyarteritis is a necrotizing inflammatory vasculitis of small- or medium-sized arteries. Thrombosis and fibrinoid necrosis of blood vessels occur. Potentially any organ in the body can be involved but the clinical symptoms are variable and often nonspecific. It is rare in children. There is a generalized disease with fever, malaise, skin rash, conjunctivitis, and respiratory symptoms. The organ systems most commonly involved are skin, peripheral nerves, joints, GI tract, and kidneys. There is also an infantile form with coronary artery involvement and heart failure.

Vascular nephropathy and segmental necrotizing glomerulonephritis may result in renovascular hypertension. Gastrointestinal ischemia results in abdominal pain and may simulate an acute abdomen and there may be hematemesis or melena.

Parasthesias are common and may involve a single nerve or poly-neuropathy.

The laboratory tests show anemia and elevated ESR. Histologic examination of biopsy specimens show an inflammatory infiltrate. The feature that confirms the diagnosis is aneurisms of the medium-sized arteries. ANCA may be positive.

Corticosteroids may suppress the clinical manifestations and help in the long-term management. Cyclophosphamide or azathioprine may be useful to reduce relapses.

Reiter's Syndrome

The features of this syndrome, also called reactive arthritis, include arthritis, ocular inflammation and urethritis. *Chlamydia trachomatis* is often associated and it is frequently seen in HLA-B27-positive individuals. Reactive arthritis may occur as part of Reiter's syndrome, or separately, and is arthritis that follows infection of a variety of organisms of the GI tract, also associated with HLA-B27 patients. The organisms include *Yersinia, Campylobacter, Salmonella,* or *Shigella* species. The arthritis occurs 10–21 days after the onset of the diarrhea.

Scleroderma

There is deposition of collagen into the skin and other tissues which results in progressive hardening. Children have the focal form known as morphea or linear scleroderma (LS). The systemic forms of systemic sclerosis (SS) and CREST (see below) syndrome are less common in children.

LS is a tight band-like constriction of the skin of the trunk or limb. If there is involvement of the area around a joint or if it is extensive, contractures may develop and growth failure may result. LS *en coup de sabre* is an area of thickening of the scalp that may extend down into the face.

SS in childhood may lead to inflammation and fibrosis of heart, lungs and kidney in addition to diffuse tightening of the skin. Although the onset is gradual, the effects can be life threatening. CREST syndrome is calcinosis, Raynaud's phenomenon, esophageal dysmotility, sclerodactyly, telangiectasia. Telangiectasia is often the initial finding. There may be life-threatening pulmonary fibrosis, swallowing dysfunction, and severe renal disease.

If there is local skin involvement, no treatment may be needed. Because the systemic disorders are rare, there is not much experience in treatment. Corticosteroids may not be very useful. D-penicillamine may be beneficial for some patients. Methotrexate and cyclosporine are under investigation.

Wegener's Granulomatosis

This is a rare vasculitis of unknown etiology that presents with fever, anorexia, and weight loss. There is a triad of necrotizing granulomatous vasculitis of the upper and of the lower respiratory tract and focal segmental glomerulonephritis. Small arteries and veins are the most affected vessels. The lesions involve the nasal mucosa and sinuses, lungs, and kidneys. Rhinorrhea, nasal mucosal ulceration, and sinusitis are seen with upper airway involvement. Pulmonary involvement leads to cough, hemoptysis, and pleurisy. Renal involvement results in hematuria. Beyond the triad, there may be eye symptoms, arthritis, and inflammation of the heart may lead to arrhythmia.

Serum antibodies that react with cytoplasmic component of neutrophils (c-ANCA) are present in 80 percent of cases. Biopsy of the lesion is necessary to make the diagnosis. There is granuloma with vasculitis. Corticosteroids on their own may not be sufficient treatment, but with cyclophosphamide in addition there may be improvement. Also azathioprine may reverse the condition. There is potential for improvement with these drugs, for a condition that used to be fatal.

28

Chapter Twenty-Eight

Dermatologic Disorders

Skin disorders are commonly associated with chronic illness in children. A lesion of the skin may be the first indication of an underlying disorder including infection or a metabolic, immune, or neurologic disorder. There are skin diseases that are dominantly dermatologic and there are systemic illnesses that have cutaneous manifestations. As in all areas, a focused history and physical examination is necessary for evaluation of a skin disorder. Inquiry should be made of the duration and progression of a lesion or rash, of symptoms which may include itching or pain, and of allergies known or medications taken.

Skin disorders tend to be described on the basis of their morphologic appearance. Table 28-1 lists the description of the skin finding. Acne is classified as papular, impetigo as vesicular, bullous or pustular, psoriasis as papulosquamous, and are examples of chronic disorders.

The most useful dermatologic tests are the potassium hydroxide preparation (KOH) and the skin biopsy. Skin scrapings are taken, often from more than one site, and blood may be drawn at the site and the scrapings placed on a glass slide. A few drops of 10 percent KOH are added and a coverslip placed over the specimen. After gently heating, the specimen is examined under low power with a light source and dermatophytes appear as septate hyphae and yeasts appear as budding spores with short non-septate hyphae. The scrapings of scabies lesions

TABLE 28-1. TYPES OF SKIN LESIONS

Macule—non-palpable skin rash < 0.5 cm
Papule—discrete raised palpable lesion < 0.5 cm
Nodule—palpable raised lesion > 0.5 cm
Papulosquamous—small elevated lesions with scaling
Plaque—coalesced papules
Erythematous—redness from increased blood flow through upper dermis
Wheal—edema in upper dermis producing raised lesion
Vesicle—blister containing clear fluid
Bulla—vesicle > 0.5 cm
Pustule—contains purulent fluid
Eczematous—lesion with oozing, crusting
Epidermal (stratum corneum)—lesion results in scaling
Lichenification—skin thickening from changes in rete ridge structure

more commonly show eggs and feces (scybala) than the mite itself.

The skin biopsy is particularly useful for the diagnosis of inflammatory and neoplastic lesions. An incision or punch biopsy is taken of the lesion with aspectic technique and local anesthesia. The tissue should be handled carefully and routine and special stains prepared for histology or immunofluorescence.

Acne Vulgaris

Acne vulgaris means common acne and is one of the commonest problems of teenagers. It is caused by increased sebum production by sebaceous glands that increases at the time of puberty. There is partial obstruction of the pilosebaceous canal and infection is associated. There is a genetic influence but other factors including endocrine, dietary, emotional, and bacterial are all inter-related.

Pilosebaceous follicles secrete sebum which increases in amount at the time of puberty because of androgenic hormone secretion. In the pilosebaceous canal, the triglycerides of sebum are cleaved into free fatty acids by lipase from the anaerobic diphtheroid *Propionobacterium acnes*. The fatty acids and pro-staglandins are irritating and chemotactic. There is partial obstruction of the follicle which results in the formation of come-dones. The closed comedo is called the "whitehead" and is a skin-colored palpable lesion without a very visible pore. The closed comedo is liable to get infected sometimes after months and results in inflammatory papules or pustules. The open comedo or "blackhead" is wider and the pore is open and filled with black material. This material is not dirt but rather compact keratin, melanin, and oxidized lipids. They are less likely to become inflamed than the closed comedo.

■ **CLINICAL FEATURES**

In early adolescence, acne tends to be comedonal with both closed and open comedones and confined to the face. By mid-adolescence, inflammatory acne with papules and pustules is the most common form and the chest and back are also involved. Although papules and pustules may be superficial, there may be deeper lesions in the lower portion of the hair canal that are much more persistent. Nodulocystic lesions, which are coalescences of adjacent pustules, may develop, especially on the lower face and neck and on the earlobes.

Acne cysts may take months to granulate and heal. Acne scars are the result of inflammatory acne. Much of the scarring from superficial lesions results from self-inflicted trauma from scratching and squeezing lesions.

There are forms of acne that have special features. Acne neonatorum may result from sebaceous gland hyperactivity from maternal hormones. Infantile acne develops after 3 months of age and resolves spontaneously by 18 months of age. Boys born with a strong family history of severe acne tend to be affected. It tends to be mild and involves the cheeks with comedones and papules. It may be related to using oils and lotions on the skin. Cosmetic acne in teenage girls is caused by oily moisturizers, foundations, and hair preparations. Cocoa butter is a common cause of comedonic acne and hair preparations may lead to acne on the forehead. Because the lesions are slow to develop, the diagnosis may not be obvious.

Acne conglobata is a particularly severe form of nodulocystic acne that occurs in 3 percent of white male adolescents. There may be large multipored open comedones with draining nodules and sinuses. The back is predominantly affected and it may also involve the face, upper arms, thighs, and buttocks. A rare form is known as acne fulminans with fever, polyarthritis, anemia, and leukocytosis. Large lesions are found on the upper chest and back.

■ MANAGEMENT

Although certain foods have been identified to worsen acne, there is little evidence that dietary restrictions make a difference. If a patient feels that chocolate, nuts, seafood, or cola drinks make their acne worse, it would be reasonable to avoid the food or drink. It definitely makes sense to avoid moisturizers and oil-based make up and use water-based make up or none at all.

Benzoyl peroxide preparations are the most commonly used acne medications. Benzoyl peroxide is an oxidizing agent with bacteriostatic properties that increases blood flow to the lesion and accelerates healing. It is keratolytic and decreases the adherence of follicular horny cells. It may cause contact allergy with itching, erythema, and periorbital edema. There are several topical treatments that include antibiotics that may be effective. Systemic antibiotics with activity against *Propionobacterium acnes* may be useful in papulopustular, cystic, and nodular acne including tetracycline (not to be used during pregnancy) and erythromycin.

Tretinoin (Retin A) is a topical vitamin A analogue that normalizes keratinization of the sebaceous follicles and decreases horny cell adhesion. It effectively promotes deplugging of comedones and prevents new microcomedone formation. As comedones are expelled, pustules may develop 3–4 weeks after starting treatment and should not be a reason to stop treatment. Photosensitivity is common and secondary hyperpigmentation may occur in African American or Asian patients.

Isotretinoin (Accutane) is a systemic vitamin A analogue that causes involution of sebaceous glands and should be reserved for very severe acne. Treatment is usually for several months and there is a persistence of effect even after the drug is discontinued. There are significant side effects including dry skin and lips, epistaxis, conjunctivitis, and elevation of triglyceride levels. It is teratogenic and should never be used during pregnancy. Effective birth control is essential for all females taking isotretinoin.

Diaper Dermatitis

This is the most common skin disorder of babies but it is not confined to infants and the principles apply to older children who require diapers. There are various disorders that have distinct types of eruptions: (1) Irritant contact dermatitis results from skin irritation by urine and stool. It is made worse by occlusion and the moisture combined with friction leads to maceration of the skin. It is worse on convex surfaces with relative sparing in the folds. It tends to occur after 3 months of age. The rash is shiny and erythematous, and pustules, nodules, and erosions are frequently present. Diarrheal stools tend to produce severe lesions in the perianal and buttock area. (2) Candidal infection is the most characteristic of the diaper rashes. It may be primary or associated with irritant dermatitis. The rash is intensely red with sharp borders and satellite pustules and papules beyond the borders. Oral thrush often accompanies candidal diaper rash. The rash commonly follows taking broad-spectrum antibiotics. (3) Seborrheic dermatitis commonly occurs at 3–4 weeks of age. The scale is yellow and greasy and other sites, for example the scalp, face, or axilla, may be involved at the same time. Secondary yeast infection is common.

Management first requires identifying which of the above is the major cause. The diaper area should be cleaned after urination by gentle drying and cleansing after bowel movements. Gentle soap should be used. Ointments such as zinc oxide or A & D ointment may prevent contact with irritants and reduce friction. Commercial wipes may exacerbate the condition. Cornstarch may be helpful, but talcum powder may cause pulmonary irritation and baking soda may cause metabolic alkalosis.

Candidal infections are best treated by keeping the area dry and application of an antifungal topical preparation. Clotrimazole or ketoconazole applied for 3 weeks usually will resolve the rash and oral or GI candida needs to be treated with nystatin or recurrence of the diaper rash may occur. Seborrheic or allergic dermatitis may benefit from treatment with topical non-fluoridated corticosteroids. Secondary infection with streptococcus or *Staphylococcus aureus* may occur in the affected area and needs to be treated.

It is important to be aware that other diagnoses may be present particularly if there is failure to respond to treatment. Metabolic, infectious, and immune disorders are all possible.

Hemangioma

Vascular skin lesions are composed of blood or lymphatic vessels. Non-proliferative lesions include salmon patches or port-wine stains. Salmon patches are nevus simplex and tend to be at the back of the neck and on the forehead (stork-bites) and tend to fade with time. Port-wine stains are red and flat and persist and may deepen in color over time. If they are on the head or face, Sturge–Weber syndrome needs to be considered if the area of distribution is the first branch of the trigeminal nerve. This disorder may have cerebral angiomatosis, seizures, and glaucoma. All children with facial lesions near the eye should be checked for glaucoma. Port-wine stains of the face may be treated with pulsed-dye laser in infancy.

Nevus vasculosa is the strawberry mark which is the commonest vascular nevus. They are benign proliferative tumors seen in 10 percent of infants that appear in the first few weeks of life, although they may be present at birth. They appear as raised, bright-red lesions with well-defined borders. Some may be deeper and are called cavernous hemangiomas and tend to be less distinct and colored blue or purple. The natural history is to resolve over time spontaneously so that they are at their peak between 6 and 12 months of age and start to regress between 12 and 18 months. After the age of 3 years, they resolve at the rate of 10 percent per year so that 50 percent are clear by 5 years and 80 percent by 8 years.

Complications from hemangiomas are unusual but there are two complications of importance. A very large lesion may have a major arteriovenous anastamosis that can lead to congestive heart failure. Occasionally, platelets can be trapped which is called Kasabach–Merritt syndrome. Also if the lesion is in a problem area, for example causing airway obstruction, treatment may be necessary. Corticosteroids, alpha interferon 2a, embolization, or pulsed-dye laser may all be considerations for treatment.

Lymphangiomas are malformations of the lymphatic system that are usually present at birth and they may increase in size and tend not to regress. Lymphangioma simplex is a solitary skin-colored lesion usually on the head, neck or proximal extremity and amenable to surgical removal. Lymphangioma circumscriptum is the most common form. They are found on the proximal extremities, neck, trunk, and oral mucosae. They may appear to be red if there are hemangiomatous elements present. Surgical removal is difficult and recurrence is common. Cavernous lymphangiomas are large cystic dilations of the deep dermis and may involve large areas. They may be on the extremities, trunk, and face. Because they have many channels they are difficult to remove and may recur. Cystic hygromas are large lymphangiomas that are in the neck, axillae, or inguinal areas. They may be unilocular but they are often extensive and difficult to remove.

Hereditary Hemorrhagic Telangiectasia

This is Osler–Rendu–Weber syndrome, an autosomal dominant condition with progressive development of mucocutaneous and visceral telangiectasia. The skin lesions usually appear after puberty and involve face, ears, forearms, and hands. The mucosa of the lips, tongue, buccal mucosa, and nasal septum are involved. Nose bleeds are the commonest presentation and gastro-intestinal bleeding occurs in half the cases. Pulmonary arteriovenous fistulas occur in 20 percent of cases.

Impetigo

Staphylococcus aureus and group A *Streptococcus pyogenes* are the most common organisms in bacterial skin infections and they may both be present. Impetigo is the term used for superficial skin infection and it occurs most commonly in young children. It is particularly associated with crowded conditions and poor hygiene. The lesions are mostly around the mouth, initially erythematous macules that evolve into vesicles or pustules. They tend to be pruritic and local spread occurs because of scratching and release of infected vesicle fluid. Lesions most commonly occur on the face, especially around the mouth and nose, less commonly on the extremities or trunk. Glomerulonephritis is a complication of group A streptococcal infection.

Because of the risk of glomerulonephritis, systemic antibiotics are indicated in addition to the topical treatment.

Psoriasis

Psoriasis affects 1–3 percent of the population and 37 percent of cases first develop the disorder during childhood, mostly during adolescence. The diagnosis is not easy and there tends to be spontaneous remissions and recurrences. The genetics appear to be in part autosomal dominant but the underlying cause is unknown. Stress, trauma, and infection tend to exacerbate the disease. The rash is characterized by well circumscribed scaly patches. The histology reveals parakeratosis, a diminished or absent granular layer and microabscesses in the epidermis. There is acanthosis, papillomatosis, and perivascular infiltrate. There is hyperproliferation of keratinocytes with impaired differentiation and increase in certain forms of keratin.

The distribution of the rash results in 4 forms that can be differentiated: (1) discrete scaly patches of the scalp, knees and elbows, and the buttocks; (2) small ovoid erythematous scaling papules that tend to be generalized and commonly follow 2–3 weeks after pharyngitis, particularly *Streptococcus*; (3) pustular psoriasis may be localized to the soles or palms or may be generalized; and (4) diffuse erythematous form with generalized desquamation and erythema.

Psoriatic arthritis is uncommon in children but can occur in the second decade. It is more common in girls and half the patients have a positive family history. The skin disease may be mild or even absent initially. Joint disease tends to be asymmetric and involve one or more joints. Rheumatoid factor is usually absent in the serum. The joint disease tends to be relatively non-destructive and responds to anti-inflammatory agents.

■ MANAGEMENT

Biopsy may be necessary to confirm the diagnosis although it may show non-specific changes particularly if there has been treatment. The management includes corticosteroids topically, with tars and anthralin as adjunct therapy. Calcipotriene, a vitamin D derivative, has been approved for children over 12 and may be beneficial in some cases.

Psoriasis is a chronic disorder characterized by relapses. Injury to the skin should be avoided as lesions may occur 1–3 weeks later (Koebner's phenomenon) in the same area. Tight clothing, especially with elastic that is constricting, and shoes should be avoided. Sunlight in small doses may be beneficial but sunburn will make the lesions worse. Infection needs to be treated. Severe cases should be managed by a dermatologist.

Verrucae

Verrucae (warts) arise on skin and mucous membranes as a result of infection with human papillomavirus (HPV) with an incubation period that is thought to be 1–6 months. HPV-1 affects the palms and fingers of the hand and the soles of the feet. Persistent rough-surfaced papules on the fingers and hand that are especially troublesome around the nails are called verruca vulgaris or "common warts." When they occur on the feet they are plantar warts (verrucae plantaris) which may be single or multiple and are often painful and difficult to eradicate. Verrucae plana are flat warts 2–5 mm mostly found on the face, arms, and legs. Genital warts (condyloma acuminata) involve the mucous membranes or anogenital area. They are caused by HPV-6 and -11 and may be transferred during passage through an infected birth canal or by sexual transmission. They tend to be moist and cauliflower shaped.

Even though infants may develop warts as long as 20 months after transmission from maternal genital warts during delivery, any child with condyloma acuminata should be considered to be a possible victim of sexual abuse.

Most warts (60–70 percent) resolve within 2 years and indication for treatment will include symptoms of pain or discomfort. Unfortunately treatment is unpredictable in outcome and recurrence is common. The most common therapy is salicylic acid and lactic acid (e.g., Duofilm). It should be applied 1–2 times daily, after soaking the wart(s), directly to the lesion and not the surrounding skin. Results can be expected within 3–4 weeks.

Cimetidine has been associated with 50–80 percent clearance rates after 2–3 months of treatment presumably a result of stimulation of immune mechanisms. Cantharidin may be useful for plantar warts but may produce a ring of satellite warts around the treated wart. Podophyllum is used for condyloma acuminata. It has renal and neuro-toxicity and should not be used in children or pregnant women.

More aggressive treatment includes cryotherapy with liquid nitrogen which is painful and pulsed-dye laser is used for difficult-to-clear warts. Carbon dioxide laser has been used for condyloma acuminata and laryngeal papillomatosis.

I

Bibliography

The source for all of the information that has been included in this book lies in the books listed here. Most of the facts, particularly the numbers and statistical data, were checked in several sources.

The books are in three categories. The more general pediatric texts are listed first and of these the prime authority has been *Rudolph's Pediatrics*. Next are the psychiatric books (including mental health and psychosocial) that contributed to different sections of Part I as well as Chapter 26. Last are the books that were more specific to a particular topic or chapter and listed under the individual chapter.

I have all of these books. It is possible that they are not all easily available but most of them are. I am very grateful to all the authors and contributors to these books.

GENERAL

Batshaw ML: *Children with Disabilities*. Baltimore: Paul H. Brookes, 1997.

Bernstein D and Shelov SP: *Pediatrics*. Baltimore: Williams & Wilkins, 1996.

Dershewitz RA: *Ambulatory Pediatric Care*. Philadelphia: Lippincott-Raven, 1999.

Gartner JC: *Common and Chronic Symptoms in Pediatrics*. St. Louis: Mosby-Year Book, Inc., 1997.

Hay WW, et al.: *Current Pediatric Diagnosis and Treatment.* Stamford: Appleton & Lange, 1997.

Jackson PL and Vessey JA: *Primary Care of the Child with a Chronic Condition.* St. Louis: Mosby-Year Book, Inc., 1996.

Nickel RE and Desch LW: *The Physician's Guide to Caring for Children with Disabilities and Chronic Conditions.* Baltimore: Paul H. Brookes, 2000.

Rudolph AM: *Rudolph's Pediatrics.* Stamford: Appleton & Lange, 1996.

Rudolph AM and Kamei RK: *Rudolph's Fundamentals of Pediatrics.* Stamford: Appleton & Lange, 1998.

Wong DL: *Whaley and Wong's Essentials of Pediatric Nursing.* St. Louis: Mosby-Year Book, Inc., 1997.

MENTAL HEALTH

Kass FI, Oldham JM, and Pardes H: *The Columbia University College of Physicians and Surgeons Complete Home Guide to Mental Health.* New York: Henry Holt, 1992.

Klykylo WM, Kay J, and Rube D: *Clinical Child Psychiatry.* Philadelphia: W.B. Saunders, 1998.

Rapoport JL and Ismond DR: *DSM-IV Training Guide for Diagnosis of Childhood Disorders.* New York: Bruner/Mazel, Inc., 1996.

Roberts MC: *Handbook of Pediatric Psychology.* New York: The Guilford Press, 1995.

Wolraich ML: *The Classification of Child and Adolescent Mental Diagnoses in Primary Care.* Elk Grove Village: American Academy of Pediatrics, 1996.

SPECIFIC

3.   Impact on the Child and Family

Beresford L: *The Hospice Handbook.* New York: Little, Brown, 1993.

Doka KJ: *Living with Life-Threatening Illness: A Guide for Patients, Their Families, and Caregivers.* San Francisco: Jossey-Bass, Inc., 1993.

Pitzele SK: *We Are Not Alone: Learning to Live with Chronic Illness.* New York: Workman Publishing, 1985.

4.   Nutrition

Ekvall SW: *Pediatric Nutrition in Chronic Diseases and Developmental Disorders.* New York: Oxford University Press, 1993.

Kirschmann GJ and Kirschmann JD: *Nutrition Almanac.* New York: McGraw-Hill, 1996.

Kleinman RE and Committee on Nutrition, American Academy of Pediatrics: *Pediatric Nutrition Handbook.* Elk Grove Village: American Academy of Pediatrics, 1998.

6. Complementary Medicine

Beinfield H and Korngold E: *Between Heaven and Earth: A Guide to Chinese Medicine.* New York: Ballantine, 1992.

Olness K and Kohen DP: *Hypnosis and Hypnotherapy with Children.* New York: The Guilford Press, 1996.

Rosenfeld I: *Dr. Rosenfeld's Guide to Alternative Medicine.* New York: Fawcett Columbine, 1996.

8. Pediatric Rehabilitation

Campbell SK: *Physical Therapy for Children.* Philadelphia: W.B. Saunders, 1995.

10. Mental Health Problems

Williamson ME: *Fibromyalgia: A Comprehensive Approach: What You Can Do About Chronic Pain and Fatigue.* New York: Walker, 1996.

12. Home Care and Technology Dependence

Dunne PJ and McInturff SL: *Respiratory Home Care: The Essentials.* Philadelphia: F. A. Davis, 1998.

Rice R: *Home Health Nursing Practice Concepts and Application.* St. Louis: Mosby-Year Book, Inc., 1996.

13. Child Abuse and Neglect

Reece RM: *Child Abuse: Medical Diagnosis and Management.* Baltimore: Williams & Wilkins, 1994.

15. Genetic Disorders

Jones KL: *Smith's Recognizable Patterns of Human Malformation.* Philadelphia: W.B. Saunders, 1997.

17. Endocrine Disorders

Saudek CD, Rubin RR, and Shump CS: *The Johns Hopkins Guide to Diabetes for Today and Tomorrow.* Baltimore: The Johns Hopkins University Press, 1997.

19. Infectious Diseases
Pickering LK and the Committee on Infectious Diseases, American Academy of Pediatrics: *Red Book 2000*. Elk Grove Village: American Academy of Pediatrics, 2000.
Pinsky L and Douglas PH: *The Essential HIV Treatment Fact Book*. New York: Pocket Books, 1992.

20. Pulmonary Disease
Hilman BC: *Pediatric Respiratory Disease: Diagnosis and Treatment*. Philadelphia: W.B. Saunders, 1993.

23. Gastrointestinal Disorders
Saibil F: *Crohn's Disease and Ulcerative Colitis*. New York: Firefly Books, 1997.

24. Hematology and Oncology Disorders
Fromer MJ: *Surviving Childhood Cancer: A Guide for Families*. Oakland: New Harbinger Publications, Inc., 1998.
Keene N: *Childhood Leukemia: A Guide for Families, Friends and Caregivers*. Sebastopol: O'Reilly & Associates, Inc., 1997.
Murphy GP, Morris LB, and Lange D: *Informed Decisions: The Complete Book of Cancer Diagnosis, Treatment, and Recovery*. New York: American Cancer Society/Viking Penguin, 1997.

25. Neuromuscular Disorders
Fenichel GM: *Clinical Pediatric Neurology*. Philadelphia: W.B. Saunders, 1997.
Lechtenberg R: *Epilepsy and the Family*. Boston: Harvard University Press, 1984.
Miller F and Bachrach SJ: *Cerebral Palsy: A Complete Guide for Caregiving*. Baltimore: The Johns Hopkins University Press, 1995.

27. Rheumatology Disorders
Klippel JH: *Primer on the Rheumatic Diseases*. Atlanta: The Arthritis Foundation, 1997.

II

Resources

The resources listed in this appendix are in order of the chapters in the book. There are medical sites, educational sites, and useful contacts. The organization is named and the address is provided with telephone and fax numbers. The email address and internet site addresses (URLs) are current at the time of publication. The choice of sites is arbitrary and based on those that seemed to be the most useful. Preference was given to those sites that were good stepping-off points to other areas of the internet. Sincere apologies for any leads that result only in blind alleys or that do not work properly. Even more apologies for sites that should have been included and were not. Unless otherwise noted the site is in the USA.

The starting point for many journeys should be the American Academy of Pediatrics. The AAP Policy Statements are a treasure-box of information:

Internet site: http://www.aap.org/policy/pprgtoc.cfm

National Headquarters:
The American Academy of Pediatrics
141 Northwest Point Boulevard
Elk Grove Village, IL 60007-1098
Telephone: 847-434-4000
Fax: 847-434-8000
Internet site: http://www.aap.org/

1. Chronic Illness in Children

United States Agency for International Development (USAID)
Ronald Reagan Building
Washington, DC 20523-0016
Telephone: 202-712-4810
Fax: 202-216-3524
Internet site:
http://www.usaid.gov/pop_health/

The National Organization for Rare Disorders, Inc.
PO Box 8923
New Fairfield, CT 06812-8923
Telephone: 203-746-6518, 800-999-6673
Fax: 203-746-6481
Internet site:
http://www.rarediseases.org/

Internet site:
http://www.disability resources.org/SPECIFIC.html

2. Health Maintenance

Internet site:
http://www.webmd.com/

Sites using WebMD

http://www.healthlinkusa.com/1.htm
http://health.excite.com/
http://health.msn.com/
http://health.yahoo.com/

Maternal and Child Health Bureau
Office of State and Community Health
Room 18-31
Parklawn Building
5600 Fishers Lane
Rockville, MD 20857
Telephone: 301-443-2204
Fax: 301-443-9354
Email: BlockGrantGuidance @hrsa.gov
Internet site:
http://www.mchb.hrsa.gov/

Internet site:
http://www.ahcpr.gov/ppip/ppchild.htm

3. Impact on the Child and Family

Center for Children with Chronic Illness and Disability
Box 721 UMHC
420 Delaware SE
Minneapolis, MN 55455
Telephone: 612-626-4032

Hospice

Children's Hospice International
2202 Mount Vernon Avenue
Suite 3C
Alexandria, VA 22301
Telephone: 703-684-0330
Fax: 703-684-0226

Internet site:
http://www.chionline.org/

Hospice Foundation of America
2001 S Street NW, Suite 300
Washington, DC 20009
Telephone: 800-854-3402
Fax: 202-638-5312
Email:
hfa@hospicefoundation.org
Internet site: http://www.
hospicefoundation.org/

4. Nutrition

Internet site:
http://www.fns.usda.gov/wic/
Internet site: http://www.
familyfoodzone.com/

The American Society for
Clinical Nutrition
9650 Rockville Pike
Bethesda, MD 20814-3998
Telephone: 301-530-7110
Fax: 301-571-1863
Email:
secretar@ascn.faseb.org
Internet site:
http://www.faseb.org/ascn

American Society for
Nutritional Sciences
9650 Rockville Pike
Suite 4500
Bethesda, MD 20815
Telephone: 301-530-7050

Fax: 301-571-1892
Email:
secretar@ascn.faseb.org
Internet site:
http://www.faseb.org/asns

American Society for Parenteral
and Enteral Nutrition (ASPEN)
8630 Fenton Street
Suite 412
Silver Spring, MD 20910
Telephone: 800-727-4567
Email: aspen@nutr.org
Internet site:
http://www.nutritioncare.org

5. Eating/Elimination Disorders

Anorexia Nervosa

National Association of
Anorexia Nervosa and
Associated Disorders
(ANAD)
PO Box 7
Highland Park, IL 60035
Hotline: 847-831-3438
Fax: 847-433-4632
Email: info@anad.org
Internet site:
http://www.anad.org/
Internet site:
http://www.aabainc.org/
home.html
Internet site:
http://www.dietitian.com/
anorexia.html

Bulimia

Internet site:
http://www.aabainc.org/
home.html
Internet site:
http://www.dietitian.com/
bulimia.html

Elimination Disorders

Internet site:
http://www.babyzone.com/
drnathan/medref/
encopresis.htm

6. *Complementary Medicine*

NCCAM Clearinghouse
PO Box 8218
Silver Spring, MD 20907-8218
Telephone: 888-644-6226
TTY/TDY: 888-644-6226
Fax: 301-495-4957
Internet site:
http://nccam.nih.gov/

Naturopathy:
http://www.
thenaturalphysician.com/

Hypnosis

American Society of Clinical
Hypnosis
130 East Elm Court, Suite 201
Roselle, IL 60172-2000
Telephone: 630-980-4740

Fax: 630-351-8490
Internet site:
http://www.asch.net/

Society for Clinical and
Experimental Hypnosis
2201 Haeder Road, Suite 1
Pullman, WA 99163
Telephone: 509-332-7555
Fax: 509-332-5907
Email: sceh@pullman.com
Internet site:
http://sunsite.utk.edu/IJCEH/
scehframes.htm

The Milton H. Erickson
Foundation, Inc.
3606 North 24th Street
Phoenix, AZ 85016-6500
Telephone: 602-956-6196
Fax: 602-956-0519
Internet site: http://www.
erickson-foundation.org

Acupuncture

Internet site: http://www.
pediatricacupuncture.com/
index.htm

Herbal

http://www.alternative
parenting.com/health/
natural_remedies/
herbal_dosage.htm

8. Pediatric Rehabilitation

Office of Special Education and Rehabilitative Services (OSERS) Communication and Media Support Services
US Department of Education
330 C Street SW, Room 3132
Washington, DC 20202-2524
Telephone: 202-205-8241
Internet site:
http://www.ed.gov/offices/OSERS/

Physical Therapy

American Physical Therapy Association (APTA)
Email: scinquiries@apta.org
Internet site:
https://www.apta.org/Home

Occupational Therapy

Disabled Sports USA (DS/USA)
451 Hungerford Drive
Suite 100
Rockville, MD 20850
Telephone: 301-217-0960,
TDD: 301-217-0693
Email: dsusa@dsusa.org
Internet site:
http://www.dsusa.org

Wheelchair Sports, USA
3595 East Fountain Boulevard
Suite L1

Colorado Springs
CO 80910-1740
Telephone: 719-574-1150
Email: wsusa@aol.com
Internet site:
http://www.wsusa.org

ABLEDATA
(assistive technology)
8630 Fenton Street
Suite 930
Silver Spring, MD 20910
Telephone: 800-227-0216,
301-608-8912 (TTY)
Fax: 301-608-8958
Email:
ABLEDATA@macroint.com
Internet site:
http://www.abledata.com/

Center for Accessible Technology
2547 8th Street, Suite 12-A
Berkeley, CA 94710
Telephone (voice/TTY):
510-841-3224
Email: info@cforat.org
Internet site:
http://www.cforat.org

9. Sensory Disorders

Blindness

American Council of the Blind (ACB)

1155 15th Street NW
Suite 1004
Washington, DC 20005
Telephone: 800-424-8666
(answer only 2–5 pm Eastern
time); 202-467-5081
Email: info@acb.org
Internet site:
http://www.acb.org/

American Foundation for the
Blind (AFB)
11 Penn Plaza, Suite 300
New York, NY 10001
Telephone: 212-502-7600
Email: afbinfo@afb.net
Internet site:
http://www.afb.org/

National Association for
Parents of the Visually Impaired
(NAPVI)
PO Box 317
Watertown, MA 02272
Telephone: 617-972-7441,
800-562-6265
Internet site:
http://www.
spedex.com/napvi/

National Library Services for
the Blind and Physically
Handicapped
1291 Taylor Street NW
Washington, DC 20542
Telephone: 202-707-5100,
202-707-0744 (TDD)

Email: nls@loc.gov
Internet site:
http://www.loc.gov/nls

National Organization of
Parents of Blind Children
(NOPBC)
1800 Johnson Street
Baltimore, MD 21230
Telephone: 410-659-9314
Email: nfb@nfb.org
Internet site: http://
www.nfb.org

Deafness

Alexander Graham Bell
Association for the Deaf and
Hard of Hearing
3417 Volta Place NW
Washington, DC 20007-2778
Telephone: 202-337-5220
(Voice /TTY)
Internet site:
http://www.agbell.org/

American Society for Deaf
Children
PO Box 3355
Gettysburg, PA 17325
Telephone: 717-334-7922
(Business V/TTY), 800-942-
ASDC (2732, Parent Hotline)
Fax: 717-334-8808
Email: ASDC1@aol.com
Internet site:
http://deafchildren.org/

National Association of the
Deaf (NAD)
814 Thayer Avenue
Suite 250
Silver Spring, MD 20910-4500
Telephone: 301-587-1788,
301-587-1789 (TTY)
Email: NADinfo@nad.org
Internet site:
http://www.nad.org

National Deaf Education
Network and Clearinghouse
Gallaudet University
800 Florida Avenue NE
Washington, DC 20002-3695
Telephone: 202-651-5051
(Voice), 202-651-5052 (TTY)
Email: clearinghouse.
infotogo@gallaudet.edu
Internet site: http://www.
gallaudet.edu/~nicd

10.   Mental Health Problems

American Academy of Child
and Adolescent Psychiatry
(AACAP)
3615 Wisconsin Avenue NW
Washington, DC 20016
Telephone: 202-966-7300
Internet site:
http://www.aacap.org/

National Alliance for the
Mentally Ill
NAMI Office of Development
2107 Wilson Boulevard
Suite 300
Arlington, VA 22201-3042
Telephone: 703-524-7600
Internet site:
http://www.covenant
house.org/cov_abo.htm

Covenant House
346 W. 17th Street
New York, NY 10011
Telephone: 800-388-3888
Email: dcmail@covcorp.org
Internet site:
http://www.covenant
house.org/cov_abo.htm

Anxiety Disorders Association
of America (ADAA)
11900 Parklawn Drive
Suite 100
Rockville, MD 20852
Telephone: 301-231-9350
Fax: 301-231-7392
Email: anxdis@adaa.org
Internet site:
http://www.adaa.org

Center for Substance Abuse
Prevention (CSAP), Substance
Abuse and Mental Health
Services Administration
(SAMHSA)

5600 Fishers Lane, Rockwall II
Rockville, MD 20857
Email: nnadal@samhsa.gov
Internet site:
http://www.samhsa.gov/csap/

13. Child Abuse and Neglect

Prevent Child Abuse America
200 S. Michigan Avenue
17th Floor
Chicago, IL 60604-2404
Telephone: 312-663-3520
Fax: 312-939-8962
Internet site: http:
//www.preventchildabuse.org/

National Clearinghouse on
Child Abuse and Neglect
Information
330 C Street SW
Washington, DC 20447
Telephone: 800-394-3366,
703-385-7565
Fax: 703-385-3206
Internet site:
http://www.calib.com/
nccanch/index.htm

International Society for
Prevention of Abuse and
Neglect
200 North Michigan Avenue
Suite 500
Chicago, IL 60601
Telephone: 312-578-1401
Fax: 312-578-1405

Email: ISPCAN@ISPCAN.org
Internet site:
http://ispcan.org/

Kempe Children's Center
1825 Marion Street
Denver, CO 80218
Telephone: 303-864-5252
Fax: 303-864-5302
Email:
Kempe@KempeCenter.org
Internet site:
http://kempecenter.org/

14. Ethical and Legal Issues

Children's Defense Fund
25 E Street NW
Washington, DC 20001
Telephone: 800-233-1200,
202-628-8787
Email:
mlallen@childrensdefense.org
Internet site: http://www.
childrensdefense.org

15. Genetic Disorders

Genetic Information and Patient
Services, Inc. (GAPS)
PO Box 67302
Phoenix, AZ 85082-7302
Internet site:
http://aspin.asu.edu/geneinfo/
Internet site: http://www.kumc.
edu/gec/support/grouporg.
html#national

Human Genome Project

Internet site:
http://www.ncbi.nlm.nih.gov/genome/guide/

Down Syndrome

National Down Syndrome Society (NDSS)
666 Broadway
New York, NY 10012
Telephone: 212-460-9330
800-221-4602
Fax: 212-979-2873
Internet site:
http://www.ndss.org/

Achondroplasia

Human Growth Foundation (HGF)
997 Glen Cove Avenue
Glen Head, NY 11545
Telephone 800-451-6434
Email: hgf1@hgfound.org
Internet site:
http://www.hgfound.org

Little People of America (LPA)
Box 9897
Washington, DC 20016
Internet site:
http://www.lpaonline.org

Arthrogryposis Multiplex Congenita

Internet site:

http://www.shrinershq.org/patientedu/arthrogryposis.html
Internet site:
http://www.sonnet.com/avenues/pamphlet.html

Cleft Lip and Palate

American Cleft Palate-Craniofacial Association
Cleft Palate Association
ACPA/CPF National Office
104 South Estes Drive
Suite 204
Chapel Hill, NC 27514
Telephone: 919-933-9044
Fax: 919-933-9604
Email: cleftline@aol.com
Internet site:
www.cleftline.org

Fetal Alcohol Syndrome

National Organization on Fetal Alcohol Syndrome
216 G Street NE
Washington, DC 20002
Telephone: 202-785-4585
Email : information@nofas.org
Internet site:
http://www.nofas.org

Fragile X

The National Fragile X Foundation
PO Box 190488
San Francisco, CA 94119

Telephone: 800-688-8765, 510-763-6030
Fax: 510-763-6223
Email: natlfx@sprintmail.com
Internet site:
http://www.FragileX.org

Klinefelter Syndrome

American Association for Klinefelter Syndrome Information and Support (AAKSIS)
2945 W. Farwell Avenue
Chicago, IL 60645-2925
Telephone: 888-466-KSIS (5747)
Email: AAKSIS@aaksis.org
Internet site:
http://www.AAKSIS.org/

Internet site:
http://www.hgfound.org

Noonan Syndrome

The Noonan Syndrome Support Group, Inc.
PO Box 145
Upperco, MD 21155
Telephone: 410-374-5245, 888-686-2224
Email:
info@noonansyndrome.org
Internet site:
http://www.noonan
syndrome.org/

Marfan Syndrome

National Marfan Foundation
382 Main Street
Port Washington, NY 11050
Telephone: 800-8-MARFAN (627326), 516-883-8712
Fax: 516-883-8040
Email: staff@marfan.org
Internet site:
http://www.marfan.org/

Osteogenesis Imperfecta

Osteogenesis Imperfecta Foundation
804 West Diamond Avenue
Suite 210
Gaithersburg, MD 20878
Telephone: 301-947-0083, 800-981-2663
Fax: 301-947-0456
Email: bonelink@oif.org
Internet site:
http://www.oif.org/

Prader–Willi Syndrome

The Prader–Willi Syndrome Association (USA)
5700 Midnight Pass Road
Suite G
Sarasota, FL 34242
Telephone: 800-926-4797, 941-312-0400
Fax: 941-312-0142
Email: pwsusa@aol.com
Internet site:
http://www.pwsausa.org/

Tay–Sachs

National Tay–Sachs and Allied Diseases Association, Inc. (NTSAD)
2001 Beacon Street, Suite 204
Boston, MA 02135
Telephone: 800-906-8723
Fax: 617-277-0134
Email: NTSAD-Boston @att.net
Internet site:
http://www.ntsad.org/

Trisomy 13 and 18

SOFT USA (Support for Trisomy)
Barb Vanherreweghe
2982 South Union Street
Rochester, NY 14624
Telephone: 716-594-4621,
800-716-SOFT (7638)
Email: barbsoft@aol.com
Internet site:
http://www.trisomy.org/

Turner Syndrome

The Turner's Syndrome Society of the United States
14450 T. C. Jester
Suite 260
Houston, TX 77014
Telephone: 800-365-9944,
832-249-9988
Fax: 832-249-9987

Email:
tssus@turner-syndrome-us.org
Internet site: http://www.turner-syndrome-us.org/

Williams Syndrome

The Williams Syndrome Association
PO Box 297
Clawson, MI 48017-0297
Telephone: 248-541-3630
Fax: 248-541-3631
Email: TMonkaba@aol.com
Internet site:
http://www.williams-syndrome.org/

Williams Syndrome Foundation
University of California, Irvine
Irvine, CA 92697-2310
Telephone: 949-824-7259
Email: hmlenhof@uci.edu
Internet site:
http://www.wsf.org/

16.   Metabolic Disorders

Inborn Errors of Metabolism

Internet site:
http://web.indstate.edu/thcme/mwking/inborn.html

Phenylketonuria

National PKU News, 6869 Woodlawn Avenue NE #116 Seattle, WA 98115
Internet site:
http://205.178.182.34/index.htm

Children's PKU Network (CPN)
1520 State Street, Suite #240
San Diego, CA 92101
Telephone: 619-233-3202
Fax: 619-233-0838
Internet site:
http://www.kumc.edu/gec/support/pku.html

Familial Hypercholesterolemia

MEDPED and the Inherited High Cholesterol Foundation
University of Utah,
410 Chipeta Way, Room 161
Salt Lake City, UT 84108
Telephone: 888-244-2465
Fax: 801-581-5402
Email:
slarri@ucvg.med.utah.edu
Internet site:
http://www.medped.org

Galactosemia

Parents of Galactosemic Children
885 Del Sol Street
Sparks, NV 89436

Email:
mesameadow@aol.com
Internet site:
http://www.galactosemia.org/

Glycogen Storage Disease

Association for Glycogen Storage
PO Box 896
Durant, IA 52747-9769
Telephone: 319-785-6038
Fax: 319-785-6038
Internet site:
http://www.kumc.edu/gec/support/glycogen.html

Hunter Syndrome, Hurler Syndrome

National Mucopolysaccharidoses/Mucolipidoses Society, Inc. (MPS)
102 Aspen Drive
Downingtown, PA 19335
Telephone: 610-942-0100
Fax: 610-942-7188
Email: info@mpssociety.org
Internet site:
http://mpssociety.org

Krabbe Disease

Krabbes Family Network
PO Box 563
East Aurora, NY 14052
Email:
webmaster@krabbes.net

Internet site:
http://www.krabbes.net

Maple Syrup Urine Disease

MSUD Family Support Group
24806 SR 119
Goshen, IN 46526
Telephone: 219-862-2992
Fax: 219-862-2012
Email:
msud-support@juno.com
Internet site: http://www.msud-support.org/

Niemann–Pick Disease

National Niemann–Pick
Disease Foundation
N1590 Fairview Lane
Fort Atkinson, WI 53538
Telephone: 1-877-CURE-NPC
(287-3672)
Internet site:
http://www.nnpdf.org/

17.   *Endocrine Disorders*

Diabetes Mellitus

American Diabetes Association
1701 North Beauregard Street
Alexandria, VA 22311
Telephone: 800-342-2383
Email: customerservice@
diabetes.org
Internet site:
http://www.diabetes.org/

Internet site:
http://www.childrenwith
diabetes.com/index_cwd.htm

Adrenal Insufficiency

National Adrenal Diseases
Foundation
505 Northern Boulevard
Great Neck, NY 11021
Telephone: 516-487-4992
Email: nadfmail@aol.com
Internet site: http://www.
medhelp.org/nadf/

**Congenital Adrenal
Hyperplasia**

MAGIC
1327 N. Harlem Avenue
Oak Park, IL 60302
Telephone: 708-383-0808
Fax: 708-383-0899
Internet site:
http://www.magic
foundation.org/cah.html

Diabetes Insipidus

Email:
diabetesinsipidus@
maxinter.net
Internet site:
http://diabetesinsipidus.
maxinter.net/

Internet site:
http://www.ndif.org/
index.html

Hypoglycemia

Internet site:
http://www.niddk.nih.gov/
health/diabetes/pubs/hypo/
hypo.htm

Internet site:
http://www.delphi.com/
diabetes/hypo.html

Hyperthyroidism,
Hypothyroidism

The American Thyroid
Association, Inc.
Townhouse Office Park
55 Old Nyack Turnpike
Suite 611
Nanuet, NY 10954
Fax: 914-623-3736
Email: admin@thyroid.org
Internet site:
http://www.thyroid.org/

Internet site:
http://home.ican.net/
~thyroid/Guides/HG09.html

18. Allergy and Immunology
Disorders

Asthma

Allergy and Asthma Network:
Mothers of Asthmatics, Inc.
2751 Properity Avenue
Suite 150
Fairfax, VA 22031

Telephone: 800-878-4403,
703-641-9595
E-mail: aanma@aol.com
Internet site:
http://www.aanma.org

Allergy, Asthma and
Immunology Online
American College of Allergy,
Asthma and Immunology
85 West Algonquin Road
Suite 550
Arlington Heights, IL 60005
Telephone: 847-427-1200
Fax: 847-427-1294
E-mail: mail@acaai.org
Internet site:
http://www.allergy.mcg.edu/

Immune Deficiency Foundation
40 W. Chesapeake Avenue
Suite 308
Towson, MD 21204
Telephone: 800-296-4433
Fax: 410-321-9165
Email:
idf@primaryimmune.org
Internet site:
http://www.primaryimmune.
org/

Severe Combined
Immunodeficiency
Email: scidemail@scid.net
Internet site:
http://www.scid.net/

19. Infectious Diseases

Internet site: http://www.
cdcnpin.org/

AIDS

National Pediatrics AIDS
Network
PO Box 1032
Boulder, CO 80306
Telephone: 800-646-1001
Email: gary@npan.org
Internet site:
http://www.npan.org/

The Elizabeth Glaser Pediatric
AIDS Foundation
2950 31st Street, #125
Santa Monica, CA 90405
Telephone: 800-499-4673,
310-314-1459
Fax: 310-314-1469
Email: Research or Grants:
research@pedAIDS.org
Fundraising and Donations:
development@pedAIDS.org
Internet site: http://www.
pedaids.org/index.html
Internet site: http://www.
thekidsaidssite.com

Children With AIDS Project of
America
PO Box 23778
Tempe, AZ 85282-3778
Telephone: 602-973-4319
Fax: 602-530-3541

Internet site:
http://www.aidskids.org/

Tuesday's Child
8501 W. Washington Boulevard
Culver City, CA 90232
Telephone: 310-204-3848
Fax: 310-204-1875
Email:
jsheeran@tuesdayschild.org
Internet site:
http://www.tuesdayschild.org/

Tuberculosis

Internet site:
http://www.cdcnpin.org/tb/
pubs/Emats.htm

Hepatitis

Hepatitis Education Project
4603 Aurora Avenue N.
Seattle, WA 98103
Telephone: 206-732-0311
Fax: 206-732-0312
Email: hep@scn.org
Internet site:
http://www.scn.org/health/
hepatitis/index.htm

20. Pulmonary Disease

Cystic Fibrosis

Cystic Fibrosis Foundation
6931 Arlington Road
Bethesda, MD 20814

Phone: 301-951-4422,
800-FIGHT CF (344-4823)
Fax: 301-951-6378
Email: info@cff.org
Internet site:
http://www.cff.org/

International Association of CF
Adults
Internet site: http://www.
iacfa.org/home.htm

Central Hypoventilation Syndrome

Congenital Central
Hypoventilation Syndrome
(CCHS) Family Support
Network
71 Maple Street
Oneonta, NY 13820
Telephone: 607-432-8872

21. Cardiac Disorders

American Heart Association
National Center
7272 Greenville Avenue
Dallas, TX 75231
Internet site: http://www.
americanheart.org/

Congenital Heart Disease

CHASER (Congenital Heart
Anomalies—Support
Education & Resources)

2112 North Wilkins Road
Swanton, OH 43558
Telephone 419-825-5575
Fax: 419-825-2880
Email:
chaser@compuserve.com
Internet site: http://www.
csun.edu/~hfmth006/chaser/

Children's Health Information
Network
1561 Clark Drive
Yardley, PA 19067
Telephone: 215-493-3068
Email: mb@tchin.org
Internet site: http://www.
tchin.org/

22. Renal Disease

Alport Syndrome Home Page
Internet site: http://www.cc.
utah.edu/~cla6202/ASHP.htm

23. Gastrointestinal Disorders

Crohn's and Colitis Foundation
of America
386 Park Avenue South
17th Floor
New York, NY 10016-8804
Telephone 212-685-3440,
800-932-2423
Fax: 212-779-4098
Email: info@ccfa.org
Internet site:
http://www.ccfa.org/

Celiac Sprue Association
CSA/USA, Inc.
PO Box 31700
Omaha, NE 68131-0700
Telephone: 402-558-0600
Fax: 402-558-1347
Email: celiacs@csaceliacs.org
Internet site:
http://www.csaceliacs.org/

Children's Liver Disease
Foundation
36 Great Charles Street
Birmingham B3 3JY
United Kingdom
Telephone: 0121 212 3839
Fax: 0121 212 4300
E-mail:
cldf@childliverdisease.org
Internet site: http://www.
childliverdisease.org/

24. Hematology and
    Oncology Disorders

American Cancer Society
Internet site:
http://www.cancer.org/

The Candlelighters Childhood
Cancer Foundation
3910 Warner Street
Kensington, MD 20895
Telephone: 800-366-2223
Fax: 301-962-3521
Email: info@candlelighters.org

Internet site:
http://www.candlelighters.org/

Leukemia and Lymphoma
Society, Inc.
1311 Mamaroneck Avenue
White Plains, NY 10605
Telephone: 914-949-5213
Fax: 914-949-6691
Internet site:
http://www.leukemia.org/

Sickle Cell Disease

Sickle Cell Disease Association
of America, Inc.
200 Corporate Pointe
Suite 495
Culver City, CA 90230-8727
Telephone: 310-216-6363,
800-421-8453
Fax: 310-215-3722
Email:
scdaa@sicklecelldisease.org
Internet site:
www.sicklecelldisease.org

Hemophilia

National Hemophilia
Foundation
116 West 32nd Street
11th Floor
New York, NY 10001
Telephone: 212-328-3700
Fax: 212-328-3777
Email: info@hemophilia.org

Internet site:
www.hemophilia.org
Hemophilia Home Page
Email: hemophilia@web-depot.com
Internet site: http://www.web-depot.com/hemophilia/

World Federation of Hemophilia
1425 René Lévesque
Boulevard West, Suite 1010
Montréal, Quebec
Canada H3G 1T7
Tel: 514-875-7944
Fax: 514-875-8916
Email: wfh@wfh.org
Internet site:
http://www.wfh.org/

25. Neuromuscular Disorders

Cerebral Palsy

United Cerebral Palsy
Associations (UCPA)
1660 L Street NW, Suite 700
Washington, DC 20036
Telephone: 800-872-5827,
Voice: 202-776-0406,
TDD: 202-973-7197
Email: webmaster@ucpa.org
Internet site:
http://www.ucpa.org

American Academy for
Cerebral Palsy and
Developmental Medicine
(AACPDM)

6300 North River Road
Suite 727
Rosemont, IL 60018-4226
Telephone: 847-698-1635
Email: sking@aaos.org
Internet site:
http://www.aacpdm.org/

Epilepsy

Epilepsy Foundation
4351 Garden City Drive
Landover, MD 20785
Telephone: 301-459-3700
Fax: 301-577-4941
Email: webmaster@efa.org
Internet site:
http://www.
epilepsyfoundation.org

Neural Tube Defect

Spina Bifida Association of
America (SBAA)
4590 MacArthur Boulevard
NW, Suite 250
Washington, DC 20007-4226
Telephone: 800-621-3141,
202-944-3285
E-mail: sbaa@sbaa.org
Internet site:
http://www.sbaa.org/

Muscle Disorders

International Myotonic
Dystrophy Organization
764 Old Westbury Road

Crystal Lake, IL 60012
Telephone: 815-477-0047
Email: myotonicdystrophy@
yahoo.com
Internet site: http://www.
myotonicdystrophy.com/

Muscular Dystrophy
Association
3300 E. Sunrise Drive
Tucson, AZ 85718
Telephone: 800-572-1717
Internet site: http://mdusa.org

Tourette Syndrome

National Tourette Syndrome
Association
42–40 Bell Boulevard
Bayside, NY 11361
Telephone: 718-224-2999
Fax: 718-279-9596
Email:
tourette@ix.netcom.com
Internet site: http://www.
tourette-syndrome.com

Werdnig–Hoffmann Disease

Families of Spinal Muscular
Atrophy
PO Box 196
Libertyville, IL 60048-0196
Telephone: 800-886-1762,
847-367-7620
Fax: 847-367-7623
Email: shelley@fsma.org
Internet site: http://www.fsma.
org/

26. Psychological Disorders

Attention-Deficit Hyperactivity Disorder

CHADD
8181 Professional Place
Suite 201
Landover, MD 20785
Telephone: 800-233-4050,
301-306-7070
Fax: 301-306-7090
Internet site:
http://www.chadd.org/

National ADDA
1788 Second Street,
Suite 200
Highland Park, IL 60035
Telephone: 847-432-ADDA
(2332)
Fax: 847-432-5874
Email: mail@add.org
Internet site:
http://www.add.org/

Mental Retardation

Internet site:
http://www.thearc.org/

Autism

Center for the Study of Autism
PO Box 4538
Salem, OR 97302
Internet site:
http://www.autism.org/

Autism Research Institute
4182 Adams Avenue
San Diego, CA 92116
Fax: 619-563-6840
Internet site:
http://www.autism.com/ari/

27. Rheumatology Disorders

Juvenile Rheumatoid Arthritis

Arthritis Foundation
1330 West Peachtree Street
Atlanta, GA 30309
Telephone: 404-872-7100
Internet site:
http://www.arthritis.org/

Lupus Erythematosis

Lupus Foundation of America
1300 Piccard Drive
Suite 200
Rockville, MD 20850-4303
Telephone: 301-670-9292
Fax: 800-558-0121
Internet site:
http://www.lupus.org/

Kawasaki Disease

The Kawasaki Syndrome
Support Group

(United Kingdom)
Sue Davidson
13 Norwood Grove
Potters Green
Coventry CV2 2FR, UK

Parents Association of
Kawasaki Disease
(Kawasaki Byo no Kodomo
wo Motsu Oya no Kai)
c/o Mr. Mitsuru Asai
Minami-ikuta 6-34-16
Tama-ku, Kawasaki-city
Kanagawa, 214 Japan
Fax: 81-044-977-8451
Internet site:
http://ourworld.compuserve.
com/homepages/kawasaki/

28. Dermatologic Disorders

American Academy of
Dermatology
930 N. Meacham Road
Schaumberg, IL 60173
Telephone: 888-462-DERM
(3376)
Internet site:
http://www.aad.org/

Index

A

Abdominal masses, 301
Abdominal pain, 308–309
Abdominal trauma, 130
Achondroplasia, 154
  clinical features, 154–155
  mangement, 155
Acne vulgaris, 406–409
  clinical features, 407–408
  management, 408–409
Acquired heart disease, 267
Acquired immunodeficiency
  syndrome (AIDS), 225, 227
  features in children and adults,
  228
Acupuncture, 54, 56–59
Acute lymphoblastic leukemia
  (ALL), 332–335
  management, 333–335
Acute non-lymphoblastic
  leukemia, 335
Acute stress disorder (ASD), 387
Acyanotic lesions, 270–273
Addison's disease, 183–184
Adolescent growth and
  development, 68
Adoption, 23–24
Adrenal gland defects, 183–187
Adrenal insufficiency, 183–187

management, 184–187
Advance directives, 142–144
Aerosol therapy, 117–118
Affective disorders, 379–382
Aid to Families with Dependent
  Children (AFDC), 17
Airway clearance techniques
  (ACTs), 118–119, 255
Alcohol, 356
Allergen avoidance, 209
Allergy, 201–223
  resources, 434–435
Alpha-thalassemia, 328–329
Alport syndrome, 289
Alternative medicine. See
  Complementary and
  alternative medicine (CAM)
Ambiguous genitalia, 196–197
Anemia, 322–325
  causes, 323
  management, 324–325
Angelman syndrome, 162–163
Anorexia nervosa (AN), 43–45
  diagnosis, 44
Antidiuretic hormone (ADH),
  195–196
α_1-Antitrypsin deficiency, 313
Anxiety disorders, 369–370, 382–388
Aortic stenosis, 273
Apnea, 247–248

ISBN 0-07-134720-8

9 780071 347204   90000

LIGHT/PEDIATRIC CHRONIC